DIETARY FACTORS
AND
BIRTH DEFECTS

Raghubir P. Sharma, Editor

PACIFIC DIVISION, AAAS
San Francisco, California
1993

From the Seventy-second Annual Meeting
of the Pacific Division of the American
Association for the Advancement of Science
held at Utah State University, Logan, Utah
June 23-27, 1991

Based on the symposium titled
*Nutritional Factors in Normal and
Abnormal Embryological Development*
organized by Ragubir P. Sharma, Center
for Environmental Toxicology, Utah
State University, and Calvin C. Willhite,
Toxic Substances Control, California
Department of Health Services, Berkeley

Library of Congress Cataloging-in-Publication Data
Dietary factors and birth defects / Raghubir P. Sharma, editor.
    "From the Seventy-second Annual Meeting of the Pacific Division
of the American Association for the Advancement of Science held at
Utah State University, Logan, Utah, June 23-27, 1991" – T.p. verso.
    Includes bibliographical references and index.
    ISBN 0-934394-08-3 (pbk. : acid-free paper)
    1. Fetal malnutrition - Compilations - Congresses.
2. Abnormalities, Human - Etiology - Congresses. 3. Malnutrition in
pregnancy - Compilations - Congresses. 4. Pregnancy - Nutritional
aspects - Congresses. 5. Teratogenesis - Congresses. I. Sharma,
Raghubir P. (Raghubir Prasad), 1940-   . II. American Association for
the Advancement of Science. Pacific Division. Meeting. (72nd:1991:
Utah State University)
    RG627.6.M34D54   1993   616'.043-dc20   93-12186 CIP

Pacific Division AAAS
California Academy of Sciences
San Francisco, California 94118

Contents

Preface   iii

Acknowledgements   v

Contributors   vii

Chapter 1. Maternal Nutrition and Pregnancy:
  An Overview – R. P. Sharma   1

Chapter 2. Nutrient Deficiencies and Pregnancy
  Outcome – S. T. Omaye   12

Chapter 3. Nutrient Factors in Juvenile Cataracts
  G. E. Bunce and J. L. Hess   42

Chapter 4. Iron Status During Pregnancy
  D. Zhang and A. W. Mahoney   73

Chapter 5. Embryonic Nutrition and Yolk Sac
  Function – M. R. Juchau, J. M. Creech-Kraft,
  Q. P. Lee, H. L. Yang and M. J. Namkung   109

Chapter 6. Retinoids and Fetal Malformations
  D. M. Kochhar and M. A. Satre   134

Chapter 7. Selenium in Nutrition and Pregnancy
  D. S. Wilson   230

Chapter 8. Teratogenic Potential of Mycotoxins
  R. V. Reddy and C. S. Reddy   270

Chapter 9. Natural Products and Congenital
  Malformations: Structure-Activity Relationships
  R. F. Keeler, W. Gaffield and K. E. Panter   310

Chapter 10. Cyanide Containing Foods and Potential
  for Fetal Malformations – *R. P. Sharma*   332

Chapter 11. Substance Abuse and Pregnancy Outcome
  R. P. Sharma and Y. W. Kim   349

Index   377

Preface

The importance of adequate nutrition during pregnancy needs no emphasis. Both a lack of, and excess of, certain dietary factors can harm the fetal health and considerably alter the pregnancy outcome. A healthy newborn is essential not just in relation to his/her immediate appearance but also for a normal development in the early neonatal phase. It has been suggested that the physical and intellectual development of a child, and even the susceptibility to disease during early life, can be related to a healthy pregnancy. Healthy pregnancy is not merely disease-free; it also requires adequate diet.

The material contained in this book is based on a symposium organized at the 1991 annual meeting of the Pacific Division of the American Association for the Advancement of Science. A revision of the contents, however, was necessary because many speakers were unable or unwilling to provide an adequate manuscript; other contributors were invited to cover topics of importance and to make the review of various dietary factors as complete as possible. It is the editor's hope that the material contained in this volume will be useful both to scientists working in this field of research and also to some extent, laymen who would like to know more about various topics covered here. The contributors of the various chapters deserve due credit; only the editor is responsible for any shortcomings. The timely cooperation of the authors is indeed highly appreciated.

The quality of information contained here could not be as

it is without the help of peer reviewers. All papers included here were prepared by well-known scientists in their fields. They were also reviewed by experts in the respective areas. A list of reviewers who devoted their time and experience to complete this project follows this section.

A sad note — during the preparation of this volume our dear friend and contributor of a chapter, Dr. Arthur W. Mahoney, passed away. Therefore, this book is dedicated to his memory.

The Editor

Acknowledgments

The editor is indebted to Dr. Alan E. Leviton of the Pacific Division of the American Association for the Advancement of Science for his excellent collaboration in organizing the symposium during the annual conference. Thanks are due to all speakers and contributors to this volume who spent a great deal of time to make this task a success and to several anonymous reviewers, members of the AAAS Pacific Division's Publications Committee, who reviewed all manuscripts and recommended their publication in this symposium volume.

The efforts of Mrs. Amy Ryan for making arrangements during the symposium and Mrs. Rosemary Parkinson in preparing the manuscripts for final publication are gratefully appreciated.

Thanks are due to various experts who provided timely peer reviews of various sections of this volume. A list of these professionals is provided below:

Narsingh D. Agnish, Hoffman-LaRoche, Nutley, NJ.

Maciej S. Buchowski, Maharry Medical College, Nashville, TN.

Bette J. Caan, Kaiser Research, Oakland, CA.

Roger A. Clemens, Carnation, Glendale, CA.

Roger A. Coulombe, Jr., Utah State University, Logan, UT.

David B. Drown, Utah State University, Logan, UT.

Kurt Gutknecht, Utah Agricultural Experiment Station, Logan, UT.

W. Chris Hawkes, U.S. Department of Agriculture, San Francisco, CA.

Craig Harris, University of Michigan, Ann Arbor, MI.

W. Brian Howard, Xavier University, New Orleans, LA.

Jodi I. Huggenvik, Utah State University, Logan, UT.

Richard Litov, Bristol-Meyers Squibb, Evansville, IN.

K. Mayura, Texas A & M University, College Station, TX.

Evelyn McGown, Letterman Army Inst. of Research, San Francisco, CA.

Russel J. Molyneux, U.S. Department of Agriculture, Al
bany, CA.
Kathleen T. Shiverick, University of Florida, Gainesville,
FL.
Marty L. Slattery, University of Utah, Salt Lake City, UT.
Dianne R. Soprano, Temple University, Philadelphia, PA.
Allen Taylor, Tufts University, Boston, MA.
Anthony T. Tu, Colorado State University, Fort Collins,
CO.

List of Contributors

Dr. G. E. Bunce
Department of Biochemistry and Nutrition
College of Agriculture and Life Science
Virginia Polytechnic Institute & State University
111 Engel Hall
Blacksburg, VA 24061-0308

Dr. J. M. Creech-Kraft
Department of Pharmacology
University of Washington
School of Medicine - SJ 30
Seattle, WA 98195

Dr. W. Gaffield
USDA Agricultural Research Service
Western Regional Research Center
Albany, CA 94710

Dr. J. L. Hess
Department of Biochemistry and Nutrition
College of Agriculture and Life Science
Virginia Polytechnic Institute & State University
111 Engel Hall
Blacksburg, VA 24061-0308

Dr. M. R. Juchau
Department of Pharmacology
University of Washington
School of Medicine - SJ 30
Seattle, WA 98195

Dr. R. F. Keeler
Poisonous Plants Research Laboratory
1150 E. 1400 North
Logan, UT 84321

Mr. Y. W. Kim
Center for Environmental Toxicology
Utah State University, UMC 5600
Logan, UT 84322-5600

Dr. D. M. Kochhar
Department of Anatomy & Developmental Biology
Thomas Jefferson University
1020 Locust Street
Philadelphia, PA 19107

Dr. Q. P. Lee
Department of Pharmacology
University of Washington
School of Medicine - SJ 30
Seattle, WA 98195

*Dr. A. W. Mahoney
Department of Nutrition and Food Science
Utah State University, UMC 8700
Logan, UT 84322-8700

Dr. M. J. Namkung
Department of Pharmacology
University of Washington
School of Medicine - SJ 30
Seattle, WA 98195

Dr. S. T. Omaye
Department of Nutrition
University of Nevada
Fleishmann Bldg., Rm. 113
Reno, NV 89557

Dr. K. E. Panter
Poisonous Plants Research Laboratory
1150 E. 1400 North
Logan, UT 84321

---

* Deceased

Dr. C. S. Reddy
Department of Veterinary Biomedical Sciences
University of Missouri
Columbia, MO 65211

Dr. R. V. Reddy
Sterling Winthrop Pharmaceuticals
81 Columbia Parkway
Rensselaer, NY 12144

Dr. M. A. Satre
Department of Anatomy & Developmental Biology
Thomas Jefferson University
1020 Locust Street
Philadelphia, PA 19107

Dr. R. P. Sharma
Center for Environmental Toxicology
Utah State University, UMC 5600
Logan, UT 84322-5600

Dr. D. S. Wilson
Department of Nutrition
University of Nevada
Fleishmann Bldg.
Reno, NV 89557

Dr. H. L. Yang
Department of Pharmacology
University of Washington
School of Medicine - SJ 30
Seattle, WA 98195

Dr. D. Zhang
Department of Nutrition and Food Sciences
Utah State University, UMC 8700
Logan, UT 84322-8700

DIETARY FACTORS

AND

BIRTH DEFECTS

Chapter 1

Maternal Nutrition And Pregnancy: An Overview

Raghubir P. Sharma

There is little argument to the fact that diet plays an important role in the outcome of a healthy pregnancy. This is not to imply that the nutritional quality of the diet that the majority of women consume during pregnancy is unhealthy; on the contrary, the quality of food and relevant dietary information is better than ever before. It is the diet of a small minority of women that may be of concern. In these cases, the overall quality of the diet is compromised by a deficiency of one or more of the essential constituents or by the presence of undesirable substances. This is largely due to the economic status of the women or a lack of information about the necessity of a healthy diet, particularly during pregnancy. The problem is most serious in much of the nonindustrialized world where both the availability of adequate food and lack of education are contributing factors. In some cases, the type or amount of diet is related to one's life style and can have an important influence on the outcome of pregnancy.

Much of the information provided in this book relates to the potential of dietary factors that cause birth defects of many types. Visible malformations in the newborn, for example, are not the only concern in pregnancy. Low birth weight is perhaps the major concern that can be considered a result of an inadequate diet during gestation (National Research Council, 1990). Intrauterine growth retardation is related to maternal weight gain during pregnancy and it is obvious that supplemental nutrition is needed for such maternal weight gain. Requirements for supplemental diet during pregnancy are briefly summarized here.

This book is intended as a source of information for both

1

researchers in this field and also an educated layman. Experts from all over the country have provided contributions and all are considered authorities in their fields. It has been pointed out that misinformation may be more harmful than a lack of information, particularly in the case of nutrition and pregnancy issues. In a survey of articles in popular magazines, Gunderson-Warner, *et al.* (1990) reported that of the 56 articles relating to pregnancy exposures, a majority of them (55.4%) were deemed as inaccurate or misleading. The information contained in a significant number of these articles (46.4%) was considered alarming, while in others (14.3%) it presented a false sense of security. Only 22 (39.3%) of the articles provided a balanced presentation. In most cases, the conclusions provided in these articles were unsupported by the scientific literature. Therefore, it is important to reference the information with the original source. An attempt has been made in all the papers presented here to include lengthy lists of bibliographic citations to document conclusions and suggestions.

The two most important considerations regarding diet during pregnancy are: (1) an adequate supply of essential nutrients, both for the mother and the fetus, and (2) avoidance of any substances in food that may be harmful to the conceptus. The main purpose of this volume is to address the latter; however, it is important to note that the former is perhaps of greater importance. Chapters included here consider nutritional deficiencies, particularly those of vitamins and trace minerals. A description of the role of iron availability during pregnancy is emphasized because this dietary essential is of greatest importance during the child-bearing period (National Research Council, 1990).

Supplements Recommended During Pregnancy

A healthy pregnancy requires adequate nutrition and additional supplements that should be included in the dietary regime. Both pregnancy and lactation require additional caloric intake needed for proper development of the fetus and also for compensating the maternal changes that occur during pregnancy. The National Research Council (1989) has established "Recommended Dietary Allowances" or "RDA" for healthy individuals. The RDA values were established in 1941 and have been constantly revised as additional scientific knowledge became available. Generally, energy requirements and major food constituents depend largely on one's size (height, weight), sex, and the nature of activity involved (especially physical work routinely performed). Pregnancy and lactation particularly affect these requirements. For a thorough discussion, readers are advised to refer to the latest (10th edition) of the Recommended Dietary Allowances. Some of that information, however, is briefly summarized here.

A pregnant woman requires an additional 300 kcal/day to her subsistence caloric requirements. For an average pregnant woman, that corresponds to 2500 kcal per day rather than 2200 kcal required daily for adequate nutrition without pregnancy. These additional calories are essential for optimal weight gain during the pregnancy. Generally, the additional calories may not be necessary during the first trimester of pregnancy unless there is a known nutritional deficit prior to and at the time of conception. During lactation, particularly if breast feeding is involved, the additional energy requirement is 500 kcal per day. In all cases, an adjustment is necessary for the size of the mother and the physical activity involved (for details, see National Research Council, 1989). The supplemental calories can be provided by various food components. However, additional protein requirements during pregnancy should also be considered. It has been recommended that a woman should consume at least 10 g of additional dietary protein each day throughout the pregnancy.

In addition to maintaining a proper balance of various major dietary constituents necessary to provide adequate energy and essential components, special attention should be devoted to trace substances, namely minerals and vitamins. Only in a few cases have the supplemental requirements of these substances during pregnancy been indicated. Table 1

TABLE 1: Average Recommended Daily Intake of Selected Vitamins and Minerals in Non-pregnant and Pregnant Women[1]

Nutrient	Non-pregnant women		Pregnant women
	19-24 yrs	25-50 yrs	
Vitamins			
A (µg)	800	800	800
D (µg)	10	5	10
E (mg)	8	8	10
K (µg)	60	65	65
C (mg)	60	60	70
Thiamine (mg)	1.1	1.1	1.5
Riboflavin (mg)	1.3	1.3	1.6
Niacin (mg)	15	15	17
Pantothenic acid (mg)	1.6	1.6	2.2
Folate (mg)	0.18	0.18	0.40
Cyanocobalamine (µg)	2	2	2.2
Minerals			
Calcium (mg)	1200	800	1200
Phosphorus (mg)	1200	800	1200
Magnesium (mg)	280	280	320
Iron (mg)	15	15	30
Zinc (mg)	12	12	15
Iodine (mg)	0.15	0.15	0.175
Selenium (µg)	55	55	65
Copper (mg)	0.5-3	0.5-3	2

[1] Adapted from National Academy of Sciences (1989).

lists some of the requirements established by the National Research Council (1989). The National Research Council (1990) has further recommended that, for pregnant women who do not ordinarily follow a sufficient dietary pattern or those in high-risk categories, a multivitamin-mineral supplement should be taken daily. The high-risk categories include pregnancies with more than one fetus, smokers, or drug or alcohol users. The suggested supplementation beginning the second trimester of pregnancy should include 30 mg iron, 15 mg zinc, 2 mg copper, 250 mg calcium, 2 mg vitamin B_6, 300 μg folate, 50 mg of vitamin C and 5 μg vitamin D. The supplements should be taken between meals or at bedtime to promote adequate absorption of these substances.

Fetal and Neonatal Development

The field of "developmental toxicology" or "teratology" includes all environmental or genetic influences that may lead to any discernible abnormalities in the offspring. If the effects are incompatible with the life of the developing organism, either at the embryonic or fetal stage, the result is usually a spontaneous abortion. These lethal effects on potential offspring, although not considered teratogenic, are nevertheless important in the overall outcome of pregnancy. Many structural defects are compatible with life and some of these may be repaired either naturally or by surgical intervention. The behavioral effects, many of which disappear with the growth of the individual, may require rehabilitation and could be permanent. It has been suggested that between 10 and 20 percent of pregnancies result in spontaneous abortions (Bloom, 1981). Of these, about a third (30-40%) can be related to genetic anomalies. A significant proportion (approximately 7%) of live births have low birth weight (<2500 g), which can be related to nutritional deficiencies. In general, noticeable malformations can be observed in 2-3% of live births, whereas mental retardation in infants may involve nearly 0.4% of children born. Birth defects are therefore still a rare phenomenon and incidence attributable to a known environmental cause can be very much less, except in selected episodes such as Minamata disease or the use of thalidomide (see later in this chapter). Chromosomal anomalies are responsible for even less (0.2%) of the malformations observed.

The mechanisms for an abnormal outcome of pregnancy are known for only a few chemical or biological causes. The mechanisms that have been described involve maternal hormonal imbalances that interfere with embryonic implantation or cause abnormal development of selected organs in the fetus. Genetic mutations or chromosomal aberrations may be responsible for a small number of structural deformities. Overall maternal nutrition, including the placental influences (transport of nutrients through the placenta) may be cause of a large number of teratologic incidences. These may lead to effects in developing fetus such as lack of normal substrates, osmotic imbalance or interference with energy utilization (including available oxygen), particularly important during the period of organogenesis. This period, most sensitive to environmental insult, is considered to be days 18-60 of gestation, or within the first two months of pregnancy. Metabolic poisons such as enzyme inhibitors also cause teratogenic effects. Certain classes of chemicals including steroid hormones and retinoic acid (see Chapter 6, this volume) induce malformations by activating or inhibiting nuclear transcription factors. Exact mechanisms for a variety of chemicals that influence expression of developmental genes are not well understood.

Dietary Factors and Birth Defects

It is assumed that nearly one in three conceptions results in resorption or stillbirth, yet the prevalence of birth defects based on dietary factors is a rare phenomenon. Exposure to chemicals can account for only a very small portion (2-3%) of deformities that may be present in the newborn. A large proportion of birth defects is believed to be caused by genetic transmission or unknown mechanisms. In many cases, infections (such as rubella) have been known to cause malformations in the fetus.

Generally, chemicals are considered as teratogens if they can induce structural anomalies indicated by one or more malformations. Some of the malformations (*e.g.*, absence of a vital organ or nervous tissue) are incompatible with life, whereas others are either repairable (naturally or after surgical intervention) or have little consequence. Recently, attention has been paid to various psychomotor dysfunctions that may not be detectable at birth but obviously result in subsequent defective development. Examples of such dysfunction are alcohol related birth defects (see Chapter 11, this volume) where learning deficits, language disorders, short attention span, etc., have been implied.

Iron is perhaps the only trace nutrient whose supplementation during pregnancy is highly recommended (National Research Council, 1990). The need for iron during pregnancy is relatively high in relation to the normal dietary requirement. Pregnant women with iron supplementation have a higher level of hemoglobin compared to those without supplementation. However, adverse effects of possible maternal iron deficiency on fetal health are considered only suggestive. A detailed consideration of iron bioavailability has been provided in Chapter 4 (this volume).

Both deficiency and excess of certain trace substances can influence the normal outcome of pregnancy. An example of such a nutrient is vitamin A or its derivatives. Deficiency of vitamin A is a known cause of fetal abnormalities. Excess of vitamin A or treatment with certain retinoids also have been shown to cause malformations. Because a large amount of information is available on this substance, and to some extent its molecular mechanisms are understood, a detailed review of this chemical is provided in Chapter 6 (this volume). However, it is suggested that normal supplementation of vitamin A during pregnancy is relatively free of any risk (Werler, *et al.*, 1990). A similar trace mineral may be selenium where both deficiency and excess can be harmful to the newborn (see Chapter 7, this volume, for details).

Prescription Drugs

Prescription drugs are perhaps a major cause of fetal malformations observed. The importance of prescription drugs as tertogens was emphasized after the thalidomide episode (Lenz, 1966). Thalidomide was used as an analgesic in Europe, Australia and Japan to combat nausea and vomiting in pregnancy. The drug was presumably responsible for malformations in as many as 10,000 children. The affected offspring were typically afflicted with amelia (absence of limbs) or phocomelia (limbs of small sizes of varying degrees). The known cases of human fetal malformations by retinoids have also resulted after the use of prescription chemicals. The same is also true for diethylstilbestrol (DES) that has been linked to post-natal incidence of cancer of the cervix (Poskanzer & Herbst, 1977). A review of these substances, however, is beyond the scope of this book and the interested reader is advised to consult the excellent reviews of Miller, *et al.* (1987).

In some cases, the presence of a substance in the diet or the use of a drug can interfere with the availability or metabolism of an essential nutrient that may be required for proper fetal growth. Examples of such substances have been discussed in terms of iodine deficiency induced by the presence of thiocyanates in food (Chapter 10) or the use of antiepileptic drugs, which are implicated in folate deficiency. A variety of antiepileptic drugs (trimethadione, valproate, carbamezapine and even phenytoin) have been associated with increased incidence of malformations in children born to mothers on therapy. The exact association is not definite and it has been reported that children born to women treated by a combination of drugs were more likely to have congenital defects than those born to mothers on a single drug therapy (Lander & Eadie, 1990). Various associated teratologic effects include spina bifida, neural tube defects, craniofacial alterations, fingernail hypoplasia and retardation of development. A deficiency of folic acid caused by antiepileptic drug therapy has been implicated but a definite association is yet to be established.

Environmental Pollutants Contaminating Food

It was not possible here to cover nonessential contaminants in food in relation to their reproductive outcome. An example of a calamity of epidemic proportions was the presence of methylmercury in contaminated fish (Smith & Smith, 1975). During the late 1950s, a disease, now called Minamata disease, occurred near Minamata Bay in Southwest Japan. The problem was related to the presence of methylmercury in local fish, which were the primary source of dietary protein for local communities (Harada, 1978). The condition was more prominent in families of fishermen who depended more on their catch than on other sources for protein. The disease afflicted people of all ages causing problems with sensory and locomotor functions of extremities. There was numbness of limbs, difficulty with hand movement, lack of coordination, weakness, and tremor. There was also slurring of speech, ataxic gait, and problems with vision and hearing. In addition to having symptoms of methylmercury poisoning in adults, the children born to a number of women in afflicted families exhibited congenital malformations. In many cases, the mothers did not exhibit apparent symptoms of mercury poisoning. A number of these mothers, however, had subclinical neurological disorders. The affected children had malformations of limbs, severe mental retardation, difficulty in speaking (dysarthria) and central and peripheral neurological disturbances. Most of the symptoms were nonreversible and persisted for years. Methylmercury easily crosses the placenta and enters the fetus; thus the condition may have worsened by consuming contaminated milk in infancy from mothers having a high body burden of methylmercury.

Lead is another environmental pollutant that has been shown to have an association with defective development of children after *in utero* exposure (Bellinger, *et al.*, 1987). Fetal exposure to levels of lead previously considered safe may be linked to impairment of infant mental development (Davis & Svensgaard, 1987). Maternal blood lead levels of 10-15 μg/dl, which did not have any observable effect on the mother herself, were linked with undesirable developmental outcomes. The effects were not structural. However, the mental development of children born to mothers with cord-blood lead levels of higher than 10 μg/dl, was significantly slower than those in the low cord-blood lead group (<3 μg/dl).

References

Bellinger, D., Leviton, A., Waternaux, C., Needleman, H., and Rabinowitz, M. (1987). Longitudinal analysis of prenatal and postnatal lead exposure and early cognitive development. *New Engl. J. Med.* 316:1037-1043.

Bloom, A. D., ed. (1981). Guidelines for Studies of Human Populations Exposed to Mutagenic and Reproductive Hazards. March of Dimes Foundation, New York. 37-110 pp.

Davis, J. M., and Svendsgaard, D. J. (1987). Lead and child development. *Nature* 329:297-300.

Gunderson-Warner, S., Martinex, L. P., Martinex, I. P., Carey, J. C., Kochenour, N. K., and Emery, M. G. (1990). Critical review of articles regarding pregnancy exposures in popular magazines. *Teratology* 42:469-472.

Harada, M. (1978). Methylmercury poisoning due to environmental contamination (Minamata disease). Pages 261-302 *in* F. W. Oehme, ed., *Toxicity of Heavy Metals in the Environment.* Part 1. Marcel Dekter, New York.

Lander, C. M., and Eadie, M. J. (1990). Antiepileptic drug intake during pregnancy and malformed children. *Epilepsy Res.* 7:77-82.

Lenz, W. (1966). Malformations caused by drugs in pregnancy. *Amer. J. Dis. Child.* 112:99-106.

Miller, R. K., Kellogg, C. K., and Saltzman, R. A. (1987). Reproductive and perinatal toxicology. Pages 195-309 *in* T. J. Haley and W. O. Berndt, eds., *Handbook of Toxicology.* Hemisphere Publishing, Washington, D.C.

National Research Council (1989). *Recommended Dietary Allowances,* 10th Ed. National Academy Press, Washington, D. C. 285pp.

National Research Council (1990). *Nutrition During Pregnancy.* National Academy Press, Washington, D. C. 454 pp.

Poskanzer, D. C., and Herbst, A. L. (1977). Epidemiology of

vaginal adenosis and adenocarcinoma associated with exposure to stilbestrol *in utero. Cancer* 39:1892-1895.

Smith, W. E., and Smith, A. M. (1975). *Minamata.* Holt, Rheinhart & Winston, New York.

Werler, M. M., Lammer, E. J., Rosenberg, L., and Mitchell A. A. (1990). Maternal vitamin A supplementation in relation to selected birth defects. *Teratology* 42:497-503.

Chapter 2

Nutrient Deficiencies And Pregnancy Outcome

Stanley T. Omaye

Just as in the adult, it can be shown that in the developing embryo and the fetus, balanced proportions of fundamental nutrients must be incorporated in the diet. A correct balance of proteins, lipids, carbohydrates and also vitamins and minerals is essential for the normal progression that leads to the birth of healthy new life. All the nutrients that are required for this ordinary progression must be derived through the placenta and, in turn, from the mother's blood. Energy for maintenance and growth comes mostly from glucose, while nitrogen for the synthesis of a myriad of different proteins in the body is secured from amino acids. In addition, minerals, vitamins, purine bases, and small quantities of essential fatty acids are extracted for their important roles in the development. At every stage of its development, the embryo is a living organism that requires nutrients for its vital workings.

The growth process consists of the consumption and combustion of massive amounts of nutrients. When the blastocyst is free and unattached to the uterus, it absorbs nutrients through its outer layer, the trophoblast, and from the discharge of the uterine glands (uterine milk). After the blastocyst becomes implanted in the uterine epithelium, placental circulation begins.

Embryo nutrition must be adequate and balanced in both macro- and micronutrients. The embryo is unable to withstand nutritional inadequacy, and it has varying requirements during differing stages of its development. Nutritional deficiency produces devastating effects qualitatively in the early stages of development and quantitatively in the subsequent stages. These effects include: growth retardation, physical malformation, and/or intrauterine exitus.

This chapter will report what is currently understood about the effects of nutrient deficiencies on the outcome of pregnancy. Because it is not often possible to examine maternal-fetal relationships directly at the molecular or cellular levels in humans, a great deal of the information presented is derived from research done on animals or taken from *in vitro* culture techniques using animal embryos (Webster, 1989; Scott, *et al.*, 1990). In animals, we have been able to manipulate the diets of pregnant females and observe the eventual outcome. Such findings have contributed significantly toward our better understanding of nutrient deficiency and the importance that nutrients play in pregnancy.

Stages of Growth and Consequences of Growth Failure

Types of Growth

Growth in all animals takes place in one of two ways. The cells within the organism either increase in number (hyperplasia) or increase in size (hypertrophy). In the first stage of growth, cells increase in number by hyperplasia; cells replicate and all are of nearly equal size. In the second stage of growth, new cells continue to be established, but the ones already present experience hypertrophy. This stage is characterized by increase in both cell number and size. The third stage is totally hypertrophic; growth in the third stage takes place only by increases in cell size. No new cells are added during this stage. The fourth stage is maturity, in which all cell growth essentially stops. Now we see further development as various enzyme systems are detailed and cell functions become integrated into various systems. Figure 1 is a schematic that illustrates the stages of cell growth based on measurements of the DNA contents of organs or tissues. It is known that the cellular DNA content is the same for any given species. Therefore, the amount of DNA in an organ or tissue sample divided by the amount of DNA per cell gives the

Stages of Cell Growth

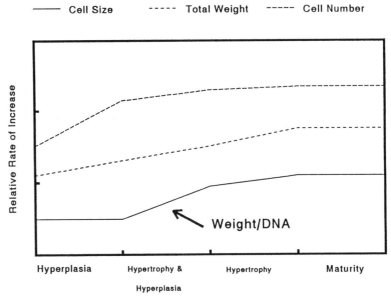

FIGURE 1. Stages of cell growth. Graphs derived from Worthington-Roberts & Williams, 1989.

number of cells present. Subsequently, the total weight of the organ can be divided by the number of cells to give an indication of the average cell mass (Worthington-Roberts & Williams, 1989).

As development proceeds with increased cell division, intracellular activity increases. Cell division requires that every organelle of the cell be duplicated. This includes the mitochondria, the ribosomes, the assorted intracellular and outer membranes, the chromosomes, and all their various enzymes and components responsible for such activities. All these organelles and suborganelles dictate synthesis and congregation from a multitude of different substances, *i.e.*, DNA, RNA, protein, lipid, as well as various micronutrients. Such synthesis and congregation require enzymes that themselves have been synthesized according to directions from the genes. These processes require considerable activity and coordination that eventually results in an astronomical number of orderly molecular events. Any impairment of early cell proliferation may ultimately become amplified many times. Hyperplasia-hypertrophy is a critical period of development which is especially vulnerable to adverse effects.

Effect of Timing and Critical Periods

As indicated above, development of all organs occurs by the processes of hyperplasia and hypertrophy. These two processes may occur simultaneously, may overlap, or may occur in sequence. There is a characteristic schedule for each developing organ. The critical period may be during cell division or when differentiation and proliferation occur, although the most conspicuous growth is noted in the times of increase in size. In order for an organ to reach its full potential, nutrient supplies must be optimal from the beginning. Limiting cell division and the final cell number that is expected in an organ can have irreversible effects, which may not be realized until the individual reaches maturity. Figure 2 illustrates the weeks of human pregnancy during which some body organs and tissues are most vulnerable to injury or lack of adequate nutrients.

Each organ and tissue is most susceptible to nutrient deprivation during its specific critical periods. The heart is well developed at 16 weeks, while the lungs are still immature 10 weeks later. Subsequently, early nutrition deprivation affects the heart most severely, while later deprivation will affect the lungs. Although the embryonic period of hyperplasia is of major importance, one must not exclude that later nutritional deprivation may also produce damage to the developing offspring. The structure of an organ may not be noticeably affected, but lack of nutrient may result in suboptimal function of that organ. Regardless of species, the consequences of any interruption of normal cell growth are dependent on the time at which it occurs. Interruption during hyperplasia will result in a decrease in the number of cells produced. If the hypertrophic stage is interrupted, cells will be smaller. Both types of interference could result in growth failure.

Critical Times of Development

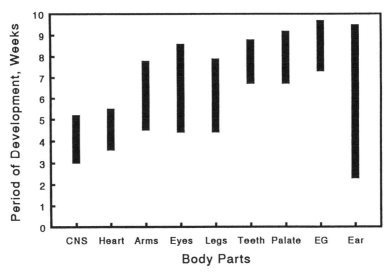

FIGURE 2. Critical times of development when certain organs or tissues are prone to adverse teratogenic effects of dietary deficiencies.

Brain development is very susceptible to lack of nutrients, especially during its growth spurt, the period in which the brain weight increases most rapidly (Winick & Rosso, 1969). This period is around midpregnancy and continues into the second year after birth (Hurley, 1980). There are also species-related differences. In contrast to the human, in the rat, neurons of the central nervous system (CNS) stop dividing before birth. Inadequate nutrition during this period may produce irreversible damage to the brain, which modifies later behavior.

Malnutrition, Undernutrition, and Pregnancy

There are two ways that researchers investigate the effects of nutrient defects on the developing embryo or fetus (Figure 3). The first is global and works from the perspective of overall inadequate or undernutrition, which can be found in many undeveloped nations. In general, global effects do not

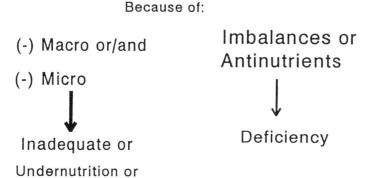

FIGURE 3.   Approaches that a lack of nutrients may effect the developing embryo or fetus.

influence the balance of nutrients, although both macro-and/or micronutrients may be effected. The second approach is a study of a single nutrient deficiency. Discrete developmental effects of single nutrient deficiencies are seldom seen in the real world, especially in humans. Discrete deficiencies can occur as a result of antinutrients, which bind or compete with a nutrient and make it unavailable. An example is avidin, found in raw egg white, which combines with the vitamin biotin and makes it unavailable for absorption. Studies of single nutrient deficiencies and their metabolic effects have been extremely useful in elucidating biochemical mechanisms.

Both approaches are readily reproduced in laboratory animal studies by imposing maternal dietary restriction during fetal growth and development. One method is simply to restrict animal's food intake so that the diet is low in calories. The other is to hold calories at an adequate level but to reduce or eliminate completely one or more essential nutrients. Global restriction has had consequences on fertility, on the weight of the embryos, and their ability to survive. Specific nutrient deficiencies may have the same results as global, but they may also induce malformations or tissue alterations (Giround, 1970).

Approximately one in every 15 infants born in the United States is a low-birth weight infant (NICHHD, 1985). These are full-term infants, not just preterm births, who are diminutive because of malnutrition. Approximately one-fourth of low-birth weight infants born in the U.S. die within the first month of life. In the world, it is estimated that almost one-sixth of all live infants are of low-birth weight.

It is difficult to observe dietary effects on fetus development. Problems include determining maternal dietary intake and controlling variables. One important study was done in 1940 by Burke. In this study (Burke, et al., 1943), mothers whose diets were classified as good or excellent according to the Recommended Dietary Allowances (RDAs) gave birth to babies rated by pediatricians who were naive to the study as superior or good health 94% of the time. Only 8% of the mothers whose diets were classified as poor gave birth to infants in good or superior health.

In a more recent study, the relationship between infant birth weight and diet quality was examined (Phillipps & Johnson, 1977). These investigators found a positive correlation between higher quality of diet and infant birth weight. This study furnished supplementary data to support the hypothesis that diet during pregnancy significantly affects the health of infants.

The irreversible effects of malnutrition are illustrated in case studies where specific nutrient deficiencies caused damage to the fetus, and adequate diets after the critical time failed to reverse the damage. This was observed in the years following the Korean War when Americans adopted Korean orphans. These children experienced several years of catch-up growth but did not completely recover from their early exposure to malnutrition (Lien, et al., 1977). In the other example, maternal fasting during pregnancy can cause later obesity in a child by depriving the brain's developing regulatory centers of glucose (Kirtland & Gurr, 1979). Clearly, it is important that optimal nutrition occurs during pregnancy to insure the likelihood of a healthy birth.

In response to alarming numbers of low-birth weight infants, many intervention studies on pregnant women have been conducted throughout the world. For example, in the United States, the number of low-birth weight infants was over 250,000 in 1985, or 7 percent of the total live births world-wide (Rolfes & De Bruyne, 1990) and in the past even greater (Petros-Barvazian & Behar, 1978).

Single Nutrient Deficiency and Pregnancy

Energy, Carbohydrates, and Fat

During the course of pregnancy, a woman consumes approximately 80,000 Kcal to the recommended 25 to 35 pounds, (RDA subcommittee, 1989). Because most of the growth of the fetus occurs in the last two trimesters, most increased consumption occurs after the first three months. This can be illustrated by studying the weights of live-born infants at differing gestational ages. Figure 4 is a composite of the calculations of Widdowson (1987), superimposed over data from Gruenwald (1966) and Iffy, *et al.*, (1975). Widdowson (1987) took the data of live-born infants and plotted their weights from 18 to 42 weeks of age. These cross-sectional data illustrated that by 28 weeks, the fetus weights were just over 1 kg; the rate of growth then accelerated up to about 33 weeks, where it peaked and slowed down for the next 7 weeks (Figure 4a). Her calculations made this clear by looking at weight in terms of velocity of gain (Figure 4b).

The primary source of energy for the fetus is carbohydrate in the form of glucose (Hay, 1991). Glucose is used early in the free blastocyst, but at a very low concentration compared to the maternal serum. From glucose, glycogen is formed in the placenta, especially during the first several weeks (Huggett, 1961). Later, from glucose, the fetus synthesizes

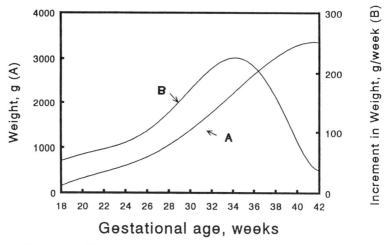

FIGURE 4. (a) Human fetus weights at birth and (b) the velocity of weekly gain. Graphs are composites from data of Gruenwald (1966) and Iffy, *et al.*, (1975) and derived from calculations of Widdowson, (1987).

glycogen which is stored mainly in the heart, liver, and skeletal muscle (Widdowson, 1968). Glucose serves as the precursor from which the fetus synthesizes fat.

In early gestation, the fetus only uses essential lipids and phospholipids derived from the maternal circulation for laying down cell membranes and nervous system. In addition, the cholesterol used by the placenta for steroid hormone synthesis is derived from the maternal plasma (Hellig, *et al.*, 1970). After 20 weeks, white fat begins to be synthesized and laid down in connective tissue; and brown adipose tissue cells accumulate fat during the latter part of gestation, but in much less quantity than white fat. Free fatty acids cross the human placenta freely, and essential fatty acids of maternal origin are found in the fetal tissues (Widdowson, *et al.*, 1975). However, the cord blood of neonates contains relatively low concentrations of the major essential fatty acids; and delay in feeding premature infants increases the incidence of essential fatty acid deficiency (Farrell, *et al.*, 1988; Farrell, *et al.*, 1985).

Burr & Burr (1929) made the first observations that female rats fed a fat-deficient diet were sterile, and/or their embryos died. This was subsequently traced to a need for essential fatty acids. Farrell and workers have found that premature infants are born with depressed linoleate levels in plasma and bronchial secretions and that delayed feeding of these infants exacerbates the essential fatty acid deficiency (Farrell, *et al.*, 1988; Farrell, *et al.*, 1985). The proportion of infants with essential fatty acid deficiency increased with age unless supplements were provided. The authors advocated adding linoleate through parenteral nutrition because of the vital role such lipids play in prostanoid metabolites (Dupont, *et al.*, 1980).

The energy requirement of the fetus is on the order of 35.6 kcal/kg/24 hrs. This value is based on the assumption that the human fetus utilizes 5 ml of oxygen/kg/min and uses glucose as primary fuel. One consequence of the use of glucose as a primary fuel is that babies of diabetic mothers have an increased rate of malformations, most frequently neural tube defects (Leck, 1979; Wheeler, *et al.*, 1982). The maternal precondition might lead to a delay in switching from anaerobic to aerobic use of carbohydrates in early uterine life, which may explain the higher neural tube defects incidence in such pregnancies (Freinkel, *et al.*, 1984). Recently, a study addressed the prospect that the teratogenic effects of a diabetic pregnancy are associated with increased embryonic activities of free oxygen radicals (Eriksson & Borg, 1991). The results of the study suggest that a high glucose concentration causes embryonic dysmorphogenesis by the generation of free oxygen radicals. An enhanced production of such radicals in embryonic tissue may be directly related to the increased risk of congenital malformations in diabetic pregnancy.

Amino Acids and Protein

Maternal amino acids are the primary source of nitrogen for fetal protein synthesis (Munro, *et al.*, 1983). Placental transport must involve an active transport mechanism, but the concentration differences from maternal and fetal plasma are not the same for each amino acid. Metabolism-resistant analogues of amino acids have been used to demonstrate the presence of amino acid transport systems in fetal tissues (Yudilevich & Sweiry, 1985). For example, some amino acids are retained by the fetus for protein synthesis in greater quantities than others. Perfusion studies on human placentas show that active transport from maternal to fetal circulation occurs only for L-isomers of amino acids (Schneider, *et al.*, 1979).

The rate of protein incorporation increases throughout gestation. The protein changes are a composite of many internal alterations because of the many different proteins in the body, such as intracellular and extracellular structural, enzymes, hormones, as well as parts of other macromolecule assembly systems, each with its own rate of development.

In animal studies, protein restriction during certain critical periods produced offspring with reduced numbers of cells at term (Zeman, 1970). Supplementation after restriction during the critical periods did not produce normal numbers of cells in the liver, heart, kidney, and brain in laboratory animals. Therefore, the effects of protein deficiency in reducing cell number in selected organs is not reversible (Zeman, *et al.*, 1973).

Micronutrients

Little is known about vitamin and mineral needs during pregnancy (Worthington-Roberts, 1985). Most of the data are from animal studies and there are few controlled observations of human subjects.

Animal studies first employed synthetic diets in which only the vitamin being studied was lacking. Sometimes it was important to modify the diet procedures by using: antibiotic or germ-free animals to exclude the effects of gut microflora, or pair-fed animals to avoid misleading conclusions. More recently, antagonists of vitamins were frequently used because the effect was fast and specific periods of embryogenesis could be targeted. Several conclusions have been drawn from animal experiments. Specific nutrient deficiencies can cause reduced birth weights, smaller litter size, increased fetal resorption, increased spontaneous abortion, and increased congenital malformations.

From the limited data available on pregnant humans, such as from those women whose self-selected diets were unbalanced, we can only speculate. However, speculation should be near correct because there is no reason to believe that the human is not similar to many of the animal models that have been studied.

B Vitamins

Thiamin deficiency in pregnant rats results in an increased number of stillbirths and low birth weight pups (Nelson & Evans, 1955; Brown & Snodgrass, 1965). There is also marked maternal weight loss and elevated maternal mortality; therefore, the general gestational disorders may be related to maternal nutrient insufficiency. Also, there is reduced fertility identified with inadequate thiamin intake prior to pregnancy.

In humans, there is no manifestation of fetal malformation resulting from maternal vitamin B_1 deficiency, but several studies have pointed to congenital beriberi. In India and Japan, thiamin deficient diets are implied as responsible for premature births and stillbirths (Bourquin & Bennum, 1957; Van Gelder & Darby, 1944).

Riboflavin deficiency can produce severe congenital malformations in animals (Warkany & Schraffenberger, 1944). Defects consist of short mandible, tibia, fibula, radius and ulna, fusion of ribs, syndactyly, cleft palate, dental and facial malformations, hydrocephaly, eye defects, and other abnormalities. In addition, increased fetal death and resorption have been observed.

There are no reports of malformation in humans associated with riboflavin deficiency (Worthington-Roberts & Williams, 1989). One study involved some 900 pregnant women who were diagnosed as riboflavin deficient. These women had a higher incidence of vomiting during pregnancy, premature delivery, and stillbirths. Unsuccessful lactation was also common. On the other hand, in a study of European women where biochemical evidence of riboflavin deficiency was found, the deficiency was not correlated with abortion, pre-eclampsia, stillbirth or low birth weight.

Niacin deficiency in rats resulted in no viable fetuses. Feeding the niacin antimetabolite, 6-amino-nicotinamide, resulted in multiple congenital malformations such as defects of the skeleton, central nervous system, eyes, urinary system, trunk and thyroid and thymus glands (Chamberlain & Nelson, 1963; Pinsky & Fraser, 1960; Schardein, *et al.*, 1967). In rats, a single injection of the antimetabolite during pregnancy produced hydrocephaly and ocular, urogenital, and vascular defects.

Inspite of pellagra in some countries, there seems to be no prevalence of malformation in humans related to niacin deficiency.

Pyridoxal. Studies in animals on vitamin B_6 deficiency have shown that spontaneous abortions are frequent, but no teratogenic action has been noted (Ross & Pike, 1956; Nelson & Evans, 1951). Convulsions occurred in the early days of the life of the offspring. On the other hand, pyridoxal deficiency caused neural tube defects in some laboratory animals (Davis, *et al.*, 1970). Offspring from mothers fed B_6-deficient diets showed poor survival, slower weight gain, reduced physical activity, and a higher incidence of errors in a maze test. Neuromuscular development and coordination were also impaired. However, B_6-deficiency created through the use of pyridoxine antagonists, caused high rates of resorption, stillbirth, and low-birth-weights. High dosages of the antagonist in the diet resulted in congenital malformations, including defects in digits, cleft palate, omphalocele, shortness of the lower jaw, and exencephaly.

In humans, low maternal blood levels of B_6 have not been shown to be associated with abnormal births. Some women with low dietary and serum levels of vitamin B_6 have produced a greater number of children with low Apgar scores compared to mother with good vitamin status.

Folic acid deficiency in animals produces multiple fetal anomalies (Nelson and Evans, 1949; O'Dell, *et al.*, 1948; Hogan, *et al.*, 1950). Malformations involve the eye, central nervous system, palate, lip, gastrointestinal system, aorta, kidney, and skeleton. Likewise, using a folate antagonist produces the same adverse effects (Nelson, *et al.*, 1956; Thiersch & Phillips, 1950). The animal work reported in the literature has demonstrated that a marginal deficiency in the pregnant rat can affect the offsprings' growth rate, and more severe deficiency states result in neonatal death (Thenen, 1991; Anon, 1991a).

Folate deficiency in pregnant women has not been proven to have an adverse effect on pregnancy outcome; however, correlations have been reported between red cell folate level and incidence of congenital malformations, small-for-gestational age babies, and third trimester bleeding. In Africa and India, folate supplementation significantly reduced the rate of premature births (Thenen, 1991; Anon, 1991a). Some prospective studies have indicated that low red cell folate levels were associated with increased congenital malformations and increased incidence of neural tube defects. Hibbard & Smithells (1965) looked at folate status in 98 mothers with malformed infants and found that, of 73 of those who had CNS malformation, there was a five-fold increase in abnormal N-formimino-L-glutamate (FIGlu) test results compared to matched controls. The FIGlu test is not now considered a reliable test of folate status. In contrast, several studies have not been able to demonstrate a relationship between folate status and malformations (Fraser & Watt, 1964; Emery, *et al.*, 1969; Hall, 1972; Schorah, *et al.*, 1983). Other investigators argue that folic acid-containing multivitamins during the first six weeks of pregnancy had a significant protective effect against the occurrence of neural tube defects (Smithells, *et al.*, 1983; Mulinare *et al.*, 1988).

There is substantial geographical and ethnic variation in the prevalence of neural tube defects. For the most part, the etiology is unknown, but most believe that it is multifactorial. Women who have had an affected pregnancy are at high risk of recurrence in later pregnancies. Yet, up to 95% neural tube defects occur in families without a previous history (Hobbins, 1991). Unfortunately, the closure of the neural tube occurs in 22 to 29 days after conception. Therefore, intervention can only be effective by starting early, *i.e.*, prior to conception.

The Medical Research Council of the United Kingdom sponsored a prospective study to determine whether folate and/or multivitamin supplementation would reduce the reoccurrence of neural tube defects (MRC, 1991; Anon, 1992). The study covered from July 1983 to April of 1991 with some 2000 pregnancies. Of the 593 women who were in the group that received folate at the level of 4 mg, six had offspring with neural tube defects, and a recurrence rate of 1% compared to 3.5% found in women who received multivitamins or no supplements. Folate supplementation reduced the relative risk of recurrence to 0.28, with 95% confidence interval of 0.12. The relative risk of the group receiving multivitamins alone (no folate) had relative risk of 0.8, which was not significantly different from 1.0. Because the dose of folate was pharmacologic (10 times the RDA), this study raises serious concerns about the recommended intake for women and prompted the U.S. Centers for Disease Control to a recommendation plan (Rush, 1992).

Concerns, such as masking B_{12} deficiency and deleterious effects on zinc metabolism have been raised in response to folate supplementations (Institute of Medicine, 1990; Simmer *et al.*, 1987). The split in scientific viewpoint has produced diverse stands between two U. S. public health agencies (Palca, 1992). Only through a better understanding of mechanisms and dose-response curve will we be able to determine whether a lower intake of folic acid could further reduce even the present low incidence of nerual tube defects (at 4 mg of folic acid).

Vitamin B_{12} deficiency in animals has been reported to cause hydrocephalus and other congenital abnormalities, including flaws of the eye, decreased nerve myelination, bone defects, and increased cellularity of the bone marrow (O'Dell, *et al.*, 1951; Jones *et al.*, 1955; Woodard & Newberne, 1966). In addition, marginal B_{12} deficiency in pregnant rats has been correlated with subnormal birth weight, slow growth rate, and reduced resistance to infection.

When pernicious anemia is found in child-bearing age women, it generally is accompanied by infertility.

Pantothenic acid deficiency in pregnant rats results in complete litter resorption (Ullrey, *et al.*, 1955; Hurley, *et al.*, 1965). Antagonists have been used to augment the deficiency state. Neural tube defects have been reported in animals with pantothenic acid deficiency (Lefebvres-Boisselot, 1951).

Biotin. Although no malformations have been seen in rats with biotin deficiency (Giround, 1970), in mice fed diets containing egg white (contains avidin, a biotin antagonist), more than 90 percent of the fetuses showed external or skeletal congenital abnormalities. The predominant malformations were micrognathia, cleft palate, and micromelia. This has been corroborated recently where the combined teratogenic effects of biotin deficiency and moderately high vitamin A were mostly attributed to the biotin deficiency (Wantanabe & Endo, 1991). They concluded that, in mice, the concentrations of vitamin A in the range of 4-10 times the level recommended by the National Research Council and biotin deficiency do not interfere with one another; also, biotin deficiency *per se* is teratogenic in mice. The same authors (Wantanabe & Endo, 1989) found that biotin-deficiency-induced malformation was species dependent. No malformations were observed in the rat, but embryonic lethality was very high in biotin-deficient hamster dams. These results suggest that a possible underlying mechanism is a difference in the efficiency of the mother-to-fetus transport of biotin among these species.

Ascorbic Acid

In female guinea pigs fed vitamin C-deficient diets, no pregnancy occurred (Martin, *et al.*, 1957). With low, inadequate vitamin C diets, there was a high incidence of spontaneous abortion and resorption rate in guinea pigs. Low birth weight and retarded development of skin and muscle have been reported for the offspring of guinea pigs fed a low vitamin C diet.

In humans, several reports have indicated that low serum vitamin C levels were associated with threatened abortion or history of previous spontaneous abortions. Smithells, *et al.*, (1976) found that four women who delivered neural tube-defective babies, from a group of 1098 pregnant women, had lower white cell vitamin C levels. In addition, it was found that women at high risk (*e.g.*, history) for neural tube defects had a higher, but not statistically significant, frequency of leucocyte ascorbate levels below the fifth percentile of normal range (Smithells, *et al.*, 1983).

Vitamin A

In pigs, offspring of sows fed diets deficient in vitamin A had a higher incidence of anophthalmia or microphthalmia (Giround, 1970). Other studies demonstrated eye defects, histological abnormalities of the genitourinary tract, diaphragmatic hernia, and cardiovascular abnormalities. Other animal studies revealed dramatically reduced reproductive efficiency, high fetal mortality, and severe congenital malformations of the skeleton and other organs.

In humans, prenatal vitamin A deficiency has been related, in several instances, to eye abnormalities and impaired vision in children. An Indian women, blind from vitamin A deficiency, gave birth to premature infant with microcephaly and anophthalmia (Sarma, 1959).

Vitamin D

Deficiency in female rats and cows produces skeletal anomalies in offspring resembling those of rickets (Grant & Goettch, 1926).

Several cases of human fetal rickets have been reported where the mother had low serum vitamin D or suffered from osteomalacia during pregnancy. Neonatal hypocalcemia is reportedly more common during months of the year when daily sunlight is minimal.

Vitamin E

Deficiency in female rats produces sterility, fetal resorption, stillbirth, and high incidence of multiple congenital malformations (Evans & Bishop, 1922; Cheng, *et al.*, 1960). This includes exencephaly, anencephaly, umbilical hernia, scoliosis, club feet, cleft lip, syndactyly and kinked tail. There is high maternal mortality following pregnancy, with lethargy, pallor, dyspnea and vaginal hemorrhage.

In humans, there has been some correlation noted between birth-weight and cord blood levels of vitamin E.

Vitamin K

Deficiency in female rats has been observed in the newborn (Brown, *et al.*, 1947). The consequence has been hypoprothrombinemia with high incidence of spontaneous abortion.

In humans, a number of cases have been reported of fetal abnormalities of women treated with anticoagulants (Tournay, 1951). There is some evidence that the use of dicoumarol during pregnancy is associated with increased fetal mortality and morbidity (Tournay, 1951).

Minerals

Iron deficiency in female rats during pregnancy resulted in the delivery of pups that were anemic during the early weeks of life. The more litters the dam delivered, the greater the severity of anemia in the young. Neonatal mortality was higher in anemic offspring.

In humans, unless the iron deficiency is severe, mean hemoglobin levels of the fetus is unaffected by maternal iron levels. Infants of anemic mothers tend to show reduced iron stores and greater tendency to develop anemia in the first years of life. There also is an increased incidence of prematurity of offspring when maternal iron is deficient. For further information on the effects of iron, the reader is referred to Chapter 4 (this volume).

Calcium: If calcium deficiency is severe and/or prolonged in pregnant rats, normal development and calcification of the fetus does not occur. In humans, calcium deficiency has been proposed to be the major etiologic factor in toxemia of pregnancy (Giround, 1970).

Iodine: Cretinism has been reported in experimental and field (wild) animals by feeding the animal diets low in iodine. Cretinism was first described in the 16th century and was associated with goiter by the 19th century. Cretinous children exhibit mental and physical retardation. In New Guinea, recent outbreaks of cretinism were reversed by providing local iodine-rich salt (Underwood, 1977).

Sodium deficiency in female rats results in reduced fertility and low birth weight pups, but later work found no fetal effects, only adverse maternal responses. Deficiency of sodium in sheep produces fetal deficiency more readily. In humans, hyponatremia has been reported in offspring of women who rigorously restricted sodium during pregnancy (Underwood, 1977).

Potassium deficiency in animals have shown minimal effects in offspring.

Magnesium: Severe magnesium deficiency in female rats resulted in no pregnancies carried to term and high resorption rates (Underwood, 1977). Many of the surviving fetuses were malformed, showing cleft lip, short tongue, hydrocephalus, micrognathia, club feet, polydactyly, syndactyly, short or curly tail, herniations, and heart, lung and urogenital anomalies. There was also impaired fetal hematopoiesis and hemolytic anemia due to red cell malformation. Fetal liver and bone marrow cell demonstrated chromosomal abnormalities.

Manganese: In several animal species, manganese deficiency resulted in offspring with abnormal skeletal growth and development results in chondrodystrophy or disproportionate abnormal skeletal growth (Underwood, 1977). There was impaired mucopolysaccharide synthesis and offspring demonstrated an ataxic condition secondary to defective morphogenesis of the vestibular portion of the inner ear. In the manganese-deficiency mouse, there was an absence of vestibular otoliths. In a study which was designed to investigate the manganese status of mothers and their offspring at delivery, 12 newborn infants with congenital malformations and their mothers were determined to have manganese levels lower than the full-term and preterm infant-mother pairs (Underwood, 1977). These findings suggest that manganese deficiency may play a role in intrauterine malformations.

Copper deficient lambs showed ataxia characterized by spastic paralysis (swayback and lamkruis), severe incoordination, blindness and anemia (Underwood, 1977). The wool was abnormal, and brains were small with insufficient myelin. Offspring of calcium-deficient female guinea pigs presented similar physical changes as lambs. Dairy cows suffered reduced fertility, decreased number of young, and slowed growth and development of their calves.

Menkes-Kinky Hair Syndrome demonstraes the impact of prenatal copper deficiency in humans. Abnormalities are seen in the development of the brain, hair, bones, and blood vessels. In a recent study, the hypothesis that thiomolybdate, a compound of molybdenum and sulfur, induces copper deficiency and related teratogenesis in chick embryos was tested (Gooneratne, *et al.*, 1989). It was shown that doses of thiomolybdate at 1 microgram or greater were embryolethal, or produced growth retardation. Also present were copper deficiency symptoms such as cardiac hypertrophy and accumulation of iron in liver and kidney. It was postulated that thiomolybdate binds copper as a copper-thiomolybdate complex, thus making less copper available for the normal physiologic growth and function of the embryo.

Zinc deficiency in female rats resulted in fetal resorption. Viable offspring of these dams were small and suffered a high incidence of congenital malformation (Hurley, 1980; Solomons, et al., 1986; Hickory, et al., 1979). Defects were many and affected every organ system. In rats or monkeys, mild to moderate deficiency was associated with delivery of offspring with abnormal learning and behavior (Hurley & Baly, 1982). Offspring of pregnant mice provided a diet moderately restricted in zinc showed depressed immune response through 6 months of age.

Epidemiologic data seem to support a relationship between zinc deficiency and CNS malformation in humans. Significant zinc deficiency has been found in Egypt, Turkey, and Iran where high rates of CNS anomalies are seen (Cavdar, *et al.*, 1980; Sever & Emanuel , 1973; Sever, 1981). In Sweden, low zinc status in pregnant women has been found to be associated with higher incidence of abnormal deliveries and malformed infants.

Recommended Dietary Allowances (RDA)

The 1989 version of the RDA for pregnant and nonpregnant adult women is summarized in Table 1 (National Research Council, 1989). RDAs for women during pregnancy are now tabulated as absolute numbers rather than as additions (except for energy) to the basic allowances as was done in prior versions. Based on the committee's findings, this is a convenience and reflects the precision with which the additional cost of reproduction is known. The values apply to healthy women and do not take into account those who may enter pregnancy in poor nutrition status or who suffer from diseases or health problems. The table illustrates our lack of knowledge because only 19 of nearly 40 nutrients known to be essential for health are listed. In that regard, it is obvious that those who attempt to take this table literally, *i.e.*, by fortified foods or pills, can be misled because of being inadequate in those not listed. This emphasizes the need to consume whole foods.

Summary

As evident from this discussion, a deficient state can have an adverse effect on the reporductive sucess, fetal develop-

TABLE 1. Recommended Dietary Allowances for
Healthy Adult Women, in Pregnancy

Nutrient	Allowance
Energy (kcal)	+300
Protein (gm)	60
Vitamin A (RE)[1]	800
Vitamin D (μg)[2]	10
Vitamin E(mg)[3]	10
Vitamin K (μg)	65
Vitamin C (mg)	70
Thiamin (mg)	1.5
Riboflavin (mg)	1.6
Niacin (mg NE)[4]	17
Vitamin B_6 (mg)	2.2
Folate (μg)	400
Vitamin B_{12} (μg)	2.2
Calium (mg)	1,200
Phosphorus (mg)	1,200
Magnesium (mg)	320
Iron (mg)	30
Zinc (mg)	15
Selenium (μg)	65
Iodine (μg)	175

[1] Retinol equivalents. 1 retinol equivalent = 1 μg retinol or 6 μg β-carotine
[2] As cholecalfiferol. 10 μg cholecaliciferol = 400 IU of vitamin D
[3] α-Tocopherol equivalent. mg d-α tocopherol = 1 α-TE
[4] 1 NE (niacin equivalent) is equal to 1 mg of niacin or 60 mg of dietary tryptophan

ment and neonatal health. There is general agreement that maternal undernutrition depresses birth weight, and there is some evidence that this undernutrition can be prevented by nutritional supplementation (Anon, 1991b). However, because of paucity of data and limitations of our knowledge of the role of nutrition relative to that of nondietary factors such as genetic, environmental, and physiological variables in determining the outcome of pregnancy, our understanding about the minimal nutrient intakes associated with satisfactory reproduction remain largely unknown (Walker, *et al.*, 1991). This applies to the roles of both pregestational and intergestational dietary practices. For example, it can be recognized that while the extremes of diet, famine, and massive obesity are known to be detrimental to the outcome of pregnancy, the consequence of marginal imbalances are less well understood.

As to individual nutrients, it was suggested (Walker, *et al.*, 1991) that "iron" is the only known nutrient for which requirements cannot be met reasonably by diet alone. Therefore, supplementation with iron may be advisable. It appears beneficial to consider folate even though folate deficiency is rare in the U.S. This is because it now appears that folic acid is essential for normal cellular proliferation, growth and mautration seen in embryogenesis. In addition, there is evidence periconceptional use of folate does protect against the occurrence of neural tube defects in some circumstances.

References

Anonymous. (1991a). Folate deficiency and pregnancy outcome. *Nutr. Rev.* 49:314-315.

Anonymous. (1991b). Nutrition during pregnancy. *Nutr. Today* 25: 13-22.

Anonymous. (1992). Folate supplements prevent recurrence of neural tube defects. *Nutr. Rev.* 50:22-24.

Bourquin, A., and Bennum, R. (1957). The preconception diet of women who have had unsuccessful pregnancies. *Amer. J. Clin. Nutr.* 5:62-69.

Brown, E. E., Fudge, J. F., and Richardson, L. R. (1947). Diet of mother and brain hemorrhages in infants rats. *J. Nutr.* 34:141-151.

Brown, M. L., and Snodgrass, C. H. (1965). Reproduction and maternal response of the rat when thiamine intake is limited. *J. Nutr.* 87:353-356.

Burke, B. S., *et al.*, (1943). The influence of nutrition during pregnancy upon the condition of the infant at birth. *J. Nutr.* 26:569-583.

Burr, G. O., and Burr, M. M. (1929). A new deficiency disease produced by the rigid exclusion of fat from the diet. *J. Biol. Chem.* 82:345-367.

Cavdar, A. O., Arcasoy, A., Baycu, T., and Himmetoglu, O.

(1980). Zinc deficiency and anencephaly in Turkey. *Teratology* 22:141-142.

Chamberlain, J. G., and Nelson, M. M. (1963). Multiple congenital abnormalities in the rat resulting from acute maternal niacin deficiency during pregnancy. *Proc. Soc Exp. Biol. Med.* 112:836-840.

Cheng, D. W., Bairnson, T. A., Rao, A. N., and Subbammal, S. (1960). Effect of variations of rations on the incidence of teratogen in vitamin E deficient rats. *J. Nutr.* 71:54-60.

Davis, S. D., Nelson, T., and Shepard, T. H. (1970). Teratogenicity of vitamin B (B_6) deficiency: Omphalocele, skeletal and neural defects and splenic hypoplasia. *Science* 169:1329-1330.

Dupont, J., Mathias, M. M., and Connally, P. T. (1980). Effects of dietary essential fatty acid concentration upon prostanoid synthesis in rats. *J. Nutr.* 110:1695-1702.

Emery, A. E. H., Timson, J., and Watson-Williams, E. J. (1969). Pathogenesis of spinal bifida. *Lancet* 2:909-910.

Eriksson, U. J., and Borg, L. A. H. (1991). Protection by free oxygen radical scavenging enzymes against glucose-induced embryonic malformations in vitro. *Diabetologia* 34: 325-331.

Evans, H. M., and Bishop, K. S. (1922). On the existence of a hitherto unrecognized dietary factor essential for reproduction. *Science* 56:650-652.

Farrell, P. M., Gutcher, G. R., Palta, M., and DeMets, D. (1988). Essential fatty acid deficiency in premature infants. *Amer. J. Clin. Nutr.* 48:220-229.

Farrell, P. M., Mischler, E. H., Engle, M. J., Brown, J., and Lau, S.-M. (1985). Fatty acid abnormalities in cystic fibrosis. *Pediatr. Res.* 19:104-109.

Fraser, J. L., and Watt, H. J. (1964). Megaloblastic anaemia in pregnancy and the puerperium. *Amer. J. Obstet. Gynecol.* 89:532-540.

Freinkel, N., Lewis, N. J., Akazawa, S., Roth, S. I., and Gorman, L. (1984). The honeybee syndrome — implications of the teratogenicity of mannose in rat-embryo culture. *New Engl. J. Med.* 310:223-230.

Giround, A. (1970). *The Nutrition of the Embryo*. Charles C. Thomas, Springfield, IL, pp. 43-56.

Gooneratne, S. R., Christensen, D. A., and Wenger, B. S. (1989). Effects of thiomolybdates in chick embryos. *Nutr. Rep. Intern.* 40:85-92.

Grant, A. H., and Goettsch, M. (1926). The nutritional requirements of nursing mothers, the effect of a deficiency of the antirachitic vitamin only in the diet of the mother, upon the development of rickets in the young. *Amer. J. Hyg.* 6:211-219.

Gruenwald, P. (1966). Growth of the human fetus. I. Normal growth and its variation. *Amer. J. Obstet. Gynecol.* 94: 1112-1119.

Hall, M. H. (1972). Folic acid deficiency and congenital malformation. *J. Obstet. Gynaecol.* 79:159-161.

Hay, W. W. Jr. (1991). Energy and substrate requirements of the placenta and fetus. *Proc. Nutr. Soc.* 50:321-336.

Hellig, H., Gattereau, D., Lefebvre, Y., and Bolte, E. (1970). Steroid production from plasma cholesterol I. Conversion of plasma cholesterol to placental progesterone in humans. *J. Clin. Endocrinol. Metab.* 30:624-631.

Hibbard, E. D., and Smithells, R. W. (1965). Folic acid metabolism and human embryopathy. *Lancet* 1:1254.

Hickory, W., Nanda, R., and Catalanotto, F. A. (1979). Fetal skeletal malformations associated with moderate zinc deficiency during pregnancy. *J. Nutr.* 109:883-891.

Hobbins, J. C. (1991). Diagnosis and management of neural-tube defects today. *New Engl. J. Med.* 324:690-691.

Hogan, A. G., O'Dell, B. L., and Whitley, J. R. (1950). Maternal nutrition and hydrocephalus in newborn rats. *Proc. Soc. Exp. Biol. Med.* 74:293-296.

Huggett, A. S. G. (1961). Carbohydrate metabolism in the placenta and in the fetus. *Brit. Med. J.* 17:122.

Hurley, L. S. (1980). *Developmental Nutrition*. Prentice Hall, Englewood Cliffs, N.J.

Hurley, L. S., and Baly, D. L. (1982). The effects of zinc deficiency during pregnancy. Pages 145-159 *in* A. S.

Prasad, ed., *Clinical, Biochemical, and Nutritional Aspects of Trace Elements*. A. R. Liss, New York.

Hurley, L. S., Volker, N. E., and Eichner, J. T. (1965). Panthothenic acid deficiency in pregnant and non-pregnant guinea-pigs with special reference to effects on the fetus. *J. Nutr.* 86:201-212.

Iffy, L., Jakobvits, A., Westlake, O., Wingate, M., Calerini, H., Konofskky, P., and Menduke, H. (1975). Early intrauterine development. I. The rate of growth of caucasian embryos and fetuses between the 6th and 28th weeks of gestation. *Pediatrics* 56:173-186.

Institute of Medicine. (1990). *Nutrition During Pregnancy*. National Academy of Sciences, Washington, D.C., pp. 412-419.

Jones, C. C., Brown, S. O., Richardson, L. B., and Sinclair, J. G. (1955). Tissue abnormalities in newborn rats from vitamin B_{12} deficient mothers. *Proc. Soc. Exp. Biol. Med.* 90:135-140.

Kirtland, J., and Gurr, M. I. (1979). Adipose tissue cellularity: A review: II. The relationship between cellularity and obesity. *Intern. J. Obesity* 3:15-55.

Leck, I. (1979). Teratogenic risks of disease and therapy. Pages 23-43 *in* M. A. Klingbert and J. A. C. Weatherall, eds., *Epidemiologic Methods for Detection of Teratogen,* Vol. 1. Karger, Basel, Switzerland.

Lefebvres-Boisselot, J. (1951). Role teratogen de la deficiency en acid panthothenique chez le rat. *Ann. Med.* 52:225-298.

Lien, N. M., Meyer, K. K., and Winick, M. (1977). Early malnutrition and "late" adoption: A study of the effects on the development of Korean orphans adopted into American families. *Amer. J. Clin. Nutr.* 30:1734-1739.

Martin, M. P., Bridgforth, E., MacGanity, W. J., and Darby, W. J. (1957). The Vanderbilt cooperative study of maternal and infant nutrition. X. Ascorbic acid. *J. Nutr.* 62:201-224.

MRC Vitamin Study Research Group. (1991). Prevention of

neural tube defects: Results of the Medical Research Council Vitamin Study. *Lancet* (338):131-137.

Mulinare, J., Cordero, J. F., Erickson, J. D., and Berry, R. J. (1988). Periconceptional use of multivitamins and the occurrence of neural tube defects. *J. Amer. Med. Assoc.* 260:3141-3145.

Munro, H.N, Pilistine, S. J., and Fant, M.E. (1983). The placenta in nutrition. *Ann. Rev. Nutr.* 3:97-124.

National Institute of Child Health and Human Development (1985). *Facts about Premature Birth.* HHS publication, no. (NIH) 461-338-841-25324. U. S. Government Printing Office, Washington, D.C.

National Research Council. (1989). *Recommended Dietary Allowances*, 10th Edition. National Academy Press, Washington, D.C.

Nelson, M. M., and Evans, H. M. (1949). Pteroylglutamic acid and reproduction in the rat. *J. Nutr.* 38:11-24.

Nelson, M. M., and Evans, H. M. (1951). Effect of pyridoxine deficiency on reproduction in the rat. *J. Nutr.* 43:281-294.

Nelson, M. M., and Evans, H. M. (1955). Relation of thiamin to reproduction in the rat. *J. Nutr.* 55:151-163.

Nelson, M. M., Wright, H. V., Asling, H. V., and Evans, H. M. (1956). Multiple congenital abnormalities resulting from transitory deficiency of pteroylglutamic acid during gestation in the rat. *J. Nutr.* 56:349-370.

O'Dell, B. L., Whitley, J. R., and Hogan, A. G. (1948). Relation of folic acid and vitamin A to incidence of hydrocephalus in infant rats. *Proc. Soc. Exp. Biol. Med.* 69:272-275.

O'Dell, B. L. Whitley, J. R., and Hogan, A. G. (1951). Vitamin B_{12} a factor in prevention of hydrocephalus in infant rats. *Proc. Soc. Exp. Biol. Med.* 76:349-353.

Palca, P. (1992). Agencies split on nutrition advice. *Science* 257:1857.

Petros-Barvazian, A., and Behar, M. (1978). Low birthweight — What should be done to deal with this global problem? *WHO Chronicle* 32:321-232.

Phillipps, C., and Johnson, N. E. (1977). The impact of quality of diet and other factors on birth weight of infants. *Amer. J. Clin. Nutr.* 30:215-225.

Pinsky, L., and Fraser, F. C. (1960). Congenital malformations after a two-hour inactivation of nicotinamide in pregnant mice. *Brit. Med. J.* 11:195.

Rolfes, S. R., and DeBruyne, L. K. (1990). *Life Span Nutrition: Conception Through Life.* West Publ. Co., San Francisco, CA., pp. 81-100.

Ross, M. L., and Pike, R. L. (1956). The relationship of vitamin B_6 to protein metabolism during pregnancy in the rat. *J. Nutr.* 58:251-268.

Rush, D. (1992). Folate supplements and neural tube defects. *Nutr. Rev.* 50:25-26.

Sarma, V. (1959). Maternal vitamin A deficiency and fetal microcephaly and anophthalmia. *Obstet. Gynecol.* 13:299-301.

Schardein, J. L., Woosley, E. T., Peltzer, M. A., and Kaump, D. H. (1967). Congenital malformation induced by 6-amino-nicotinamide in rabbit kids. *Exp. Molec. Path.* 6:335-346.

Schneider, H., Mohlen, K. H., and Dancis, J. (1979). Transfer of amino acids across the in vitro perfused human placenta. *Pediatr. Res.* 13:236-240.

Schorah, C. J., Wild, J., Hartley, R., Sheppard, S., and Smithells, R. W. (1983). The effect of periconceptional supplementation on blood vitamin concentrations in women at recurrence risk for neural tube defects. *Brit. J. Nutr.* 49:203-211.

Scott, J. M., Kirke, P. N., and Weir, D. G. (1990). The role of nutrition in neural tube defects. *Ann. Rev. Nutr.* 10:277-295.

Sever, L. E. (1981). Caution on preventing neural-tube defects. *Brit. Med. J.* 283:1605.

Sever, L. E., and Emanuel, I. (1973). Is there a connection between maternal zinc deficiency and congenital malformation of the central nervous system in man? *Teratology* 7:117-118.

Simmer, K. Iles, C. A., James, C., and Thompson, R. P. H. (1987). Are iron-folate supplements harmful? *Amer. J. Clin. Nutr.* 45:122-125.

Smithells, R. W., Seller, M. J., Harris, R., Fielding, R. W., and Schorah, C. J. (1983). Further experience of vitamin supplementation for prevention of neural tube defect recurrences. *Lancet* 1:1027-1031.

Smithells, R. W., Sheppard, S., and Schorah, C. J. (1976). Vitamin deficiencies and neural tube defects. *Arch. Dis. Child.* 51:944-950.

Solomons, N. W., Helitzer-Allen, D.L., and Villar, J. (1986). Zinc needs during pregnancy. *Clin. Nutr.* 5:63-71.

Thenen, S. W. (1991). Gestational and neonatal folate deficiency in rats. *Nutr. Res.* 11:105-116.

Thiersch, J. B., and Philips, F. S. (1950). Action of 4-aminopteroylglutamic acid on the early pregnancy of rats and mice. *Fed. Proc.* 9:346.

Tournay, R. (1951). Possible dangers of dicumarol treatment during pregnancy. *Arch. Hosp.* 23:25-27.

Ullrey, D. E., Becker, B. E., Terrill, S. W., and Notozold, R. A. (1955). Dietary levels of pantothenic and reproductive performance of female swine. *J. Nutr.* 57:401-414.

Underwood, E. J. (1977). *Trace Elements in Human and Animal Nutrition.* Academic Press, New York, N.Y.

Van Gelder, D. W., and Darby, F. U. (1944). Congenital and infantile beriberi. *J. Pediat.* 25:226-235.

Walker, A. R. P., Walker, B. F., and Labadarios, D. (1991). Nutritional needs in pregnancy: Why is the state of knowledge still speculative? *Nutr. Today* 26:18-24

Warkany, J., and Schrafenberger, E. (1944). Congenital malformations induced in rats by maternal nutritional deficiency. VI. The preventive factor. *J. Nutr.* 27:477-484.

Watanabe, T., and Endo, A. (1989). Species and strain differences in teratogenic effects of biotin deficiency in rodents. *J. Nutr.* 119:255-261.

Watanabe, T., and Endo, A. (1991). Biotin deficiency per se is teratogenic in mice. *J. Nutr.* 121:101-104.

Webster, W. S. (1989). The use of animal models in understanding human teratogens. *Congenital Anomalies* 28: 295-302.

Wheeler, F. C., Gollmar, C. W., and Deeb, L. C. (1982). Diabetes and pregnancy in South Carolina: Prevalence, perinatal mortality, and neonatal morbidity in 1979. *Diabetes Care* 5:561-565.

Widdowson, E. M. (1968). Growth and composition of the fetus and newborn. Pages 1-25 *in* Assali, N. S., ed., *Biology of Gestation.* Academic Press, New York.

Widdowson, E. M. (1987). Fetal and neonatal nutrition. *Nutr. Today* 22:16-21.

Widdowson, E. M., Dauncey, M. J., Gairdner, D. M. T., Jonxis, J. H. P., and Pelikan-Filipkova, M. (1975). Body fat of British and Dutch infants. *Brit. Med. J.* 1:653-655.

Winick, M., and Rosso, P. (1969). The effect of severe early malnutrition on cellular growth of the human brain. *Pediatric Res.* 3:181-184.

Woodard, J. C., and Newberne, P. M. (1966). Relation of vitamin B_{12} and one carbon metabolism to hydrocephalus in the rat. *J. Nutr.* 88:375-381.

Worthington-Roberts, B. (1985). Preconceptional and prenatal nutrition: Part II-Vitamins, minerals, alcohol and caffeine. *J. Can. Diet Assoc.* 46:176-181.

Worthington-Roberts, B., and Williams, S. R. (1989). *Nutrition in Pregnancy and Lactation.* Times Mirror/Mosby, St. Louis, MO.

Yudilevich, D. L., and Sweiry, J. H. (1985). Transport of amino acids in the placenta. *Biochim. Biophys. Acta* 822: 169-201.

Zeman, F. J. (1970). Effect of protein deficiency during gestation on postnatal cellular development in the young rat. *J. Nutr.* 100:530-538.

Zeman, F. J., Shrader, R. E., and Allen, L. H. (1973). Persistent effects of maternal protein deficiency in postnatal rats. *Nutr. Rep. Intern.* 7:421-436.

Chapter 3

Nutrient Factors In Juvenile Cataract

George Edwin Bunce and John L. Hess

A cataract is an opaque region appearing in the normally clear mammalian lens in a location that interferes with vision. The only treatment for cataract is surgical removal of the entire lens and use of eyeglasses, contact lenses or intraocular implants to compensate for the lost focusing power. Fortunately, such procedures restore useful vision in better than 90% of the cases.

Cataract is primarily a disease of the elderly. In the Framingham Eye Study, the prevalence of senile cataract was found to be 4.5%, 18.0% and 45.9% of persons who were 52-64, 65-74, and 75-85 years of age, respectively (Kahn, *et al.*, 1977). Congenital cataracts represent a major cause of childhood blindness, 14-40% dependent on the study, but when considered among the causes of blindness for all age groups the prevalence of congenital cataract is less than 10% (NIH Publ. 83-2473, 1983). Congenital cataracts are subdivided into two categories: genetic and non-genetic. Genetic cataracts in humans have been difficult to study because of the limited number of patients in any given lineage and because of their heterogeneity with regard to loci and underlying mechanism. Genetic cataracts have been studied in several mouse models (*i.e.*, Nakano, Emory, Philly, Fraser). It is considered likely that human equivalents to the mouse models do exist. Non-genetic congenital cataracts may occur in response to various viral infections (notably *Rubella*), metabolic disorders, chemical teratogens and deficiencies or excesses of some nutrients as will be described. There is always a high possibility of the existence of synergistic relationships.

Embryology, Anatomy and Transparency of the Mammalian Lens

In the embryo, lens induction is a multi-step process in which the presumptive lens ectoderm is successively exposed to several inductor tissues (Harding & Crabbe, 1984). A scheme for the development of the lens is illustrated in Figure 1. The neural groove runs longitudinally in the center of the embryonic plate bounded on either side by neural ridges. The optic pits mature into primary optic vesicles after complete closure of the neural tube. At the 4.5 mm embryonic stage in man, the primary optic vesicles give rise to the secondary optic vesicles. The lens vesicles separate by the 10 mm stage to form a sphere whose wall consists of a single layer of epithelium. The cells of the posterior wall undergo differentiation and elongation filling the lumen and becoming primary fiber cells. Their nuclei and other subcellular organelles disappear. Epithelial cells at the equator differentiate into secondary fiber cells, a process that occurs throughout life, forming successive layers of cells around the primary fibers.

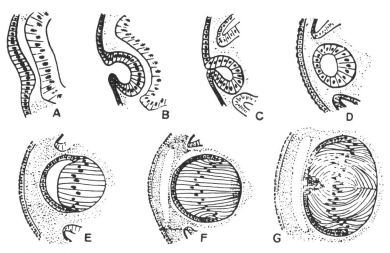

FIGURE 1. Scheme to show the development of the lens. A – lens thickening; B – lens pit; C – lens pit closing; D – lens vesicle; E – elongation of cells of posterior wall of lens vesicle; F – obliteration of cavity of lens vesicle by cells of posterior wall; G – formation of lens sutures by the meeting of the fibers developed in the equatorial region. *Reproduced from Mann (1964), by permission of the publishers.*

Thus, the cells at the very center of the lens become known as the embryonal or fetal nucleus and are among the oldest surviving cells in the adult body. The central core of the adult lens is the nucleus and is overlaid by the cortex. A monolayer of epithelial cells remains over the anterior hemisphere. These cells are metabolically active and play a critical role in ion balance and oxidant defense in the mature lens. The entire lens is enclosed within a capsule secreted by the epithelial cells and the fiber cells.

The unique quality of the lens is, of course, its transparency. This property requires that the tissue possess a highly ordered structure and a nearly uniform refractive index. Fiber cells contain α-, β-, and γ-crystallins organized spatially in a repeating lattice. The α- and β-crystallins exist in polymeric assemblies, whereas the γ-crystallins remain monomeric. Modern techniques of molecular biology have revealed that crystallins are products of gene duplication and divergent evolution from ancestors of different function. These fascinating relationships have been recently reviewed (Wistow & Piatigorsky, 1988). Events that cause loss of order and induce abrupt discontinuities in refractive index are the physical bases for increased light scattering and loss of transparency.

The principal perturbations capable of producing opacities in mature lenses are localized changes in water content and formation of random protein aggregates. Osmotic injury may result from defects in cation transport processes, increases in membrane permeability, or accumulation of osmolytes. The increase of sodium and water can promote the formation of vacuoles or water clefts and culminate in the rupture of fiber cell membranes. Protein aggregation most often occurs as a consequence of chemical modification of lens proteins leading to crosslinking and unfolding. The absence of protein synthetic capacity in fully differentiated lens fiber cells means that adduct formation or loss of protein can not be effectively repaired. The cumulative impact of nonenzymatic oxidation of cellular proteins, nucleic acids and lipids by hydrogen peroxide, superoxide anion, singlet oxygen and hydroxyl radical is conceded to play an important biochemical role in the pathogenesis of senile cataract (Spector, 1984). One must, however, keep in mind that, in adults, the time scale for spontaneous senile cataract emergence is likely to be a significant fraction of an animal's lifetime, but that congenital cataract arises because of insults occurring within much briefer periods. Developmental events require the precise and timely expression of genes necessary for cellular differentiation and organ development. An interruption in this sequence can rarely be repaired. Thus, in considering nutrient factors in juvenile cataract, we must examine the interactions of nutrition and embryology in addition to those events known to be of importance in senile opacities. Also, we shall consider both prenatal and early postnatal nutrition as appropriate to this review.

The study of nutritional influences upon embryonic development is complicated. Let us first consider the possible outcomes of malnutrition in the mother. The most extreme indication of an abnormal event is fetal death. With a lesser level of stress, congenital abnormalities of form or function may appear. A third outcome of nutritional influence on prenatal development is low birth weight. The severity, timing and duration of stress are crucial to the effect on the fetus. The nutritional environment of the fetus is conditioned by the homeostatic and hormonal responses of the mother and the efficiency of placental nutrient transfer. Further, the nutrition of the post-partum suckling mammal is a function of the effect of maternal diet on milk quantity and quality. Typically, scientists use a reductionist approach in the attempt to minimize the number of factors that might confuse interpretation. Thus, animal experiments are performed in which specific single factors are restricted and all other nutrients provided in optimal amounts. Such precision is rarely encountered in human pregnancies. Moreover, nutrient interactions are the rule rather than the exception and the consequences of multiple, mild deficiencies can be quite different from those encountered with singular dietary alterations. In the material to follow, we shall attempt to present a comprehensive citing and interpretation of those studies that have consistently linked nutrient substances with abnormalities of the juvenile lens.

Nutrients with Broad Impact on Organ Development

A. Nutrients that Participate in Regulation of Gene Expression.

Vitamins A and E and Zinc

The first demonstration that the absence of a nutritional factor could produce congenital malformations in a mammal was made by Hale (1933). A single sow, fed a vitamin A-deficient ration for five months before breeding and for the first 40 days of pregnancy, gave birth to a litter of 11 piglets exhibiting cleft palate, hernias and small or missing eyes. The effect of vitamin A deficit as a function of time period was thoroughly explored by Warkany and his colleagues 20 years later (Wilson, *et al.*, 1953). Female rats were fed diets lacking vitamin A and then treated with vitamin A on specific days of gestation. Abnormalities occurred in numerous sites including eyes, heart, lungs and kidneys. This experiment established the general principle that the timing of the teratogenic insult relative to the stage of development was critical to the type of defect produced. Thus, female rats given vitamin A supplementation on the 10th, 11th or 12th day of gestation showed no eye defects but anophthalmia and microphthalmia occurred in 4%, 17% and 28%, respectively, of the offspring when the vitamin A dose was provided on the 13th, 14th or 15th day of gestation. Hypervitaminosis A will also severely interfere with the orderly development of many organs including the eye. Rats subjected to excessive vitamin A from the 5th to the 8th day showed anophthalmia. From the 8th to the 11th day, both anophthalmia and microphthalmia were evident. If the treatment was applied from the 18th to the 21st day, however, only cataract formation was observed (Giroud & Martinet, 1956). We now know that cells contain specific protein receptors for vitamin A and its metabolites and that the ligand receptor complexes are able to bind to

DNA and suppress or induce gene expression (Weinberger & Bradley, 1990).

Vitamin E was linked to reproductive success when it was found that a strict dietary deficiency of vitamin E caused male rats to become sterile and female rats to resorb spontaneously their fetuses. When amounts of vitamin E just sufficient to maintain pregnancy were administered, a high incidence of multiple congenital abnormalities was observed including exencephaly, anencephaly, hernia, scoliosis, club feet, cleft lip and syndactly (Cheng, *et al.*, 1960), but microphthalmia was found in only two of 112 embryos. Bunce & Hess (1976) detected small nuclear cataracts at weaning in seven of 111 progeny (6%) when rats were fed throughout gestation and lactation a diet in which the sole limiting nutrient was vitamin E at a level of 0.1 mg dl-tocopheryl acetate/100 g diet. In this instance, no other anomalies were seen. Callison & Orent-Keiles (1951) found that many of the offspring of rats deprived of vitamin E had eye abnormalities, principally microphthalmia and retinal changes suggestive of retrolental fibroplasia. Ferguson, *et al.* (1956) observed a "cloudiness" in the central portion of lenses from eggs laid by turkey hens fed a practical-type diet of low vitamin E content. At the histological level, the lens epithelium displayed degeneration and proliferation. Jensen & McGinnis (1956) confirmed the existence of nuclear cataracts in hatched turkey poults from hens fed a low vitamin E ration during laying and established the incidence to be 5%.

Vitamin E, a collective term for a small group of related tocopherols, is the major lipid-soluble antioxidant and free radical quencher responsible for protecting membranes against peroxidation. As noted above, oxidation of lens membrane lipids and proteins is considered to be a major factor in the progression of events that culminate in senile cataract. The multiple anomalies described in the offspring of vitamin E-deficient rats, however, suggest a general failure in enzyme induction during development. Hauswirth & Nair (1972) summarized observations of several authors that suggested that the cell nucleus is the locus of important biological actions of vitamin E and presented evidence for concentration of administered vitamin E within the nuclear fraction. Recent identification of the substantial structural homology among receptor proteins for steroids, thyroid hormones and vitamins A and D has given rise to a concept of a superfamily of lipid-activated, regulatory proteins that integrate numerous metabolic activities. These proteins are crucial to pattern formation and spatial organization in embryonic development (Wahli & Martinez, 1991; Weinberger & Bradley, 1990). The existence of so-called "orphan" receptors, additional regulatory proteins with similar structural domains, implies that other lipophilic ligands remain to be discovered. Vitamin E would seem to be a very strong candidate in this regard.

An interesting interaction between vitamin E and tryptophan has been described. Chaves, *et al.* (1964) reported the occurrence of unilateral and bilateral cataract and microphthalmia in about 30% of the progeny of female rats fed throughout pregnancy and lactation a diet in which cowpeas (*Vigna sinensis*) and cashew nuts were the sole sources of protein at a total protein content of 10%. In a subsequent joint study, Bunce, *et al.* (1972) showed that although the original diet failed to provide the NRC recommended level (for the rat) of numerous nutrients, only supplementation with either vitamin E or a mixture of L-methionine, L-tryptophan and niacin prevented the eye lesions. The vitamin E content of the original diet was found by analysis to be 0.1 mg/100 g diet. The NRC recommended level for gestation in the rat is 3 mg/100 g diet. In a further study, Bunce & Hess (1976) prepared a control, semipurified diet that met all of the minimum nutrient requirements of the rat and used pure L-amino acids (12.4 g/100 g diet) in place of protein. When this diet was adjusted to provide only 75 mg L-tryptophan (200 mg/100 g diet is the NRC recommended minimum), nuclear cataracts were observed in 42 of 126 (33%) offspring representing 11 out of 19 litters. No cataracts were found at this level of tryptophan, however, when the tocopherol content was increased to 40 mg/100 g diet and only 7/111 (6%)

when L-tryptophan was added at a level of 500 mg/100 g diet while leaving the vitamin E content low. As will be seen in a later section, tryptophan deficiency is cataractogenic in weanling rats as well. Since tryptophan is vulnerable to oxidative destruction, the sparing effect of vitamin E on tryptophan is consistent with its antioxidant properties.

A deficiency of zinc in the maternal diet produces a wide variety of gross congenital malformations in the rat. A thorough study by Hurley and associates (1971) showed that virtually every organ system was affected. Malformations of the nervous system were especially noteworthy. In full-term fetuses of rats given the zinc-deficient diet from conception to term, 47% had brain anomalies and 42% had microphthalmia or anophthalmia; cataract was not mentioned among the lesions. The widespread presence of zinc metalloenzymes in the pathways for synthesis of DNA, RNA and protein has led some to suggest that deficits in the levels of these enzymes are responsible for these developmental anomalies. The recent discovery of the zinc finger motif as one of the three major DNA binding sequences in proteins that regulate gene expression, however, provides the basis for an alternative hypothesis (Miller, *et al.*, 1985). The observed defects may be a consequence of significant disarray in the gene inductions required for development and differentiation. Bilateral cataract has been occasionally observed in acrodermatitis enteropathica, the genetic disease of zinc malabsorption (Cameron & McClain, 1986; Racz, *et al.*, 1979). Once mammals pass beyond the gestational stage of eye development, zinc does not appear to be of special importance to the maintenance of lens transparency. An interesting association between cataract and dietary zinc has been observed in fish. These studies were begun in response to the sudden widespread appearance of cataract in 65-85% of salmon and trout reared in commercial fish hatcheries following substitution of whitefish meal for herring meal in practical rations. Ketola (1979) found that a single supplement of 150 ppm of zinc as zinc sulfate was sufficient to prevent this phenomenon. The original whitefish meal ration contained 60 ppm of zinc but was rich in both calcium and soybean meal, the latter being a source of phytate. Together, calcium and phytate form a complex with zinc that greatly diminishes its availability. Ogino & Yang (1978) reported a 50% incidence of cataract in rainbow trout after eight weeks of consuming an egg albumin based diet providing only 1 ppm zinc and lacking phytate. The unusual sensitivity of the young fish lens to zinc deficiency merits further study.

B. Nutrients that Participate in DNA Synthesis.
Folic Acid and Vitamin B_{12}

The importance of folic acid during pregnancy in mammals has been studied extensively. Many of the studies have been performed using folic acid antagonists in combination with a low dietary supply of folate. Numerous congenital defects have been recorded including hydrocephalus, syndactyly, skeletal malformations, cleft palate and multiple defects of the face, brain and eyes. In an early study by Nelson, *et al.* (1955), the most frequently encountered eye defect was the Morgagnian-type cataract in association with microphthalmia, anophthalmia and "open eyes" (abnormal development of the eyelids). Grainger, *et al.* (1954) fed pregnant rats a corn-wheat-gluten diet known to be rachitogenic and deficient in both riboflavin and vitamin B_{12} and observed a high incidence (14-25%) of skeletal defects and hydrocephalus and "small or missing eyes" in 6-15% of the offspring. Supplementation of this diet with riboflavin had no effect on the incidence of either hydrocephalus or eye defects, but both were virtually abolished by the addition of vitamin B_{12}. Based on morphological comparisons, Woodward & Newberne (1967) concluded that the congenital hydrocephalus produced by either a deficiency of vitamin B_{12} or by administration of folate antagonists had a similar pathogenesis. Folate is required in purine biosynthesis. Vitamin B_{12} is an essential cofactor for the reaction which regenerates tetrahydrofolate from its predominate metabolite methylfolate. The absence of vitamin B_{12} results in the accumulation of folate in this metabolic cul-de-sac from which it can not escape (known as the methylfolate trap). Strict vegetarians are at risk of developing vitamin B_{12} deficiency since it is not present in fruits, vegetables and grains. It has also been reported that megadoses (1 gram) of vitamin C may adversely affect the availability of vitamin B_{12} (Hines, 1975).

C. Vitamins with a Principal Role in Bioenergetics.
Riboflavin, Niacin, Pantothenic Acid, Thiamine

The fetal consequences of a maternal deficiency of riboflavin have been listed by Hurley (1980) to include bone deformities, fused or missing digits (syndactyly), cleft palate, hydrocephaly and eye defects. It should be noted that a relatively mild deficiency in the mother is sufficient to bring about a high degree of teratogeny. Administration of the riboflavin antimetabolite, galactoflavin, increased the number of soft tissue defects including microphthalmia. Experimental riboflavin deficiency was the first nutrient to be associated with cataract in dietary experiments with weanling rats (Salmon, et al., 1928). Subsequent studies have reported a wide disparity in incidence of riboflavin-related cataract ranging from 0 to 85%. Cataract as an outcome of riboflavin dietary deficit has been confirmed in other species such as the pig (Miller, et al., 1954), cat (Gershoff, et al., 1959) and salmonids (Poston, et al., 1977). There is little doubt of riboflavin's significance in the maintenance of lens transparency. It is likely that the biochemical effect of riboflavin deficit on cataract in post partum animals is a consequence of its role in the oxidant defense system as a cofactor in the enzyme glutathione reductase rather than as a participant in the mitochondrial electron transport chain.

Study of niacin deficiency is complicated by the ability of most species to utilize tryptophan to a limited degree as a niacin precursor. Pike (1951) prepared a tryptophan-free experimental diet (acid-hydrolyzed casein) containing 10 mg nicotinic acid/100 g diet; added back increments of 0.01-0.2% L-tryptophan and fed it to female rats throughout gestation.

The young were removed at term and incidence of congenital cataract was determined by histological examination. Of 11 young from dams fed 0.01-0.025% tryptophan, seven were found to have cataract. No cataracts were detected in 10 young when the maternal diet contained 0.2% tryptophan. When nicotinic acid was omitted from this diet, three cataracts were reported among 11 fetuses examined. The number of animals was small and the results somewhat ambiguous but the work has been cited as evidence for cataract associated with a maternal deficit in dietary niacin. Administration of 6-aminonicotinamide (6-AN), a potent niacin antimetabolite, produces a specific and severe niacin deficient state. When female rats or mice were treated with 6-AN during gestation, numerous teratogenic anomalies were recorded with eye defects listed as a minor component (Chamberlain & Nelson, 1963; Matschke & Fagerstone, 1977).

Experimental maternal deficiencies of pantothenic acid, either in the absence or presence of a chemical antagonist, have yielded a similar picture of multiple and extensive malformations of a variety of organs, anophthalmia and microphthalmia being the principal ocular manifestations (Giroud, 1970). It is interesting that papers describing the effect of an experimental maternal deficiency of thiamine report a high rate of stillbirths and low birth weight young but do not list congenital anomalies (Brown & Snodgrass, 1965; Nelson & Evans, 1955). One may propose from these results of studies on water-soluble vitamins that severe depletion of those with cofactor roles in mitochondrial electron transport or acetate metabolism may broadly limit the timely and sufficient generation of ATP for urgent developmental needs *in utero*. In some instances, the lens may be among those organs which display injury.

Nutrients with Singular Impact on the Lens

Tryptophan, Calcium, Selenium, Sugars

Given the facts that lens fiber cells have the highest density of protein of any body tissue and that this density is a factor of importance to lens transparency, one might well expect that a deficit of dietary protein could lead to congenital cataract. In fact, lens pathology has been linked most closely to limitations in specific amino acids; *i.e.*, imbalances, rather than to general restriction in total protein. Most of these studies have been performed on weanling rats rather than with pregnant animals. The amino acids that appear to be the most important in this regard are the aromatic amino acids, but especially tryptophan.

Curtis, Hauge & Kraybill (1932) reported that feeding weanling rats diets in which the protein source was known to be low in tryptophan regularly produced a "white opaqueness of the eye and lens." Subsequent studies have verified the cataractogenic potential of a low-tryptophan intake by young rats (Totter & Day, 1942) and guinea pigs (von Sallman, *et al.*, 1959). Ohrloff, *et al.* (1978) fed tryptophan-free diets to young rats and saw posterior subcapsular cataract within 21 days. They then added back the missing amino acid and noted the resumption of normal fiber growth and the migration of the opacific region toward the center of the lens. They also examined the crystallins of the posterior region by isoelectric focusing and noted differences in some but not all of these structural components. They interpreted these results as indicating a selective effect upon protein synthesis. Schaeffer & Murray (1950) used a technique of delayed supplementation of tryptophan. The maximum efficiency of protein synthesis occurred when all of the required amino acids were provided simultaneously. They observed that the provision of a tryptophan supplement several hours after each tryptophan-free meal was ineffective in preventing cataract. They concluded that interference in protein synthesis was the primary disturbance that caused the cataract. The minimum requirement for L-tryptophan for normal growth by the weanling rat is 0.14% (Young & Munro, 1973). Bunce, *et al.* (1978) utilized a diet containing pure L-amino acids (12.44 g/100 g diet) as the only source of nitrogen for protein synthesis. After ten days on a zero intake of tryptophan, the level of this amino acid was raised to 0.05%. Extensive regions of both nuclear and cortical opacification appeared within 7-9 weeks of the beginning of the study in 80% of the test animals. Both body weight and lens wet weight were diminished on this regimen but lens protein concentration and ratios of soluble and insoluble proteins remained constant up to the seventh week. MacAvoy & van Heyningen (1976) studied the histological changes that appeared in rats when a soya-gelatin protein delivering 0.09% L-tryptophan was the primary nitrogen source of an otherwise complete diet. Although cataracts were not grossly visible after 10 weeks, abnormalities in the number, distribution and morphology of nuclei in the lens bow were apparent within 4 weeks and were followed by altered epithelial cell differentiation. It may be that a relative deficit of L-tryptophan during the period of intense lens growth results in inefficient synthesis of some number of critical tryptophan-rich proteins thereby upsetting the normal metabolic activity in this organ.

What of the other indispensable amino acids? The most systematic study was performed by Hall, *et al.* (1948). These workers employed a basal diet consisting of an amino acid mixture that supplied three times the minimum requirement of each of the essential amino acids except the one being tested, a salt mixture, cod liver and cottonseed oils, choline chloride, water soluble vitamins (although niacin was not among those listed) and sucrose and fed it to weanling rats for three weeks. When either tryptophan, phenylalanine or histidine were withheld, the lens displayed haziness, separation of the superficial fibers, widening of the sutures, diffuse granular opacities in the cortex, the appearance of a refractile line separating cortex and nucleus and in some instances dense nuclear opacities. Obvious cataract was absent and only the milder changes were seen when the diets lacked threonine, leucine, isoleucine, valine, methionine, lysine or all amino acids. Omission of arginine was without effect in this time frame. Quam, *et al.* (1987) observed cataracts of both eyes in two of nine female kittens fed diets containing either 2.0 or 2.5 g L-histidine/kg diet for 128 days (the recommended level is 3 g/kg diet). It would appear that fish lenses are especially sensitive to a methionine deficit. When a commercial soy protein isolate was used as the sole source of dietary protein in a practical diet for fingerling Atlantic salmon, grossly discernible bilateral cataracts were visible in 90% of the fish after 12 weeks and growth was only 25% of normal. Poston, *et al.* (1977) completely prevented cataract and restored growth to near normal by supplementing this diet with 0.9% DL-methionine.

A few studies have been performed in which very low intakes of total protein have been imposed for long periods of time without significant harm to the lens. As noted in the previous paragraph, withholding all indispensible amino acids for three weeks in weanling rats yielded lens haziness, separation of fibers and widening of the sutures but no opacities were present (Hall, *et al.*, 1948). McLaren (1958) maintained 147 Wistar rats from weaning into advanced maturity on diets containing only 2 or 4% protein and did not observe a single cataract in animals that were severely reduced in body weight. In a similar study, Bagchi (1959) fed a ration consisting of maize starch, 92%; casein, 3%; salt mixture, 3%; and yeast, 2% to rats beginning at weaning and lasting for up to 350 days. The lenses of these animals were free of cataract based on both slit lamp and histological evaluation. Kauffman & Norton (1966) divided 31 weanling pigs into four groups and fed them diets containing either 0, 5, 10 or 16% protein by adjusting the ratios and quantities of soybean meal and corn. After 146 days, the surviving animals were killed and the lens, brain, heart, liver, and muscle were analyzed for total nitrogen. The nitrogen content of the lens did not diminish even on the nitrogen-free diet whereas brain nitrogen declined to 90% of control and the other organs to 10-25% at this extreme level of deprivation. It would seem that in weanling animals, very low intakes of protein can be tolerated without cataractogenic outcome so long as an amino acid imbalance is avoided.

The use of excessive amounts of certain amino acids can have a harmful effect on the lens. Alam, *et al.* (1966) reported the production of cataract in young rats fed a 6% casein diet containing 3% of added L-tyrosine. Additional supplementation with 0.8 or 1.25% L-threonine delayed but did not prevent cataract; inclusion of 0.2% L-tryptophan, however, completely prevented the lens opacities. They concluded that these cataracts were the outcome of tryptophan deficiency rather than tyrosine toxicity. Phenylalanine excess has been implicated as a cause of cataract in the rat (Bowles, *et al.*, 1950). This result may also reflect a secondary production of tryptophan deficit since tyrosine, phenylalanine and tryptophan share a common cellular uptake pathway. Laszczyk (1975) injected varying amounts of glutamic acid into 250 Leghorn hen eggs at 50 hours of incubation. Only 50% of the embryos survived and histological examination of the lenses of the live chicks revealed pathological changes in 77% of the lenses. Abnormalities ranged from slight modifications in epithelial structure to complete destruction of cells and fibers. Kawamura & Azuma (1990) administered monosodium glutamate (5 mg/g body weight) by subcutaneous injection into rats on days nine and ten post partum. By four months of age, cataracts had appeared in 75% of the test animals and the size and weight of the lenses were reduced.

Compared to the weanling animal, the developing fetus might be less vulnerable to the effects of amino acid imbalances in the maternal diet through release of amino acids into the maternal plasma following catabolism of body proteins. Experimental results, however, tend to show that a maternal tryptophan deficit is also damaging to the lens in utero. Pike (1951) fed female rats a 14.7% acid-hydrolyzed casein diet that contained less than 25 mg tryptophan/100 g diet but was supplemented with 0.15% L-cystine and 10 mg% niacin. Histological examination of lenses from the fetuses at 21 days post conception revealed abnormalities suggestive of cataract in seven of 11 pups. Chaves, *et al.* (1964) reported the appearance of uni- and bilateral nuclear cataract and microphthalmia in about 30% of the progeny of female rats fed throughout pregnancy and lactation on a 10% protein diet in which cowpeas (*Vigna sinensis*) and cashew nuts (3:1 ratio) served as the sole sources of amino acids. Subsequent investigation of this phenomenon revealed a synergistic relationship between vitamin E and tryptophan as discussed in an earlier section. This diet, which contained 75 mg tryptophan/100 g diet and 12.4% protein, was cataractogenic in the absence but not the presence of a supplement of vitamin E (30 mg/100 g diet). When, however, tryptophan was offered at 65 mg/100 g diet and the total amino acid content of the diet was doubled to 24.8% (Bunce, *et al.*, 1984), nuclear opacities (mostly of the pinhead variety) were detected in 88 of 98 rat pups and the protective effect of the vitamin E supplement was not evident (75 pups with cataract out of a total of 107 animals). Normal lens development occurred in the circumstance of a comparable reduction of sulfur-containing amino acids, L-Phe, L-Tyr, or L-Lys (less than 50% of the rat RDA) at the 12.4 g% level of total amino acids even in the absence of a vitamin E supplement. With the exception of lysine, the imposition of these amino acid deficits on the maternal diet reduced mean pup weight at postpartum day 23 from 38 ± 3 g to 15-24 g depending on the particular amino acid withheld. Mean lens wet weight was also lowered from 19.1 ± 0.4 mg to a range from 13.0-17.9 mg. The percent of lens protein in the insoluble fraction (primarily membrane proteins at this stage in life) dropped from 13.1 to 5.4-10.5.

In summary, it would appear that, in rats, a severe limitation of the dietary supply of tryptophan during the entire period of gestation and lactation or the first few weeks post weaning is cataractogenic. This outcome can be exacerbated by amino acid imbalances that further compromise tryptophan availability or by a simultaneous deficiency in vitamin E. Deficits of phenylalanine, tyrosine and histidine may also possess the potential for harm under the appropriate conditions. The importance of a balanced supply of amino acids for lens development during gestation may be underscored by the observation that many of the various genetic muscular dystrophies include cataract as a common component of the syndrome.

Lens opacities may accompany hypocalcemic tetany and rickets (Brooks, 1975) in human subjects and have been found in young rabbits reared on a diet containing adequate vitamin D but less than 0.005% calcium (Swan & Salit, 1941). Lenses maintained in organ culture in medium lacking calcium showed increased membrane leakiness and swelling (Throft & Kinoshita, 1965). A thorough review of the biochemistry of hypocalcemic cataract is available (Delamere & Paterson, 1981). Most investigations on the effect of dietary calcium on fetal development have concentrated on the skeletal system. When rats were fed a calcium deficient diet beginning on the day of mating, the young were able to maintain normal bone calcification at the expense of the maternal skeleton. Production of more prolonged or severe depletion of maternal calcium led to a high percentage of fetal deaths and incomplete fetal bone calcification. Lens abnormalities were not reported at either level of maternal calcium intake (Hurley, 1980).

A specific effect of dietary calcium on juvenile cataract was discovered unexpectedly during a study in China on the comparison of "vegetarian vs. omnivorous" diets (Chang, *et al.*, 1941a, 1941b, 1941c, Chen, *et al.*, 1941). The "vegetarian" diet consisted of whole wheat, 35%; millet, 30%; roasted soybeans, 15%; peas, 15%; and soybean or sesame oil, 5 percent. The only mineral supplement was 1 g NaCl/100 g diet. The "omnivorous" diets were prepared through the substitution of cod liver oil for soybean or sesame oil; and the addition of milk powder or dried beef muscle, yeast, wheat bran, and McCollum Salt Mixture No. 185 in place of a proportion of the soybeans and peas. The "vegetarian" rats were inferior to the "omnivorous" rats in body weight and in size of litters but their life spans equaled (males) or exceeded (females) those of their counterparts. After an alert individual noted the presence of cataract in some of the "vegetarian" animals, a systematic evaluation was conducted over a 2-year span. Examination of 356 "vegetarian" rats from five generations by means of an ophthalmoscope through dilated pupils showed an overall incidence of 71% cataract. One hundred and sixteen "omnivorous" controls were completely free of lens lesions. The cataracts were of the subcapsular punctate type affecting primarily the posterior subcapsular layer and were usually bilateral. The authors reported parathyroid hypertrophy and hypocalcemia (6.4-8.9 mg/100 ml serum) in the "vegetarian" population. The cataracts were prevented either by exposing the rats to UV irradiation or by increasing dietary calcium. Cataracts were never seen in the Fo generation although their degree of hypocalcemia and parathyroid hypertrophy was equally severe to that of the F1 rats.

The essentiality of selenium to permit normal activity of the enzyme glutathione peroxidase and the importance of oxidant stress in the promotion of age-related cataract suggested that cataract might be an outcome of selenium deficiency. Sprinkler, *et al.* (1971), Lawrence, *et al.* (1974) and Whanger & Weswig (1975) examined this possibility and determined that cataracts did eventually occur but only after severe and prolonged deprivation, sometimes requiring extending the deficiency state into the second generation. Selenium excess, on the other hand, poses a grave and specific risk for cataract when administered subcutaneously or intraperitoneally as sodium selenite to rats younger than 18-20 days old (Ostadalova, *et al.*, 1978). A single dose of 20-30 nmoles/g body wt results in virtually 100% bilateral nuclear cataracts within 3-4 days postinjection. Fatalities are rare and no other pathology has been reported at this dose level although we have noted a significant decline in subsequent body weight gain. Lens selenite increases by threefold within 24 hours and returns to normal within 7-10 days (Bunce & Hess, 1981). Selenite is reduced to hydrogen selenide by glutathione but free radicals appear to be generated during this process in quantities sufficient to damage the various components of the calcium homeostasis system (Huang, *et al.*, 1989, Seko, *et al.*, 1989). The resultant increase in lens calcium activates calpain II that attacks lens crystallins and membrane proteins leading to loss of structural order and consequent opacity (Bunce, *et al.*, 1984, David & Shearer, 1984). Administration of the same dose of selenite to rats beyond the age of 21 days has no effect on the clarity of the lens. Moreover, selenite supplementation (4.5 ppm) of the diets of female rats for 8 weeks prior to and throughout gestation had no negative affects on the progeny (Bergman, *et al.*, 1990). However, selenium toxicosis has been associated with congenital malformations in chicken and duck embryos; which showed anomalies of the extremities and the beak, hydrocephaly, anophthalmia, and microphthalmia (Hoffman & Heinz, 1988; Ohlendorf, *et al.*, 1988); and in pigs and sheep; which displayed abnormalities of the feet (Mensink, *et al.*, 1990; Underwood, 1977). Thus, selenite excess would appear to have the potential to be a dietary factor capable of generating congenital cataract but only under special circumstances or perhaps as one of several concurrent challenges.

Glucose readily enters lens epithelial and underlying fiber cells where it is metabolized by the familiar pathways of glycolysis and the hexose monophosphate shunt. In the event of an abnormal load of glucose or other monosaccharides such as galactose or xylose, excess sugar can be reduced to the sugar alcohols that tend to accumulate due to their relatively poor diffusibility. The resultant osmotic disequilibrium may progress through vacuolization and eventual rupture of the swollen cells with consequent opacity (Kinoshita, 1974). Such sugar cataracts appear in infancy and childhood in humans only in conjunction with metabolic disease. Galactosemia is a disease caused by a lack of one of three enzymes within the galactose pathways. Absence of UDP galactotransferase is associated in the newborn with hypergalactosemia and hypoglycemia. If untreated, mental retardation and cataract will occur in infancy. Early withdrawal of galactose from the diet, however, will protect the newborn from systemic manifestations of this disease including the ocular lesion (Sidbury, 1969). When the missing enzyme is galactokinase, the condition may escape notice and the patient may reach early adulthood before cataract is detected. Heterozygotes for galactokinase account for a percentage of adults who develop presenile (< 50 years of age) cataract. Absence of a third galactose enzyme, galactose epimerase, has not been associated with cataract. Lens opacities are a well known complication of diabetes, both insulin dependent and insulin independent. Proper clinical management can minimize its occurrence in infants.

Congenital Cataract of Unknown Etiology

From time to time, reports appear in the literature describing congenital cataracts of unknown etiology in various species. Such reports merit inquiry to ascertain the identity of the agents involved. One should never ignore the benefits of serendipity. Indeed, our own studies on the appearance of nuclear opacities in the progeny of female rats fed vegetable protein-based diets arose from just such an unexpected observation by Nelson Chaves and his colleagues in Brazil (Chaves, *et al.*, 1964). We list below two examples of presently unsolved mysteries of which we are aware.

Wolf pups, when intended to be sold as pets or used in exhibits, must be removed from the dam at an early age in order to minimize the imprinting of the wild instinct. This practice obviously necessitates a suitable artificial formula. Vainisi, *et al.* (1981) reported that 12 wolf pups from seven litters developed posterior subscapular cataract after they were removed from their mother and fed a commercial canine milk-replacement product (Esbilac-Borden). Pups left with the bitch or a foster German Shepherd exhibited normal lenses. Some of the cataractous lenses recovered transparency after the pups were able to begin consumption of a commercial dry dog food. Supplementation of the milk-replacement product with either arginine or lactose prevented the cataract but supplements of vitamin C, tryptophan, methionine, or corn oil were ineffective. The authors noted that four wolf pups taken from the bitch at five days of age and raised on goat milk also developed dense opacities. The milk-replacement product was used in dogs without complaint by the vast majority of customers and the producer could not duplicate its putative cataractogenic effect except in one instance when the litter was placed on Esbilac within 24 hours of birth. Martin & Chambreau (1982), however, described the occurrence of mild cataracts in six of twelve mixed breed puppies raised from 48 hours post partum to weaning on the product. Glaze & Blanchard (1983) described mild opacification in lenses of six of eight Samoyed puppies begun on the artificial formula within 24 hours of birth. It thus appeared that the use of Esbilac was associated with occasional congenital cataract. In general, it also seemed that the problem was more likely to occur in larger breeds and in animals begun on the formula soon after birth. Vainisi, *et al.* (1981) suggested that the opacities in the wolf pups were attributable to arginine deficiency and that the lactose supplement somehow enhanced arginine availability. We suggest an alternative hypothesis, transient hypoglycemia. Arginine is a poor candidate as a limiting cataractogenic amino acid. As noted in an earlier section, arginine was the only essential amino acid that had no effect on lens morphology when it was omitted from the diet of young rats for three weeks. The suggestion that lactose might enhance arginine uptake is speculative and we know of no supporting data. Lactose and arginine, however, do share one metabolic attribute in common; they are both sources of glucose. Neonatal hypoglycemia has been associated with cataract in human infants of low birth weight or complicated deliveries (Brooks, 1975), and the opacity is reversible if the hypoglycemia is rapidly corrected. Moreover, the canine neonate is particularly susceptible to fasting hypoglycemia (Atkins, 1984). Its liver glycogen stores are quickly depleted, and its small muscle mass limits the availability of gluconeogenic precursors. Supplements of either arginine, an efficient gluconeogenic amino acid, or lactose, a ready source of glucose and galactose, may well have enabled stressed wolf pups to escape the consequences of hypoglycemia.

Another interesting occurrence of non-genetic congenital cataract has been reported in cattle in Britain (Ashton, *et al.*, 1977). The initial observation was made in Leicestershire in a herd of 100 pedigree Friesian cows with a high standard of health management and recording. When blindness in calves was first noticed by the owner, it was thought to be of hereditary origin. Subsequent ophthalmoscopic examination of the herd, however, revealed that the problem was not restricted to progeny of a suspect bull. Lens abnormalities were detected in 14 out of 31 calves. In the following three years, bilateral nuclear cataract was found in 59 of 192 calves. Equal numbers of male and female calves were affected and the dams were found to be normal in all instances. The cataract was confined to the nucleus and the cortex was usually perfectly clear. Soon congenital cataracts were found in similar proportions in other herds, predominantly Friesians, throughout England, Wales and Ireland. France & Shaw (1990) examined a herd of 60 pedigree Friesians in Somerset, England. Cataract was the only unusual recognized problem in an otherwise healthy herd. In 1985, approximately 90% of calves on this farm were born with grossly or ophthalmoscopically visible cataract. The proportion fell to 20% in 1986 and rose to about 40% in the 1987 calving. This herd was selected for further blood evaluation. Of 23 cows that delivered between July and August 1988, six gave birth to calves with normal lenses whereas the remaining 17 produced calves with bilateral nuclear cataracts. No differences were detected in blood glucose, calcium, or urea in samples collected from the dams in December 1987, and February, June, and October 1988. Ashton, *et al.* (1977) noted that the proportion of cataractous calves was particularly high during the months of June to September inclusive and this assessment was confirmed by Clay (1977). These cows would have been served between September and December and would have consumed a high concentrate ration during the first trimester. Lens development occurs in the bovine fetus during this period. Clay (1977) also observed that congenital cataract was rare in calves born to heifers. This may be related to the fact that replacement heifers entering a herd are fed concentrate for only a couple of weeks prior to parturition. The cause of congenital nuclear cataract in cattle in Britain remains an intriguing mystery. It does not appear to be genetic. It is not possible to state whether it is nutritional or toxic (or perhaps both) in origin.

Summary and Conclusions

The timing, duration and severity of nutritional stresses are crucial factors with regard to effects upon the eye and lens. When the stress is imposed during the embryonic period, the eye may under some circumstances be a singular target but most often anophthalmia, microphthalmia and/or cataract will appear in association with many other defects. Those nutrients most prominent in their effects on embryonic differentiation are those with roles in regulation of gene expression (excess or deficit of vitamin A, deficiencies of vitamin E or zinc), nucleic acid synthesis (deficiencies of folate or vitamin B_{12}) and production of cellular energy (deficiencies of riboflavin, niacin, or pantothenic acid). The more mature and differentiated lenses of post partum and newly weaned animals must still engage in synthesis of lens crystallins and defend against oxidant stress and osmotic injury. A total protein deficit can be tolerated rather well but deficiencies of aromatic amino acids (especially tryptophan) when imposed either pre- or immediate post-partum can result in cataract. Vitamin E may be helpful in sparing tryptophan from oxidation and riboflavin is necessary for full effectiveness of the glutathione defense system. A prolonged hypocalcemic state leads to cataract by increasing lens membrane permeability. Dietary excess of galactose or diseases of galactose or glucose metabolism can produce osmotic cataract in young as well as older animals. Subcutaneous injection of selenite produces an oxidant challenge to the preweaning rat lens that is severely cataractogenic but its importance as a dietary stress is uncertain.

References

Alam, S. Q., Becker, R. V., Stucki, W. P., Rogers, Q. R., and Harper, A. E. (1966). Effect of threonine on the toxicity of excess tyrosine and cataract formation in the rat. *J. Nutr.* 89:91-96.

Ashton, N., Barnett, K. C., Clay, C. E., and Clegg, F. G.

(1977). Congenital nuclear cataracts in cattle. *Vet. Record* 100:505-508.

Atkins, C. E. (1984). Disorders of glucose homeostasis in neonatal and juvenile dogs: Hypoglycemia-Part 1. *Compendium Cont. Educ.* 6:197-208.

Bagchi, K. (1959). The effects of dietary protein on the sulfhydryl content of crystalline lens. *Indian J. Med. Res.* 47:184-198.

Bergman, K., Cekan, E., Slanina, P., Gabrielsson, J., and Hellenäs, K.-E. (1990). Effects of dietary sodium selenite supplementation on salicylate-induced embryo- and feto-toxicity in the rat. *Toxicology* 61:135-146.

Bowles, L. L., Hall, W. K., and Sydenstricker, V. P. (1950). Ocular changes in the rat resulting from high levels of tyrosine and phenylalanine in the diet. *Anat. Rec.* 106: 265-266.

Brooks, M. H. (1975). Lenticular abnormalities in endocrine dysfunction. Pages 285-301 *in* J. G. Bellows, ed., *Cataract and Abnormalities of the Lens.* Grune & Stratton, New York.

Brown, M. L., and Snodgrass, C. H. (1965). Effect of dietary level of thiamine on reproduction in the rat. *J. Nutr.* 85:102-106.

Bunce, G. E., Cassi, P., Hall, B., and Chaves, N. (1972). Prevention of cataract in the progeny of rats fed a maternal diet based on vegetable proteins. *Proc. Soc. Exp. Biol. Med.* 140:1103-1107.

Bunce, G. E. and Hess, J. L. (1976). Lenticular opacities in young rats as a consequence of maternal diets low in tryptophan and/or vitamin E. *J. Nutr.* 106:222-229.

Bunce, G. E., and Hess, J. L. (1981). Biochemical changes associated with selenite-induced cataract in the rat. *Exp. Eye Res.* 33:505-514.

Bunce, G. E., Hess, J. L., and Batra, R. (1984a). Lens calcium and selenite-induced cataract. *Curr. Eye Res.* 3:315-320.

Bunce, G. E., Hess, J. L., and Davis, D. (1984b). Cataract formation following limited amino acid intake during gestation and lactation. *Proc. Soc. Exp. Biol. Med.* 176: 485-489.

Bunce, G. E., Hess, J. L., and Fillnow, G. M. (1978). Investigation of low tryptophan induced cataract in weanling rats. *Exp. Eye Res.* 26:399-405.

Callison, E. C., and Orent-Keiles, E. (1951). Abnormalities of the eye occurring in young vitamin E-deficient rats. *Proc. Soc. Exp. Biol. Med.* 76:295-297.

Cameron, J. D., and McClain, C. J. (1986). Ocular histopathology of acrodermatitis enteropathica. *Brit. J. Ophthalmol.* 70:662-667.

Chamberlain, J. G., and Nelson, M. M. (1963). Congenital abnormalities in the rat resulting from single injections of 6-aminonicotinamide during pregnancy. *J. Exp. Zool.* 153: 285-300.

Chang, C-Y., Chen, T-T., and Luo, T-H. (1941a). Further observations on cataract, parathyroid hypertrophy and hypocalcemia in vegetarian rats. *Chinese J. Physiol.* 16: 251-256.

Chang, C-Y., Chen, T-T., Wu, H., and Luo, T-H. (1941b). Cause of cataract, parathyroid hypertrophy and hypocalcemia in vegetarian rats. *Chinese J. Physiol.* 16:257-261.

Chang, C-Y., Wu, H., and Chen, T-T. (1941c). Life span of rats on vegetarian and omnivorous diets. *Chinese J. Physiol.* 16:229-240.

Chaves, N., Barreto, S. P., Leal, M. R. B. P., Lapa, A. G., Costa, L. P., Mayer, R., and Costa, S. (1964). Reproduction, growth and ocular alterations in rats fed with vegetable mixtures of different protein levels. *Proc. Seventh Intern. Cong. Trop. Med. Malaria* 4:8-12.

Chen, T-T., Chang, C-Y., and Luo, T-H. (1941). Cataract in vegetarian rats. *Chinese J. Physiol.* 16:241-250.

Cheng, D. W., Bairnson, T. A., Rao, A. N., and Subbammal, S. (1960). Effect of variations of rations on the incidence of teratogeny in vitamin E deficient rats. *J. Nutr.* 71:54-60.

Clay, C. E. (1977). *A study of congenital nuclear cataract in cattle.* Ph.D. Thesis. University of Cambridge, England.

Curtis, P. B., Hauge, S. M., and Kraybill, H. R. (1932). The nutritive value of certain animal protein concentrates. *J. Nutr.* 5:503-512.

David, L. L., and Shearer, T. R. (1984). Calcium activated proteolysis in the lens nucleus during selenite cataractogenesis. *Invest. Ophthalmol. Vis. Sci.* 25:1275-1283.

Delamere, N. A., and Paterson, C. A. (1981). Hypocalcemic cataract. Pages 219-236 *in* G. Duncan, ed., *Mechanisms of Cataract Formation in the Human Lens.* Academic Press, New York.

France, M. P., and Shaw, J. M. (1990). Blood glucose, calcium and urea in cows from a herd with congenital nuclear cataract. *Vet. Record* 126:484-485.

Ferguson, T. M., Rigdon, R. H., and Couch, J. R. (1956). Cataracts in vitamin E deficiency. An experimental study on the turkey embryo. *Arch. Ophthamol.* 55:346-355.

Gershoff, S. N., Andrus, S. B., and Hegsted, D. M. (1959). The effect of the carbohydrate and fat content of the diet upon the riboflavin requirement of the cat. *J. Nutr.* 68:75-88.

Giroud, A. (1970). *The Nutrition of the Embryo.* Charles C. Thomas, Springfield, IL.

Giroud, A., and Martinet, M. (1956). Tératogènese par hautes doses de vitamine A en fonction des stades du développement. *Arch. Anat. Microscop.* 45:7-98.

Glaze, M. B., and Blanchard, G. L. (1983). Nutritional cataracts in a Samoyed litter. *J. Amer. Anim. Hosp. Assoc.* 19:951-954.

Grainger, R. B., O'Dell, B. L., and Hogan, A. G. (1954). Congenital malformations as related to deficiencies of riboflavin and vitamin B_{12}, source of protein, calcium to phosphorous ratio and skeletal phosphorous metabolism. *J. Nutr.* 54:33-48.

Hale, F. (1933). Pigs born without eyeballs. *J. Heredity* 24:105-106.

Hall, W. K., Bowles, L. L., Sydenstricker, V. P., and Schmidt, H. F., Jr. (1948). Cataracts due to deficiencies of phenylalanine and histidine in the rat. A comparison with other types of cataracts. *J. Nutr.* 36:277-296.

Harding, J. J., and Crabbe, M. J. C. (1984). The lens: Development, proteins, metabolism and cataract. Chapt. 3, pages 207-492 *in* H. Davson, ed., *The Eye*, Vol. 1b, 3rd. ed. Academic Press, London.

Hauswirth, J. W., and Nair, P. P. (1972). Some aspects of vitamin E in the expression of biological information. *Ann. NY Acad. Sci.* 203:111-122.

Hines, J. D. (1975). Ascorbic acid and vitamin B_{12} deficiency. *J. Amer. Med. Assoc.* 234:24.

Hoffman, D. J., and Heinz, G. H. (1988). Embryotoxic and teratogenic effects of selenium in the diet of mallards. *J. Toxicol. Environ. Health* 24:477-490.

Huang, L-L., Hess, J. L., and Bunce, G. E. (1989). Protection against cataract formation by antioxidants in rats receiving chronic, low doses of selenite. *Invest. Ophthalmol. Vis. Sci.* 30 (Suppl.):330.

Hurley, L. (1980). *Developmental Nutrition.* Prentice-Hall, Englewood Cliffs, NJ.

Hurley, L. S., Gowan, J., and Swenerton, H. (1971). Teratogenic effects of short-term and transitory zinc deficiency in rats. *Teratology* 4:199-204.

Jensen, L. S., and McGinnis, J. (1956). Studies on the vitamin E requirement of turkeys for reproduction. *Poultry Sci.* 6:715-721.

Kahn, H. A., Leibowitz, H. M., Granley, J. P., Kini, M. M., Colton T., Nickerson, R. S., and Dawber, T. R. (1977). The Framingham Eye Study. I. Outline and major prevalence findings. *Amer. J. Epidemiol.* 106:17-32.

Kauffman, R. G., and Norton, H. W. (1966). Growth of the porcine eye lens during insufficiencies of dietary protein. *Growth* 30:463-470.

Kawamura, M., and Azuma, N. (1990). Morphological studies on cataract and small lens formation in neonatal rats treated with monosodium-L-glutamate. *Invest. Ophthal. Vis. Sci.* 31 (Suppl.):206.

Ketola, H. G. (1979). Influence of dietary zinc on cataracts in rainbow trout (*Salmo gairdneri*). *J. Nutr.* 109:965-969.

Kinoshita, J. H. (1974). Mechanisms initiating cataract formation-Proctor lecture. *Invest. Ophthalmol.* 13:713-724.

Laszczyk, W. A. (1975). Development of cataract as the effect of glutamic acid administration to chick embryo. *Ophthalmol. Res.* 7:432-439.

Lawrence, R. A., Sunde, R. A., Schwartz, G. L., and Hoekstra, W.G. (1974). Glutathione peroxidase activity in rat lens and other tissues in relation to dietary selenium intake. *Exp. Eye Res.* 18:563-569.

MacAvoy, J. W., and van Heyningen, R. (1976). Changes in the cells of the lens bow and epithelium of tryptophan deficient rats. *INSERM Colloq.* 60:245-250.

Mann, I. (1964). *The Development of the Human Eye.* Grune and Stratton, New York. 209 pp.

Martin, C. L., and Chambreau, T. (1982). Cataract production in experimentally orphaned puppies fed a commercial replacement for bitch's milk. *J. Amer. Anim. Hosp. Assoc.* 18:115-119.

Matschke, G. H., and Fagerstone, K. A. (1977). Teratogenic effects of 6-aminonicotinamide in mice. *J. Toxicol. Environ. Hlth* 3:735-743.

McLaren, D. S. (1958). Growth and water content of the eyeball of the albino rat in protein deficiency. *Brit. J. Nutr.* 12:254-259.

Mensink, C. G., Koeman, J. P., Veling, J., and Gruys, E. (1990). Haemorrhagic claw lesions in newborn piglets due to selenium toxicosis during pregnancy. *Vet. Record* 126: 620-622.

Miller, E. R., Johnson, R. L., Hoefer, J. A., and Luecke, R. W. (1954). The riboflavin requirement of the baby pig. *J. Nutr.* 52:405-413.

Miller, J., McLachlan, A. D., and Klug, A. (1985). Repetitive zinc-binding domains in the protein transcription factor IIIA from *Xenopus* oocytes. *Eur. Molec. Biol. Organiz. J.* (*EMBO J.*) 4:1609-1614.

National Institutes of Health Publication No. 83-2473 (1983).

Vision Research. Report of the cataract panel. U. S. Dep. Health & Human Services.

Nelson, M. M., and Evans, H. M. (1955). Relation of thiamine to reproduction in the rat. *J. Nutr.* 55:151-163.

Nelson, M. M., Wright, H. W., Asling, C. W., and Evans, H. M. (1955). Multiple congenital abnormalities resulting from transitory deficiency of pteroylglutamic acid during gestation in the rat. *J. Nutr.* 56:349-369.

Ogino, C., and Yang, G-Y. (1978). Requirement of rainbow trout for dietary zinc. *Bull. Japanese Soc. Sci. Fisher.* 44:1015-1018.

Ohlendorf, H. M., Kilness, A. W., Simmons, J. L., Stroud, R. K., Hoffman, D.J., and Moore, J. F. (1988). Selenium toxicosis in wild aquatic birds. *J. Toxicol. Environ. Hlth.* 24:67-92.

Ohrloff, C., Stoffel, C., Koch, H.-R., Wefers, U., Bours, J., and Hockwin, O. (1978). Experimental cataracts in rats due to tryptophan-free diet. Albrecht v. Graefes. *Arch. Ophthalmol.* 205:73-79.

Ostadalova, I., Babicky, A., and Obenbarger, J. (1978). Cataract induced by administration of a single dose of sodium selenite to suckling rats. *Experientia* 34:222-223.

Pike, R. L. (1951). Congenital cataract in albino rats fed different amounts of tryptophan and niacin. *J. Nutr.* 44: 191-204.

Poston, H. A., Riis, R. C., Rumsey, G. L., and Ketola, H. G. (1977). The effect of supplemental dietary amino acids, minerals and vitamins on salmonids fed cataractogenic diets. *Cornell Vet.* 67:473-509.

Quam, D. D., Morris, J. G., and Rogers, Q. R. (1987). Histidine requirement for kittens for growth, hematopoiesis and prevention of cataracts. *Brit. J. Nutr.* 58:521-532.

Racz, P., Kovacs, B., Varga, L., Ujlaki, E., Zombai, E., et al. (1979). Bilateral cataract in acrodermatitis enteropathica. *J. Pediatr. Ophthalmol. Strabismus* 16:180-182.

Salmon, W. D., Hays, R. M., and Guerrant, N. D. (1928). Etiology of dermatitis of experimental pellagra in rats. *J. Infect. Dis.* 43:426-441.

Schaeffer, A. J., and Murray, J. D. (1950). Tryptophan determination in cataract due to deficiency or delayed supplementation of tryptophan. *Arch. Ophthalmol.* 43:202-216.

Seko, Y., Saito, Y., Kitahara, J., and Imura, I. (1989). Active oxygen generation by the reaction of selenite with reduced glutathione *in vitro*. Pages 70-73 *in* A. Wendel, ed., *Selenium in Biology and Medicine*. Springer-Verlag, New York.

Sidbury, J. B., Jr. (1969). Investigations and speculations on the pathogenesis of galactosemia. Page 14 *in* David Y.-Y.-Hsia., ed., *Galactosemia*. Charles C. Thomas, Springfield, IL.

Spector, A. (1984). The search for a solution to senile cataracts-Proctor Lecture. *Invest. Ophthalmol.* 25:130-146.

Sprinkler, L. H., Harr, J. R., Newberne, P. M., Whanger, P. D., and Weswig, P. H. (1971). Selenium deficiency lesions in rats fed vitamin E supplemented rations. *Nutr. Rep. Intern.* 4:335-340.

Swan, K. C., and Salit, P. W. (1941). Lens opacities associated with experimental calcium deficiency. *Amer. J. Ophthal-mol.* 24:611-614.

Throft, R. A., and Kinoshita, J. H. (1965). The effect of calcium on rat lens permeability. *Invest. Ophthalmol.* 4: 122-128.

Totter J. R., and Day, P. L. (1942). Cataract and other ocular changes resulting from tryptophan deficiency. *J. Nutr.* 24:159-166.

Underwood, E. J. (1977). *Trace Elements in Human and Animal Nutrition.* Academic Press, New York. 302 pp.

Vainisi, S. F., Edelhauser, H. F., Wolf, E. D., Cotlier, E., and Reeser, F. (1981). Nutritional cataracts in timber wolves. *J. Amer. Vet. Med. Assoc.* 179:1175-1180.

Von Sallman, L., Reid, M. E., Grimes, P. A., and Collins, E. M. (1959). Tryptophan-deficiency cataract in guinea pigs. *Arch. Ophthalmol.* 62:662-672.

Wahli, W., and Martinez, E. (1991). Superfamily of steroid nuclear receptors: positive and negative regulators of gene expression. *Federation Amer. Soc. Exp. Biol. J. (FASEB J.)* 5:2243-2249.

Weinberger, C., and Bradley, D. J. (1990). Gene regulation by receptors binding lipid-soluble substances. *Ann. Rev. Physiol.* 52:823-840.

Whanger, P. D., and Weswig, P. H. (1975). Effects of selenium, chromium and antioxidants on growth of eye cataracts, plasma cholesterol and blood glucose in selenium deficient vitamin E supplemented rats. *Nutr. Rep. Intern.* 12:345-358.

Wilson, J. G., Roth, C. B., and Warkany, J. (1953). An analysis of the syndrome of malformations induced by maternal vitamin A deficiency. Effects of restoration of vitamin A at various times during gestation. *Amer. J. Anat.* 92:189-217.

Wistow, G. J., and Piatigorsky, J. (1988). Lens crystallins: The evolution and expression of proteins for a highly specialized tissue. *Ann. Rev. Biochem.* 57:479-504.

Woodward, J. C., and Newberne, P. M. (1967). The pathogenesis of hydrocephalus in newborn rats deficient in vitamin B_{12}. *J. Embryol. Exp. Morph.* 17:177-187.

Young, V. R., and Munro, H. N. (1973). Plasma and tissue tryptophan levels in relation to tryptophan requirements. *J. Nutr.* 103:1756-1763.

Chapter 4

Iron Status During Pregnancy

Dejia Zhang and Arthur W. Mahoney[1]

Iron deficiency and anemia are prevalent in pregnant women in both developing and developed countries. The incidence of iron deficiency in pregnant women was reported to vary from 10-70% in different areas, populations, and races. The dietary iron intake of pregnant women is usually not enough to meet their requirements for pregnancy. Although women can absorb more iron from foods when they are pregnant (especially in late pregnancy), total iron intake, in most cases, may still not be enough for the needs of both mother and fetus. Maternal iron status may affect infant iron status when the mother's iron intake is lacking and iron stores are exhausted. Iron deficient pregnant women may also experience more fetal complications than iron sufficient women. Mothers with a poor iron status may be at a higher risk to bear low birth weight infants. This is possibly due to the lack of oxygen transfer from mother to the fetus. On the other hand, a high maternal hemoglobin level is also related to low birth weight. It is proposed that a high hemoglobin level indicates a failure of hemodilution that can increase blood viscosity. High blood viscosity may then prevent nutrients passing through the placenta, causing low birth weight. Reports on the effects of iron-supplementing pregnant women on mother and fetus are conflicting, which may be secondary to various uncontrolled factors in the experiments such as iron status of pregnant women. Pregnant women could be categorized into three groups regarding their iron status: (1) iron sufficient (for both fetus and mother), (2) slightly iron deficient (sufficient for fetus, deficient for

---

[1]Dedicated to the memory of Dr. Arthur W. Mahoney who passed away on June 14, 1992.

mother), and (3) iron deficient (deficient for both fetus and mother) status. Iron supplementation is recommended for the women in groups 2 and 3. Perspectives for future research are also discussed.

Iron Requirements of Pregnant Women

It is estimated that a pregnant woman may need about 1200 mg iron in her whole pregnancy. This includes iron lost to the fetus and placenta, at delivery, maternal blood red cell expansion, and basal daily loss (0.8 mg/day) (Table 1). Except for basal daily iron loss, most iron required is in the last two trimesters. Plasma volume has little change before 10 weeks and expansion starts at about the second trimester. Taylor and Lind (1979) demonstrated a plasma rise of 220 ml at 12 weeks, which increased to 1100 ml at 36 weeks gestation. Assuming each gram of hemoglobin (Hb) to contain 3.35 mg iron, it may need 405 mg iron to maintain the Hb concentration at 11 g/dl with a 1100 ml blood volume expansion.

TABLE 1. Iron Requirements of Pregnancies (mg)

	WHO (1970)	Hallberg (1988)
Transfer to fetus and placenta	330	350
Lost at delivery	200	250
Maternal red cell mass expansion	500	450
Basal iron loss	220	240
Total	1220	1290

Prevalence of Iron Deficiency in Pregnant Women

Iron deficiency is prevalent in both developing and developed countries. The most vulnerable population groups are infants, teenagers, women of menstruation age and the elderly. Based on hematological data for persons aged 1 through 74 years in the second National Health and Nutrition Examination Survey (NHANES II), 1976-1980, the Expert Scientific Working Group estimated that 14.2% of females aged 15-19 and 9.6% females aged 20-44 have an impaired iron status. A ferritin model was used for the above estimation in which low iron status was defined by serum ferritin less than 12 µg/ml, transferrin saturation less than 16% and erythrocyte protoporphyrin more than 70 µg/dl RBC (Expert Scientific Working Group, 1985). Using a mean cell volume (MCV) model, an indicator of late changes of impaired erythropoiesis, 4.9% of females aged 15-19, and 5.4% of females aged 20-44 were estimated to be of impaired iron status. In this model, instead of serum ferritin values, MCV less than 80 fl was used as one of the three criteria (Expert Scientific Working Group, 1985). Using different methods and criteria, Dallman, *et al.* (1984) studied NHANES II data from 1976-1980 and estimated that the prevalence of anemia was highest in teenage girls (5.9%), young women (5.8%) and infants (5.7%). According to the pattern of laboratory abnormalities, they found iron deficiency predominated as a cause of anemia in young women and infants.

Because young women are more vulnerable to iron deficiency, pregnancy may impose additional risk to iron deficiency anemia. Since being diagnosed, iron deficiency anemia has been found prevalent in pregnant women and is still a worldwide health problem. VanNagell, *et al.* (1971) summarized in a review that the incidence of anemia during pregnancy and the immediate postpartum period varied between 10 to 20% depending on the location and economic status of the patients studied. In 1951, Lund surveyed 4,015 pregnant women and found 20% had an Hb level of 10 g/dl or less and 90% of these women were iron deficient. In a study of 1,052 pregnant women at a New York hospital, 49% of the patients were mildly anemic (Hb between 10 and 12 g/dl; hematocrit between 30 and 35%, or erythrocytes between 3,500,000 and 3,750,000/cm^3) and 22.8% of the cases were moderately or severely anemic (Hb <10 g/100 ml; hematocrit <30%, or erythrocytes below 3,500,000/cm^3) (Benjamin, *et al.* 1966). In 1968, the Council on Foods and Nutrition of the American Medical Association summarized several studies and reported that from 15 to 58% pregnant women examined were anemic (Council on Foods and Nutrition, American

Medical Association, 1968). White (1970) reported that in approximately 1000 teen-age pregnant girls of 15 or younger, 35.7% had a Hb level between 10-10.9 g/dl, 18.1% between 9-9.9 g/dl, and 6.9% below 9 g/dl. A total about 60% of the girls had Hb concentrations less than 11.0 g/dl, a generally recognized normal value for pregnant women. Most anemia in pregnant women is caused by iron deficiency. Based on serum concentration of iron, folic acid and vitamin B_{12}, among 239 women, 130 were diagnosed anemic and among the anemic women, 80% were classified as iron deficient, 64.4% were as folic acid deficient, and 30.8% were as vitamin B_{12} deficient (Benjamin, et al. 1966).

Iron deficiency in pregnancy continues as an unsolved problem. Hercberg, et al. (1987) reported an incidence of anemia at 55% in a group of pregnant Beninese women (total 126 women) according to the criteria of the World Health Organization (1972). About 73% of pregnant women were found iron deficiency as defined by a low serum ferritin concentration (<12 μg/l) combined with either a low transferrin saturation (<16%), or a high erythrocyte protoporphyrin level (>3 μg/g Hb), or both. Yepez, et al. (1987) found that 46% of pregnant Ecuadorian women living at an altitude of 2800 m were iron deficient according to the WHO references after adjusting to altitude. Iron deficiency was present in 67% of pregnant women and in 31% of menstruating women in Chad (Prual, et al. ,1988). In Karachi, Pakistan, 38% of 206 pregnant women were found to be iron deficient (Agha, et al., 1988). Lamparelli, et al. (1988) reported that from a population of 224 pregnant women in Johannesburg, 19% of women in the third trimester of pregnancy were anemic as judged by Hb levels less than 11g/dl, while 64% had a saturation of transferrin value of less than 16% and 68% a serum ferritin level less than 12 μg/l. Iron stores of those women were calculated using the method suggested by Cook & Monsen (1976) with a correction for hemodilution. Mean iron stores in the first trimester were determined at 228 mg, with 38% of women having absent iron stores. In the second and third trimesters, the figures were 74 and 92 mg, respectively. Their figures may be more conservative, because the assumption for hemodilution they used may underestimate the blood expansion.

Ho, *et al.* (1987a) determined serum ferritin level in 240 normal full-term pregnant women in Taiwan and found that 15.4% had sub-clinical iron deficiency and 13% had clinical anemia at termination of pregnancy. In another group of 198 pregnant Chinese women, 114 (52%) had some degree of iron depletion (Ho, *et al.* 1987b).

Iron deficiency at the end of gestation is common among women in the developed countries. The percentage of iron deficient anemia reported in the western world varied from 20 to 60% as reviewed by Ulmer & Goepel (1988).

Iron Intake of Pregnant Women

From the data of NHANES II, Murphy & Calloway (1986) estimated nutrient intakes of 1,066 young women 18 to 24 years of age using data from 24-hour dietary recalls. They found that mean iron intake was 10.4 mg/day, in which 3.3 mg iron/day was from meat, fish and poultry. The mean dietary iron intake of these women was about two thirds of the newly established recommended dietary allowance (RDA), 15 mg/day (National Research Council, 1989). It is reasonable to assume that these women may continue the same dietary pattern if they become pregnant. Dietary intake of pregnant women may decrease in 1st trimester and increase in 3rd trimester. Compared to RDA of iron intake for pregnant women, 30 mg/day, dietary iron intake of these women is not enough to meet their needs for pregnancy.

Iron intake of pregnant women was reported to be low from several studies. Schofield, *et al.* (1989) reported that the mean intake of iron by pregnant women was consistently below the current RDA. In a study group of 265 British women from 1st trimester of pregnancy to 2 months postpartum, iron intake of the women in London ranged from 10.5 to 12.5 mg/day and, in Edinburgh, 8.4 to 10.7 mg/day.

Dietary iron intake is even lower in the developing countries and in socioeconomically disadvantaged populations. Lehti (1989) reported that the iron intake of pregnant and lactating Amazonian women of low socioeconomic status was very low compared with current recommendations. About two-thirds of pregnant women out of 500 had their dietary iron intakes below 8 mg/day. Only about 4% of them had an iron intake of more than 15 mg/day. However, the majority of the women had acceptable Hb and hematocrit values. Only about 4% of them had a Hb below 9 g/dl or a hematocrit below 30%. The author explained this occurrence as an adaptation to low iron intake leading to increased iron absorption in these women. In our view, setting the Hb level at 10 g/dl and including serum ferritin and transferrin saturation values as iron status indicators may sharply increase the number of women who had impaired iron status.

Iron Absorption and Metabolism

Pregnant women have a physiological adjustment for iron absorption. As the pregnancy progresses, the requirement for iron increases. This may cause pregnant women to absorb more iron from their diets. Whittaker, *et al.* (1991) and Apte & Iyengar (1970) studied iron absorption of pregnant women at different stages and found that iron absorption continuously increased as pregnancies progressed (Table 2).

Iron metabolism of the fetus is very different from infants and adults. McLean, *et al.* (1970) studied iron metabolism using goats and found that the iron turnover of the fetus in uteri is many times the value reported for an adult man (0.6 ± 0.2 mg/d/dl). The difference between the goat fetus and the newborn goat is also significant (Table 3). This may indicate the existence of a very dynamic system operating *in uteri*. Two fetuses with very low hematocrit (29 and 27%) had very rapid plasma iron disappearance half-time. This may relate to a more rapid utilization of iron for erythropoiesis under this circumstance.

TABLE 2. Dietary Iron Absorption of Women in Different Pregnant Stages[2]

Gestation period (in wks)	Hb g/dl	PCV %	S-Fe µg/dl	TIBC %	Tf-Satu %	S-ferritin µg/l	Fe intake mg	Fe Abs. mg	Fe Abs. %	Ref.[3]
8-16	12.7	39	69	318	22.4		22.2	2.4	7.4	1
12	12.4		106		26	34			7.6	2
24	11.6		84		16	15			21.1	2
28-32	9.9	31	34	496	6.8		23.9	8.9	37.9	1
36	11.0		45		7	7			37.4	2
36-39	10.5	35	36	470	7.6		28.7	9.9	34.5	1
12 pp	12.8		100		23				26.3	2

[2] Abbreviations: Hb: hemoglobin; pcv: packed cell volume; S-Fe: serum Fe; TIBC: total iron-binding capacity; T-satu: transferrin saturation; S-ferritin: serum ferritin; pp: postpartum.

[3] References: 1. Whittaker, et al. (1991); 2. Apte & Iyengar (1970).

TABLE 3. Ferrokinetics in the Fetus and Newborn of Goats[4]

	Age hrs	Hct %	Serum Fe µg/dl	Plasma disappearance half-time (min.)	Plasma turnover (mg/d/dl whole blood)
Fetus	Term	32	297	22	16.1
Newborn	24-48	37	131	75	1.2

[4] Modified from McLean *et al.* (1970). Mean of four goats.

Relationship of Iron Status Between Mother and Infant

Reports from studies on the relationship of iron status between mother and infants are controversial, with the main dispute focusing on the effect of maternal iron status on fetal iron status. Clearly, the fetus takes advantage of using the iron in the mother-fetus system for its benefit. This is evidenced by cord blood iron levels that were much higher than mothers' serum iron levels at delivery (Okuyama, *et al.*, 1985). The controversial point is whether this privilege taken by the fetus is limited to some point or independent of maternal iron status. The inconsistent results from various reports indicate that the phenomenon of the fetus taking iron is unlimited until maternal iron stores are depleted. At this point, the mother starts to compete for iron to maintain her basic physiological requirements. Varied conditions, such as maternal iron status, iron index used, and the time of determination, may account for the conflicting results on the relationship of the iron status of mother and fetus.

The mechanism of transferring iron from mother to fetus is not clear. Okuyama, *et al.* (1985) suggested that ferritin in the placenta may be more actively involved in iron metabolism beyond it's iron storage function as previously known. The fetus can take up optimal amounts of iron from the mother whose iron stores may be low. This iron transfer through the placenta is against a concentration gradient, an advantage to fetal requirements rather than mothers' (Fletcher & Suter, 1969). This phenomenon has been shown by many studies. Ajayi (1988) found that the mean cord ferritin concentration in neonates was more than three times higher than that of their mothers (136 vs. 38 μg/l). Hussain, *et al.* (1977) found a mean serum ferritin level of 58 μg/l at term in 51 pregnant women compared to a mean of 183 μg/l in their newborns. Milman, *et al.* (1987) found a mother serum:fetus cord blood serum ferritin ratio of 21 vs. 128 μg/l in 85 healthy iron-supplemented mothers at parturition and in 74 of their term newborns. In another study (Rios, *et al.*, 1975), newborn serum ferritin levels were more than 5 time higher than their mothers'. Other hematological indexes such as Hb concentration, hematocrits, serum iron level, total iron-binding capacity, and transferrin saturation also indicated that the newborns had a better iron status than their mothers.

However, the privilege for the fetus to take up iron is limited to some extent by maternal iron status. Ahayi (1988) found that infants of mothers having low iron stores (ferritin level <20 μg/l) had significantly lower serum ferritin levels than infants of iron sufficient mothers. In 115 paired maternal and cord specimens, when maternal serum ferritin levels were below 10 μg/l, cord ferritin levels were also low (144 μg/l) as compared to cord ferritin levels (218 μg/l) from mothers with serum ferritin levels more than 30 μg/l (Kelly & McDougall, 1978). Serum iron, serum ferritin and transferrin saturation values of newborns from mothers of low iron status were low compared to that of the newborns from the mothers with high iron status (Rios, *et al.*, 1975). Hercberg, *et al.* (1987) found that the newborns from iron-deficiency mothers had lower Hb (16.6 vs. 18.3 g/dl), mean corpuscular volumes (102.1 vs. 108.2 fl) and serum ferritin levels (263 vs. 308 μg/l) compared to their counterparts from iron-sufficient mothers. Ilyes, *et al.* (1985) found that a group of mothers with a mean serum ferritin level of 6.5 μg/l, had infants with a mean cord ferritin level of 98.5 μg/l. This was lower than the mean cord ferritin level (147 μg/l) for the infants whose mother had a mean serum ferritin level of 38 μg/l. In a long term study, Colomer, *et al.* (1990) followed the iron status of 156 newborns from birth to one year. Infants were categorized into two groups, one with the mother having normal iron status at delivery and the other with the mother being iron deficient defined by their ferritin levels <12 μg/l and Hb <11 g/dl. They found that more infants from the mothers with low iron status had developed anemia (30%) than the infants of normal iron status mother (6%). They suggested a positive relationship between a newborn's low iron status and mother's iron deficiency during pregnancy. In some studies, the positive correlations of maternal blood Hb, serum ferritin, serum iron and erythrocyte protoporphyrin with their respective cord blood values were significant but weak (Yepez, *et al.* 1987; Daouda, *et al.* 1991). This indicates that the population in these experiments were at a turning point from unlimited fetus privilege to limited iron uptake from the mother. The correlation curve may be not a linear but a binomial curve. Because iron turnover is much faster in the fetus than in the mother, maternal iron deficiency anemia may affect, in a significant way, both the plasma iron transport rate to the fetus and the distribution of iron in the various fetal pools without affecting the fetal hemoglobin concentration (McLean, *et al.*, 1970).

Maternal erythropoiesis activity and fetal iron requirement may exhaust the iron stores before the fetal demand for iron is met. Fenton, *et al.* (1977) studied 154 pregnant women and randomly assigned them to two groups with or without iron supplementation. They found that iron supplemented pregnant women had much higher serum ferritin levels than their unsupplemented counterparts (41 vs. 13 μg/l), indicating an iron depletion in the mothers without iron supplementation. Although iron therapy did not prevent the sharp drop of maternal iron stores, it did maintain them above the iron deficient level. Also, it was found that 33 babies from mothers with serum ferritin level less than 12 μg/l at term had a mean cord ferritin of 174 μg/l that was significantly lower than the mean of 245 μg/l found in the 96 babies of mothers who had serum ferritin levels of 12 μg/l or more. This indicates that when maternal iron stores are depleted, the privilege of fetal uptake of iron from the mother is limited.

Iron deficiency in infants may affect their brain function. Iron supplementation has immediate (within 14 days) and long-term (over 3 months) benefits on behavior and psychomotor development (Parks & Wharton, 1989). The mechanisms for this may involve a number of enzymes and neurotransmitters in which iron is essential. Levels of neurotransmitters such as noradrenaline, serotonin and dopamine are altered during iron deficiency. Neonatal and postnatal iron supplementation may prevent poor infant development caused by iron deficiency.

Very few studies have been done on the mechanisms of how newborns obtain much higher Hb and ferritin levels than their mothers. Some clues may come from studies on protein absorption. Wapnir (1990) reported that fetuses absorb protein differently from adults. The adult human gastrointestinal tract, under normal conditions, is generally an effective barrier to the absorption of large molecules such as protein. In contrast, the fetal and neonatal gut normally allows for the entry of macromolecules. Two important factors contribute to the relatively high rate of intact protein absorption of the immature gut. One is the late developmental maturation sequence of proteolytic enzymes, which may not attain full activity until the end of lactation. The second factor is a greater permeability to macromolecules, apparent during the neonatal period. Even when the intestinal epithelium has not yet differentiated, the macromolecules may be absorbed. Ferritin in amniotic fluid can be swallowed and absorbed intact by the fetus. Consequently, equilibrium force may pull ferritin from the mother to amniotic fluid and then to the fetus.

Maternal Iron Status and Fetal Complications

Iron deficiency of pregnant women is related to several fetal complications, such as prematurity, congenital anomalies and stillbirth. In the 1960s, Klein (1962) reported that the incidence of prematurity in women with their Hb less than 10 g/dl was nearly double that of women having Hb more than 10 g/dl. This relationship was confirmed by Abramowicz & Kass (1966) who found that the more profound the anemia, the higher the rate of prematurity.

From a study of 486 iron deficient mothers with serum iron

levels less than 60 µg/dl in the third trimester, Roszkowski, *et al.* (1966) found that the incidence of stillbirth and neonatal death was 2.5 times of that in the control group. They also found that the incidence of congenital anomalies in the infants of iron deficient mothers was 2.8 times higher than that of control groups with more than one third of the cases having pathologic placental changes. Similar results found in iron deficient women having Hb less than 7.4 g/dl have shown an incidence of stillbirth three times higher than in control women (MacGregor, 1963). The incidences of stillbirth and prematurity were significantly reduced when iron was supplemented before 30 weeks of gestation.

Recent research has also shown that low hematologic values in pregnant women is related to fetal defects. A significant correlation between low serum ferritin levels and the incidence of preterm labor was found in 300 west German women (Ulmer & Goepel, 1988). Among women with serum ferritin levels below 10 µg/l, 52.3% had preterm labor, compared to only 9.5% of the women with serum ferritin levels above 20 µg/l. In another study of Goepel, *et al* (1988), premature labor contractions were experienced by 48% of pregnant women with serum ferritin values below 10 µg/l, while occurring in only 11% of the women with serum ferritin values exceeding 20 µg/l. It is hypothesized that apart from insufficient oxygen supply to the fetus, hypoperfusion of the placenta occurs and, as a consequence, ischemic decidual necrosis results and may lead to the release of prostaglandines that may induce labor contraction. Other mechanisms may also be involved, such as deficiency of iron related enzymes.

Recently, high hematologic values were also found to be related to fetal defects. Thus, a U-shape relationship is shown when plotting the percent of fetal defects against maternal hematologic values. Using the hematologic data and pregnancy outcome data from more than 50,000 consecutive pregnancies followed in the National Collaborative Perinatal Project of the National Institute of Neurological Disorders and Stroke, Garn, *et al.* (1981) reported that fetal death and prematurity were high for both extremes of hematologic values (Table 4). They also found the "optimal" Hb and Hct values were lower for blacks and higher for whites. Excluding the factors of smoking, maternal toxemia, and the trimester of registration, the U-shaped relationship between fetus defects and maternal hematologic values did not change.

Other researchers have also reported negative effects of

TABLE 4. Percent of Unfavorable Outcome by
Maternal Pregnancy Hemoglobin[5]

Unfavorable pregnancy outcome	Maternal hemoglobin midpoint (g/dl)						
	8	9	10	11	12	13	14
Whites							
Medical abnormality (3849)	34.4	33.4	30.5	25.6	22.7	22.8	25.3
Fetal death (633)	5.0	2.4	2.2	2.4	4.1	6.7	13.2
Low birth weight (1677)	13.8	11.5	9.7	8.9	9.0	11.4	11.0
Prematurity (2899)	21.5	19.8	17.6	15.0	14.7	18.6	22.3
Blacks							
Medical abnormality (4234)	22.0	24.2	23.7	23.7	24.1	25.9	27.6
Fetal death (563)	2.6	1.6	2.0	2.7	5.4	9.7	14.5
Low birth weight (3134)	15.9	124.9	15.5	15.9	17.9	22.4	30.4
Prematurity (5611)	30.2	28.1	28.4	27.5	28.9	32.5	40.8

[5] From Garn, *et al.* (1981), with permission of the publishers. Numbers in parenthesis are the numbers of the subjects in that category.

high Hb levels in women on pregnancy outcome. In a study of 4690 pregnant women, Mau (1977) found that pregnant women with a high Hb in 3rd trimester gave birth to prematures, dystrophic, and low birth weight infants more frequently than those with low Hb levels. Koller, *et al.* (1980) evaluated a series of 15 cases with intrauterine fetal death of unknown cause, and found that before start of labor, 10 cases had Hb levels 2 standard deviations (SD) above the mean. While in a series of 16 cases of late abortion where the fetus was alive until labor started, only one had a Hb level 2 SD higher than the mean. They suggested that with high Hb levels during pregnancy, hemodilution may have failed and high viscosity of the mother's blood may impede the uteroplacental circulation, causing placental infarction, growth retardation and ultimately fetal death.

Maternal Iron Status and Low Birth Weight

Reports on the the relationship between maternal iron and birth weight are controversial. Both low and high hemoglobin concentrations and serum iron levels of pregnant women were reported to be related to low birth weight. Deficiencies of many nutrients in the mother, such as protein, may be more important than iron for the outcome of low birth weight. A non-correlation between maternal iron status and low birth weight will not exclude this relationship. However, an established correlation between them is meaningful.

In the study of Garn, *et al.* (1981) mentioned above, in more than 50,000 consecutive pregnancies, both high and low Hb and hematocrits were related to low birth weight (Table 4). The mechanisms for these two opposite relationship are different.

It is suggested that reduced efficiency in the transport of oxygen, carbon dioxide and nutrients may be involved with low birth weight for iron deficient mothers. The placental weight was significantly higher in iron deficient (600 g) compared to non-iron-deficient women (548 g) (Daouda, *et al.*, 1991). The placenta:birth weight ratios were 0.197 in iron-deficient mothers and 0.184 in non-iron-deficient mothers, respectively. Large placental weight and a high ratio of placental to birth weight were also found to be associated with anemia and iron deficiency during pregnancy in a survey of 8684 women (Godfrey, *et al.*, 1991). This may indicate a compensation by increasing the placental size if less oxygen is transported to the fetus in low iron mothers. Beischer (1971) studied 732 pregnant women with severe anemia (Hb <8 g/dl) in Melbourne, Thailand, India, Singapore and New Guinea, and found a significant positive correlation between maternal anemia and placental weight (Table 5).

Inadequate oxygenation of the fetoplacental unit, as a consequence of maternal anemia, may evoke a physiologic response resulting in compensatory placental hypertrophy and may also cause some pathological change. Rusia, *et al.* (1988) studied the placentae of iron-deficient and non-iron-

TABLE 5. Birth Weight and Placental Weight in Patients with Hb Values 10 g/dl or Above (No Anemia) and Below 8 g/dl[6]

	Melbourne		Singapore		India		Thailand	
	No Anemia	Anemia	No Anemia	Anemia	No Anemia	Anemia	No Anemia	Anemia
Average birth weight (g)	3317	3140	3231	3133	2570	2469	2971	2719
Average placental weight (g)	553	585	517	561	476	521	530	566
PW:BW ratio[7]	0.16	0.18	0.16	0.18	0.18	0.21	0.17	0.20

[6] From Beischer (1971), with permission.
[7] Placental weight vs. birth weight ratio.

deficient mothers and found that iron deficient women had a high number of infarction in their placentae. The presence of basement membrane thickening, fibrinoid necrosis, villous fibrosis, and calcification in the placentae of iron-deficient women was significantly higher than in non-iron-deficient women (Table 6). Placental alkaline phosphatase activity decreased progressively with increasing severity of anemia and acid phosphatase activity increased significantly in iron deficient women, thereby matching the situation of hypoxia. The hypoxia and altered tissue pH directly cause an increase of acid phosphatase (lysosomal enzyme) and indirectly cause degenerative changes in the syncytiotrophoblast with decreased alkaline phosphatase. The association between iron deficiency during pregnancy and increased placental weight as well as high ratio of placental weight to birth weight may indicate that maternal nutritional deficiency may cause discordance between placental and fetal growth. This may have important implications for the prevention of adult hypertension, which appears to have its origin in fetal life.

In a recent study, Barker, *et al.* (1990) found that low birth weight was highly correlated with hypertension happening about 50 years later. The authors studied the blood pressure of 499 men and women born in Preston, Italy during 1935 - 43, along with the records of their placental and birth weights. They found that mean systolic pressure rose by 15 mm Hg as

TABLE 6. Fetus Outcomes and Placental Histopathologic Changes Categorized According to Maternal Hematological Values[8]

Parameter	Group I	Group II	Group III
Maternal Hb (g/dl)	12.8	9.5	5.2
Serum ferritin (µg/l)	31.7	45.1	11.2
Birth weight (g)	2795	2729	2183
Placental weight (g)	370	338	273
Fetoplacental ratio	7.8	8.3	9.7
	Percent of histopathologic changes		
Syncytial knots	44 (7)	20 (4)	75 (12)
Fibrinoid necrosis	19 (3)	40 (8)	65 (12)
Basement membrane thickening		35 (7)	43 (7)
Villous fibrosis		5 (1)	25 (7)
Calcification	13 (2)		62 (10)
Blood vessel abnormality			12 (2)

[8] Modified after Rusia, *et al.* (1988). Figures in parentheses represent number of women.

placental weight increased from less than 1 pound to more than 1.5 pounds and fell by 11 mm Hg as birth weight increased from less than 5.5 pounds to more than 7.5 pounds. They suggested that this relationship may be a result of hypoxia secondary to low Hb caused by iron deficiency. In response to hypoxia, the fetus may redistribute cardiac output, which favors perfusion of the brain. Reduced blood flow to the trunk induced in a fetus that is small in relation to its placenta could have irreversible consequences, perhaps by influencing arterial structure.

Very low birth weigh infants may be more vulnerable to iron depletion. In 81 Canadian infants of birth weight less than 1500 g, 54% at 12 months and 74% at 15 months had serum ferritin levels below 10 µg/l (Friel, *et al.*, 1990). These infants were fed with iron fortified formula (13 mg/l) for at least 6 months, starting at 2 months of age, and then about 90% of them were given iron fortified cereal (30 mg/100g). Both types of iron supplementation did not stop the drop of serum ferritin levels. This leads to a greater consideration of iron deficiency in these infants when non-iron fortified solid foods are introduced. It is not known to what degree iron depletion may affect infant development. Iron dependent enzymes are sensitive to iron deficiency and a decreased level of iron in tissue may alter neurologic development. The mechanism of iron depletion in very low birth weight infants are not clear. Consuming less foods at the same age as term infants (Friel, et al., 1990) may be part of the cause. Delayed development in absorptive and metabolic systems may be another cause.

A high hemoglobin level of the mother was also associated with low birth weight. Knottnerus, et al. (1990) studied pregnancy outcome of 796 Dutch women and found that those having a Hb level higher than 13 g/dl during weeks 31-32 of gestation had a significant higher percentage of low birth weight babies than the mothers having Hb levels between 11.3 to 12.9 g/dl (15 vs 4%). Koller, et al. (1979) found an inverse correlation between birth weight and the lowest Hb level reached during the pregnancy as well as the Hb level in late pregnancy. In their study, seven women who had a significantly high Hb level in late pregnancy gave birth to babies below the 2.5th percentile. The same group of researchers (Sagen, et al., 1984) later studied 877 apparently normal pregnancies and found the mothers who had high hemoglobin levels, both in the early third trimester and at term, had smaller newborns than those who had low Hb levels. However, the birth weights (averaging 3150 g) of the mother had high Hb were above the criteria for low birth weight (2500 g). In Sagen's study, the mothers having high Hb also had less body weight gain which may also be highly related to low birth weight.

The correlation between high Hb level of the mother and low birth weight may not be the cause and result relationship. It is suggested that a failure of blood volume expansion in pregnant women may be the cause of both a high Hb level and low birth weight. Dunlop, et al. (1978) determined Hb concentration, hematocrit, serum urate concentration, and fractional reabsorption of urate in 9 patients who gave birth to small-for-date infants and in 25 control patients who gave birth to normal weight infants. They found that the women who produced low birth weight infants had all above determined values significantly higher than the control women (Table 7).

Urate is filtered at the glomerulus and the filtrate is then modified by reabsorption. It is thought that secretion is directly related to serum urate concentration and reabsorption may be modified by alteration in extracellular fluid. Their data suggest that depletion of extracellular fluid volume, more specifically being the failure of blood volume expansion may be the factor causing both a high Hb level and low birth weight.

TABLE 7. Hematologic and Urate Values of Pregnant Women[9]

Measurements	LBW group	NBW group	P value
Serum urate concentration (μmol/1)	302.0	241.0	<0.05
Fractional reabsorption of urate (%)	92.48	89.18	<0.005
Hemoglobin (g/dl)	12.7	11.5	<0.001
Hematocrit (%)	37.6	34.2	<0.001

[9] From the data of Dunlop, et al. (1978). LBW: low birth weight; NBW: normal birth weight.

Iron Supplementation of Pregnant Women

Dietary iron intake of pregnant women is apparently not enough to support the needs of the mother and fetus. The National Academy of Sciences (National Research Council, 1989) recommended a RDA for pregnant women of 30 mg iron per day which is 15 mg more than for menstruating women. Since dietary iron intake of pregnant women is insufficient, iron supplementation is suggested as a way of promoting pregnancy process. However, the effect of iron supplementation on pregnant women is in dispute.

Guldhalt, et al. (1991) found that iron supplementation did improve the iron stores of pregnant women for blood volume expansion and infant growth. In their study, ferritin levels of pregnant women taking vitamin and mineral supplements (only 15 mg ferrous iron per day) sharply dropped from about 70 to 30 pmol/l from the 20th to 28th week gestation and remained at that level till the 36th week of gestation. However, when another group of pregnant women were supplemented with 100 mg ferrous iron per day, the drop of serum ferritin was slowed down. Ferritin levels dropped from 65 pmol/l at the 20th week to 50 pmol/l at the 28th week, and then raised up to 55 pmol/l at the 36th week. Puolakka, *et al.* (1980) randomly divided 32 pregnant women into two groups with or without iron supplementation. The supplemented women received 100 mg iron as ferrous sulphate twice a day. Hematological values were determined every four weeks starting from 16 weeks gestation until delivery and then at 5 days, and 1, 2 and 6 months past delivery. Mean serum ferritin level of iron supplemented women was significantly higher compared to the women without iron supplementation (Figure 1). Bone marrow iron stores were also determined, and significantly correlated with serum ferritin levels during and after pregnancy (Table 8). The authors advised routine iron supplementation to the women of that population.

Taking into account the variation caused by blood expansion of pregnant women, a measure of red cell mass has been used to determine changes of the blood-oxygen carrying system and the effect of iron supplementation on iron status of pregnant women. In calculating red cell mass, blood volume needs to be determined and then, red cell volume is calculated as the result of multiplication of blood volume and hematocrit. Taylor & Lind (1979) found that, in 42 pregnant women, average blood volume increased from 2340 ml during the non-pregnant stage to 3480 ml at the 36th week of pregnancy, almost an one third increase (Table 9). Compared to the non-pregnant stage, Hb concentrations at the 36th week decreased about 0.7 g/dl in iron supplemented and 2.2 g/dl in non-supplemented women. However, red cell mass was increased 350 ml in iron supplemented and 180 ml in non-supplemented women. Their data indicate that Hb concentrations of pregnant women may not truly reflect their real iron status, and iron supplementation improves the iron status of the pregnant women, even those having their Hb levels above 11 g/dl.

A recent survey of the Women, Infants, and Children (WIC) program showed that WIC infants consumed more

TABLE 8. Percentage of Distribution of Bone Marrow Iron
Contents of Iron-treated and Non-treated Pregnant Women[10]

Bone marrow stainable iron	Iron treated			Non-iron treated		
	Early pregnancy	Late pregnancy	2 months post partum	Early pregnancy	Late pregnancy	2 months post partum
Absent	35	43	7	20	80	80
Sparce	30	14	13	33	20	10
Sufficient	35	43	57	40	0	10
Plenty	0	0	23	7	0	0

[10] Adapted from Puolakka *et al.* (1980).

iron-fortified infant formula than non-WIC infants and, as a result, had higher daily intakes of iron and vitamin (Batten, *et al.* 1990). From 24-hour dietary recall data, mean iron intake from birth to 11 months of age were 21.4 mg/day for WIC (n = 178) and 13.5 mg/day for non-WIC (n = 84) infants, respectively. Among eligible women, participation in WIC is associated with a 16% to 20% decreased incidence of low birth weight infants. Mean birth weight appears to rise approximately 1-2%. WIC mothers appear to experience

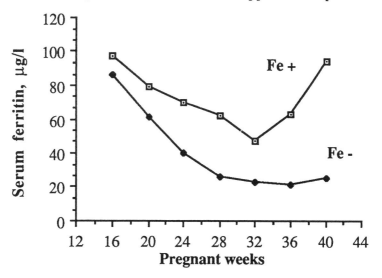

FIGURE 1. Serum ferritin levels during pregnancy in iron-treated (Fe+) and non-treated (Fe-) pregnant women. From the data of Puolakka, *et al.* (1980).

greater benefits the longer they participate in the program. Except for iron, improvement of other nutrients has also accounted for better birth outcome.

Because high Hb level is reported to be related to low birth weight, iron supplementation may be questioned to have an increasing risk of low birth weight. To study this, Hemminki & Rimpela (1991) randomly assigned 2912 pregnant women into two groups of non-routine iron and routine iron supplementation. Pregnant women in the routine iron supplementa-

TABLE 9. Plasma Volume, Red Cell Mass and Hb Concentration in the Pregnant and Non-pregnant State[11]

	Non-supplemented			Iron supplemented		
	Non-preg	12 wks	36 wks	Non-preg	12 wks	36 wks
Plasma volume, ml	2340	2540	3478	2336	2577	3384
Red cell mass, ml	1240	1138	1420	1256	1159	1605
Hb concentration, g/dl	13.3	12.0	11.1	13.4	12.1	12.7

[11] Modified from Taylor & Lind (1979).

tion group were recommended to take a once-daily dose of 100 mg elemental iron starting at the latest after the 16th week and continued throughout the pregnancy. For the non-routine iron supplementation women, if packed cell volume (PCV) below 0.30 in two visits, they were recommended to take 50 mg iron twice a day for two months or until the packed cell volume increased to 0.32. After 33 weeks gestation, the prerequisite for starting iron treatment was raised to a PCV 0.31. Among the routine iron supplemented women, except for a sharp drop from the 12th week to 20th week, PCV slightly increased up to the 36th week, while the non-routine iron supplemented women maintained a low PCV until the 36th week. No significant difference in birth weight was found between these two groups indicating that iron supplementation did not increase the risk of low birth weight. This study has also shown that more women who were routinely iron supplemented (260 women) have PCV of more than 0.39 compared to the non-routine iron supplemented women (182 women) (Table 10). This suggests that increased PCV reaching to more than 0.39 in about 80 routinely iron supplemented women may be a result of iron supplementation assuming the beginning iron status was similar between two groups as a result of random assignment. Among the rest, the proportion of the women with high PCV attributed to a failure of hemodilution is unknown. It is reasonable to assume that they are the same in the two groups. Thus, the proportion of failure of hemodilution in the routinely iron supplemented women was reduced. This coincided with the result that the routinely iron supplemented women gave birth to infants about 100 grams heavier than their counterparts (3522g vs. 3421g). Combining these two characters, it can be proposed that increased incidence of low birth weight in mothers with high PCV is a result of failure of hemodilution and not high iron levels. Unfortunately, there is no way of separating those women with normal hemodilution from the women of failure of hemodilution who had PCV of more than 0.39. Otherwise, our proposal will be more evident. The mechanism of failure of hemodilution causing low birth weight was proposed as a high viscosity of the blood that may reduce the fetal metabolism.

Effect of Iron Supplementation on Serum Zinc in Pregnant Women

Iron supplementation may affect serum zinc levels of pregnant women. However, the research results are conflicting. Dawson, et al. (1989) found that prenatal oral iron supplementation at 18 mg/d resulted in depressed maternal serum zinc concentrations between the first trimester and 12 wk postpartum. Zinc levels decreased from 1.5 µg/ml at prestudy to 0.98 µg/ml at 40 weeks of gestation (34% decrease). At the 4th week postpartum, serum Zn levels increased back to 1.5 µg/ml, a level similar to that before pregnancy. The women without iron supplementation maintained serum zinc levels around 1.5 µg/ml throughout gestation. Serum zinc levels above 0.8 µg/ml are considered normal (Sauberlich, 1983) and the reduction of zinc levels from 1.5 to 0.98 µg/ml

TABLE 10. Birth Weight by Packed Cell Volume
in Mothers During 28th Week[12]

| | Packed cell volime in | | | | | | | |
| | Non-routine iron women (n=1319) | | | | Routine iron women (n=1299) | | | |
	≤0.32	0.33-0.35	0.36-0.38	≤0.39	≤0.32	0.33-0.35	0.36-0.38	≥0.39
No. of mothers	162	462	513	182	58	395	586	260
Mean birth weight (g)	3690	3581	3574	3421	3556	3618	3601	3522
Birth weight <2500g, %	1.9	2.6	2.1	7.7	5.2	1.3	2.4	5.0

[12] From Hemminki & Rimpela (1991), with permission.

may not indicate a zinc deficiency. The authors suggested that inadequate dietary or supplemented Zn intake coupled with immature Zn metabolism and iron supplementation may jointly contribute to a severe inadequacy of maternal Zn stores and a high frequency of low birth weight, premature rupture of the membranes, congenital malformations, and fetal mortalities associated with teen-age pregnancies. The negative effect of iron supplementation on Zn retention in human pregnancy was also reported by Hambridge, et al. (1983) and Aggett & Harries (1979). It was hypothesized that increased ingestion of elemental Fe depressed the Zn bio-availability by competition in the bowel wall (Meadows, et al., 1983; Solomons & Jacob, 1981).

Some other researchers reported that iron supplementation did not affect Zn retention. Breskin et al. (1983) found that during pregnancy, serum zinc levels dropped from 0.97 µg/ml within 20 days of ovulation to 0.49 µg/ml at 240 days of gestation and back to 0.57 µg/ml 6 weeks postpartum in breast feeding mothers and 0.93 µg/ml in non-breast feeding mothers. Iron and vitamin supplementations did not affect serum zinc levels. They concluded that supplementation with 15 to 25 mg of elemental zinc and no more than 60 mg of elemental iron is related to increased serum zinc concentrations during the 1st trimester of pregnancy. Supplementation with more than 60 mg of iron may lower serum zinc levels. Sheldon, et al. (1985) reported that prenatal oral Fe supplementation had no effect on serum Zn concentrations. Hambridge, et al.

(1987) studied the effect of iron supplementation on zinc status in 20 pregnant women and found that when 261 mg iron/day was given, mean serum zinc level was slightly decreased from 0.63 to 0.59 µg/ml at 1 week with no further decline at 4 weeks after iron therapy. No control group was included in this study and a possible physiologic decline of zinc levels in normal pregnancy cannot be excluded.

Beneficiaries of Iron Supplementation

Who is the beneficiary of iron supplementation; mother, fetus or both? This totally depends on maternal iron status during pregnancy. Pregnant women can be categorized into three groups with regards to their iron status. The mother's iron stores and regular dietary iron intakes will: (1) meet the requirements of both mother and fetus, (2) meet fetal iron requirements but not mother's, and (3) meet neither fetal nor maternal iron requirement.

In the first group of pregnant women categorized above, iron supplementation is not necessary. Their iron stores are high before pregnancy, they have enough available iron from their diets and/or they have well adjusted mechanisms of iron absorption when they need more iron. Iron supplementation will not change either fetal or maternal iron status. In this group, the mother's serum ferritin levels will not correlate with their newborns, as reported by some authors (Hussain, et al., 1977; Siimes & Siimes, 1986; Wong & Saha, 1990).

In the second group, iron stores and income are sufficient for the fetus but not sufficient for maternal needs. Iron supplementation will benefit the mother. Van Eijk, et al. (1978) compared a group of women given 100 mg iron/day as ferrous sulfate from 3rd month of gestation until delivery and a group without iron supplementation. They found that at term, the iron supplemented mothers had higher Hb, serum iron and serum ferritin levels than the mothers without iron supplementation. The recovery of iron stores in the unsupplemented mothers, indicated by serum ferritin, were slower than supplemented mothers 12 weeks after delivery. However, cord blood Hb, serum iron and serum ferritin levels of their new-borns were similar between the two groups and were much higher than their mothers.

In the third group of women, iron stores and income are insufficient both for fetuses and mothers. Agha, *et al.* (1988) categorized women into two groups according to their Hb values being less than 11 g/dl or greater than or equal to 11 g/dl. They found that the newborns in the group of mothers having low Hb levels at term had cord blood hematologic values lower than the newborns from the mothers with high Hb levels (Table 11). The difference in cord ferritin between two groups was not significant, which may indicate that the cord ferritin had a large variation, and the sample size was relatively small. Iron supplementing the women having low iron status in this population will benefit both fetus and mother.

Supplementation or Treatment

There is no agreement whether iron should be routinely supplemented to all pregnant women or given to those with low iron status. Gofin, *et al.* (1989) studied the outcome of both these practices. They supplemented 478 women from

TABLE 11. Hematologic Values of Mothers and their Newborns[13]

Mothers Hb conc. (g/dl)	Mothers ferritin (μg/l)	Cord ferritin (μg/l)	Cord Hb conc. (g/dl)	Baby's birth weight (kg)
<11 (133)[14]	25.5	122.9	14.6	2.7
≥11 (59)	38.2	152.2	16.7	3.0
Significance	p<0.01	NS	p<0.001	p<0.01

[13] Modified from Agha *et al.* (1988).
[14] The value in the parenthesis is the number of subjects.

the 4th month of pregnancy with either 305 mg ferrous fumarate or 500 mg ferrous calcium citrate plus 5 mg folic acid per day, and treated another group of 392 women with 100 to 1,000 mg either ferrous calcium citrate or ferrous sulphate or ferrous gluconate per day if their Hb levels fell between 10 to 12 g/dl. From second to third trimester, mean

Hb level decreased by 0.9 and 1.1 g/dl and hematocrit decreased by 2.1 and 3.3% in iron supplemented and treated groups, respectively. They did not determine the iron status of the newborns nor maternal serum ferritin, a more precise iron status indicator. This limited the interpretation of their data. According to the information to date, treatment of women with diagnosed anemia and iron deficiency is recommended. Routine iron supplementation to all pregnant women may not be the best solution to this problem. Guldholt, *et al.* (1991) recommended a serum ferritin level of 36 µg/l in mid-pregnancy as a guide in deciding whether or not an iron supplementation is needed.

Another question in iron supplementation is what is a suitable dose amount. There has not been an experiment specifically designed to study the dose-response of iron supplementation. In most of the studies to date, about 100 mg iron/day was supplemented to pregnant women and in most cases, maternal iron status at term was improved. These doses are much higher than the RDA value (30 mg/day) (Food & Nutrition Board, National Research Council, 1989). Are these high doses necessary or may a lower dose have the same benefit to mother and fetus? More research is needed to ascertain what is a suitable dose. This might not be a single value and may vary according to the iron status of the pregnant woman.

Foods Containing High Bioavailable Iron for Pregnant Women

The recommended optimum dietary requirement for iron during pregnancy is 30 mg per day (Food & Nutrition Board, National Research Council, 1989). Because dietary iron may not be enough to meet the iron requirements of pregnant women, sufficient iron intake may be achieved either by iron supplementation (as in mineral-vitamin pills) or by including foods with highly bioavailable iron in the diet. The major factors that determine the iron absorption are the physiological need for iron and the amount of bioavailable iron consumed. During iron deficiency or anemia, the absorption of iron increases compared to that during normal health (Zhang & Mahoney, 1989). The same may be applicable during pregnancy. Meat is an excellent source of dietary iron since it contains heme iron, which is absorbed intact via a specific receptor(s) in intestines and the absorption is independent of dietary inhibiting factors (Zhang, *et al.*, 1989, 1991). Meat, beef, pork, lamb, fish and chicken, can also enhance dietary nonheme iron absorption (Cook & Monsen, 1976).

Iron can also be provided by vegetables, preferably the leafy vegetables like spinach (Zhang, *et al.*, 1985), which has approximately 30 mg of iron per kg on fresh weight basis according to USDA Handbook 8. Although the nonheme iron from vegetables is less absorbed compared to heme iron in meat, the high iron contents of these vegetables make them significant dietary iron sources (Black, *et al.*, 1986). Nonheme iron absorption can be affected by dietary inhibitors and enhancers. Among inhibitors, most considered are phytate and polyphenol that may bind iron in an insoluble form inhibiting its absorption. The most powerful enhancer is ascorbic acid that may reduce iron to valence 2 and reduce stomach pH to keep the iron in a soluble form ready for absorption (Carpenter & Mahoney, 1992). Some vegetables may contain both enhancers and inhibitors. The ways they may react with each other and with iron are not clear. Vegetables and cereals contain nonheme iron that may require specific carriers in the intestines for absorption (Zhang, *et al.*, 1989). The absorption of nonheme iron increases as the body need rises.

Highly soluble inorganic iron such as ferrous sulfate is a good iron source, especially during iron-deficiency. Inorganic iron may be easily absorbed via passive diffusion with no specific carrier required. Once inside the cells of the intestinal lumen, the iron entry into circulation requires transferrin (the specific iron transport protein) and is regulated by the iron requirement of the body rather than the form of iron consumed. Iron containing supplements should best be taken with or after meals so as to avoid irritation caused by inorganic forms of iron.

Dairy products are good protein and calcium sources but are not rich sources of iron. However, fortification of products like cheese with iron has been successfully attempted. Zhang & Mahoney (1990) have found that fortification of Cheddar cheese with either inorganic iron (ferric chloride) or iron-protein complexes resulted in products indistinguishable in cheese quality compared to the unfortified products. Excellent bioavailability of iron from fortified dairy products was reported (Zhang & Mahoney, 1989).

Research Perspectives

Human pregnancy is a very complicated physiological process. This creates difficulties in studying the influence of any single factor that may be involved in this process. Regarding the relationship between iron and fetal defects, many aspects are unclear. Listed are some suggestions for perspective research that may help to clarify the relationship between maternal iron status and fetal outcomes.

(1) For a pregnant female of low iron status, iron supplementation is recommended. However, what level is considered as a low iron status for pregnant women and when iron supplementation should be initiated are not certain. Such a study should include mothers of varying iron status who will be supplemented with the same amount of iron. Comparisons of iron status of mothers at term and fetuses among the mothers of varying iron status may reveal the optimal iron status for initiating iron supplementation.

(2) Another important question is what is the optimal level of iron supplementation. The U.S. RDA recommends 30 mg/day for pregnant women; however, most researchers have used about 100 mg/day in their studies to evaluate the effects of supplementation. The outcomes of mother and fetus treated with various levels of iron supplementation should be determined and used as a base for defining supplementation levels.

(3) Hemoglobin concentration as an indicator of iron status

for pregnant women is affected by hemodilution. Serum ferritin may also be affected by blood volume change. More research is needed to find more reliable indicator(s) of iron status, or some indices that may be used for adjustment of blood volume.

(4) It is commonly accepted that failure of hemodilution is the cause of impaired pregnancy outcome and high hemoglobin levels of pregnant women. However, the experimental data to support this hypothesis are weak and more research is needed to reveal this relationship.

(5) Iron transport from mother to fetus after 20 weeks gestation is against iron concentration. The mechanism for this transportation is unknown.

(6) Research on the possibility of increasing dietary iron intake to improve mother and infant iron status and pregnancy outcomes is lacking. Increasing intake of foods with highly available iron such as meats, increasing dietary iron absorption enhancers such as ascorbic acid, and eating more iron fortified foods, such as iron fortified cereals, drinks and cheeses (in marketing research step) may have benefits to the pregnant women and their babies.

References

Abramowicz, M., and Kass, E. H. (1966). Pathogenesis and prognosis of prematurity. *New Engl. J. Med.* 275:878-885.

Aggett, P. J., and Harries, J. T., (1979). Current status of zinc in health and disease states, *Arch. Dis. Child.* 54:909-917.

Agha, F., Hasan, T. J., Khan, R. A., and Jafarey, S. (1988). Iron stores in maternal and cord blood. *Asia-Oceania J. Obstet. Gynaecol.* 14:405-409.

Ajayi, O. A. (1988). Iron stores in pregnant Nigerians and their infants at term. *Eur. J. Clin. Nutr.* 42:23-28.

Apte, S. V., and Iyengar, L. (1970). Absorption of dietary iron in pregnancy. *Amer. J. Clin. Nutr.* 23:73-77.

Barker, D. J., Bull, A. R., Osmond, C., and Simmonds, S. J. (1990). Fetal and placental size and risk of hypertension in adult life. *Brit. Med. J.* 301:259-262.

Batten, S., Hirschman, J., and Thomas, D. (1990). Impact of the special supplemental food program on infants. *J. Pediatr.* 117:S101-109.

Beischer, N. A. (1971). The effects of maternal anemia upon the fetus. *J. Reprod. Med.* 6:262-265.

Benjamin, F., Bassen, F. A., and Meyer, L. M. (1966). Serum levels of folic acid, vitamin B12, and iron in anemia of pregnancy. *Amer. J. Obst. Gynecol.* 96:310-315.

Black, A. M., Mahoney, A. W., Hendricks, D. G., and Farley, M. A. (1986). Meal pattern of available iron; ascorbic acid; and meat, fish, poultry intakes by school children. *Nutr. Res.* 6:619-626.

Breskin, M. W., Worthington-Roberts, B. S., Knopp, R. H. Brown, Z., Plovie, B., Mottet, N. K., and Mills, J. L. (1983). First trimester serum zinc concentrations in human pregnancy. *Amer. J. Clin. Nutr.* 38:943-953.

Carpenter, C. E., and Mahoney, A. W. (1992). Contributions of heme and nonheme iron to human nutrition. *Critical Rev. Food Sci. Nutr.* 34:333-367.

Colomer, J., Colomer, C. Gutierrez, D., Jubert, A., Nolasco, A., Donat, J., Fernandez-Delgado, R., Donat, F., and Alvarez-Dardet, C. (1990). Anaemia during pregnancy as a risk factor for infant iron deficiency: Report from the valencia infant anaemia cohort (VIAC) study. *Paediat. Perinat. Epidem.* 4:196-204.

Cook, J. D., and Monsen, E. R. (1976). Food iron absorption in human subjects. III. Comparison of the effect of animal proteins on nonheme iron absorption. *Amer. J. Clin. Nutr.* 29:859-867.

Council on Foods and Nutrition, American Medical Association. (1968). Iron deficiency in the United States. Report of the committee on iron deficiency. *J. Amer. Med. Assoc.* 203:407-412.

Dallman, P. R., Yip, R., and Johnson, C. (1984). Prevalence and causes of anemia in the United States, 1976 to 1980. *Amer. J. Clin. Nutr.* 39:437-445.

Daouda, H., Galan, P., Prual, A., Sekou, H., and Hercberg, S.

(1991). Iron status in Nigerien mothers and their newborns. *Intern. J. Vit. Nutr. Res.* 61:46-50.

Dawson, E. B. Albers, J., and McGanity, W. J. (1989). Serum zinc changes due to iron supplementation in teen-age pregnancy. *Amer. J. Clin. Nutr.* 50:848-852.

Dunlop, W., Furness, C., and Hill, L. M. (1978). Maternal haemoglobin concentration, haematocrit and renal handling of urate in pregnancies ending in the births of small-for-dates infants. *Brit. J. Obstet. Gynaecol.* 85:938-940.

Expert Scientific Working Group. (1985). Summary of a report on assessment of the iron nutritional status of the United States population. *Amer. J. Clin. Nutr.* 42:1318-1330.

Fenton, V., Cavill, I., and Fisher, J. (1977). Iron stores in pregnancy. *Brit. J. Haematol.* 37:145-149.

Fletcher, J., and Suter, P. E. N. (1969). The transport of iron by the human placenta. *Clin Sci.* 36:209-220.

Friel, J. K., Andrews, W. L., Matthew, J. D., Long, D. R., Cornel, A. M., Cox, M., and Skinner, C. T. (1990). Iron status of very-low-birth-weight infants during the first 15 months of infancy. *Can. Med. Assoc. J.* 143:733-737.

Garn S. M., Ridella, S. A., Petzold, A. S., *et al.* (1981). Maternal hematologic levels and pregnancy outcomes. *Semin Perinatol.* 5:155-162.

Godfrey, K. M., Redman, C. W. G., Barker, D. J. P., and Osmond, C. (1991). The effect of maternal anaemia and iron deficiency on the ratio of fetal weight to placental weight. *Brit. J. Obstet. Gynaecol.* 94:886-891.

Goepel, E., Ulmer, H. U. and Neth, R. D. (1988). Premature labor contractions and the value of serum ferritin during pregnancy. *Gynecol. Obstet. Invest.* 26:265-273.

Gofin, R., Adler, B. and Palti, H. (1989). Effectiveness of iron supplementation compared to iron treatment during pregnancy. *Public Health* 103:139-145.

Guldhalt, I. S., Trolle, B. G., and Hvidman, L. E. (1991). Iron supplementation during pregnancy. *Acta Obstet. Gynecol. Scand.* 70:9-12.

Hallberg, L. (1988). Iron balance in pregnancy. Pages 115-

127 *in* H. Berger, ed. *Vitamins and Minerals in Pregnancy and Lactation.* Raven Press, New York.

Hambridge K. M., Krebs, N. F., Jacobs, M. A., *et al.* (1983). Zinc nutritional status during pregnancy: A longitudinal study. *Amer. J. Clin. Nutr.* 37:429-442.

Hambridge, K. M., Krebs, N. F., Sibley, L., and English, K. (1987). Acute effects of iron therapy on zinc status during pregnancy. *Obstet. Gynecol.* 70:593-596.

Hemminki, E., and Rimpela, U. (1991). Iron supplementation, maternal packed cell volume, and fetal growth. *Arch. Dis. Child.* 66:422-425.

Hercberg, S., Galan, P., Chauliac, M., Masse-Raimbault, A., Devanlay, M., Bileoma, S., Alihonou, E., Zohoun, I., Christides, J., and De Courcy, G. P. (1987). Nutritional anaemia in pregnant Beninese women: Consequences on the haematological profile of the newborn. *Brit. J. Nutr.* 57:185-193.

Ho, C. H., Yuan, C. C., and Yeh, S. H. (1987a). Serum ferritin levels and their significance in normal full-term pregnant women. *Intern. J. Gynecol. Obstet.* 25:291-295.

Ho, C. H., Yuan, C. C., and Yeh, S. H. (1987b). Serum ferritin, folate and cobalamin levels and their correlation with anemia in normal full-term pregnant women. *Eur. J. Obstet. Gynecol. Reprod. Biol.* 26:7-13.

Hussain, M. A. M., Gaafar, T. H. Laulight, M., and Hoffbrand, A. V. (1977). Relation of maternal and cord blood serum ferritin. *Arch. Dis. Child.* 52:782-784.

Ilyes, I, Jezerniczky, J., Lovacs, J., Dvoracsek, E., and Csorba, S. (1985). Relationship of maternal and newborn (cord) serum ferritin concentrations measured by immunoradiometry. *Acta Paediat. Hung.* 26:317-321.

Kelly, A. M., and McDougall, A. N. (1978). Observations on maternal and fetal ferritin concentrations at term. *Brit. J. Obstet. Gynaecol.* 85:338-343.

Klein, L. (1962). Premature birth and maternal prenatal anemia. *Amer. J. Obstet. Gynecol.* 83:588-590.

Knottnerus, J. A., Delgado, L. R., Knipschild, P. G., Essed,

G. G. M., and Smits, F. (1990). Haematologic parameters and pregnancy outcome. *J. Clin. Epidemiol.* 43:461-466.

Koller, O., Sagen, N., Ulstein, M., and Vaula, D. (1979). Fetal growth retardation associated with inadequate haemodilution in otherwise uncomplicated pregnancy. *Acta Obstet. Gynecol. Scand.* 58:9-13.

Koller, O., Sandvei, R., and Sagen, N. (1980). High hemoglobin levels during pregnancy and fetal risk. *Intern. J. Gynaecol. Obstet.* 18:53-56.

Lamparelli, R. D. V., Bothwell, T. H., Macphail, A. P., Van Der Westhuyzen, J., Baynes, R. D., and Macfarlane, B. J. (1988). Nutritional anaemia in pregnant coloured women in Johannesburg. *S. Afr. Med. J.* 73:477-481.

Lehti, K. K. (1989). Iron, folic acid and zinc intakes and status of low socio-economic pregnant and lactating Amazonian women. *Eur. J. Clin. Nutr.* 43:505-513.

Lund, C. J. (1951). Studies on the iron deficiency anemia of pregnancy. *Amer. J. Obstet. Gynecol.* 62:947-963..

MacGregor, M. W. (1963). Maternal anaemia as a factor in prematurity and perinatal mortality. *Scot. Med. J.* S:134-140.

Mau, G. (1977). Hemoglobin changes during pregnancy and growgh disturbances in the neonate. *J. Perinat. Med.* 5: 172-177.

McLean, F. W., Cotter, J. R., Blechner, J. N., and Noyes, W. D. (1970). Ferrokinetics in pregnancy. 1. Fetus and newborn. *Amer. J. Obstet. Gynecol.* 106:699-702.

Meadows, N. J., Grainger, S. L., Ruse, W., Keeling, P. W., and Thompson, R. P. (1983). Oral iron and the bioavailability of zinc. *Brit. Med. J.* 287: 1013-1014.

Milman, N., Lbsen, K. K., and Christensen, J. M. (1987). Serum ferritin and iron status in mothers and newborn infants. *Acta Obstet. Gynecol. Scand.* 66:205-211.

Murphy, S. P., and Calloway, D. H. (1986). Nutrients intakes of women in NHANES II, emphasizing trace minerals, fiber, and phytate. *J. Amer. Diet. Assoc.* 86:1366-1372.

National Research Council. 1989. *Recommended Dietary*

Allowances, 10th Edition. National Academy Press, Washington, D.C. 285 pp.

Okuyama, T., Tawada, T., Furuya, H., and Villee, C. A. (1985). The role of transferrin and ferritin in the fetal-maternal-placental unit. *Amer. J. Obstet. Gynecol.* 152:344-350.

Parks,Y. A., and Wharton, B. A. (1989). Iron deficiency and the brain. *Acta Pediatr. Scand., Suppl.* 361:71-77.

Prual, A., Galan, P., De Bernis, L., and Hercberg, S. (1988). Evaluation of iron status in Chadian pregnant women: Consequences of maternal iron deficiency on the haematopoietic status of newborns. *Trop. Geogr. Med.* 40:1-6.

Puolakka, J. Janne, O., Pakarinen, A., Jarvinen, P. A., and Vihko, R. (1980). Serum ferritin as a measure of iron stores during and after normal pregnancy with and without iron supplements. *Acta Obstet. Gynecol. Scand.*, Suppl. 95:43-51.

Rios, E., Lipschtz, D. A., Cook, J. D., and Smith, N. J. (1975). Relationship of meternal and infant iron stores as assessed by determination of plasma ferritin. *Pediatrics* 55:694-699.

Roszkowski, K., Wojcicka, J., and Zaleska, K. (1966). Serum iron deficiency during the third trimester of pregnancy; maternal complications and fate of the neonate. *Obster. Gynecol.* 28:820-825.

Rusia, U., Bhatia, A., Kapoor, S., Madan, N., Nair, V., and Sood, S. K. (1988). Placental morphology and histochemistry in iron deficiency anaemia. *Indian J. Med. Res.* 87:468-474.

Sagen, N., Nilsen, S. T., Kim, H. C., Bergsjo, P., and Koller, O. (1984). Maternal hemoglobin concentration is closely related to birth weight in normal pregnancies. *Acta Obstet. Gynecol. Scand.* 63:245-248.

Sauberlich, H. E. (1983). Current laboratory tests for assessing nutritional status. *Surv. Synth. Path. Res.* 2:120-133.

Schofield, C., Stewart, J., and Wheeler, E. (1989). The diets of pregnant and post-pregnant women in different social groups in London and Edinburgh: calcium, iron, retinol, ascorbic acid and folic acid. *Brit. J. Nutr.* 62:363-377.

Sheldon, W. L., Aspillaga, M. O. Smith, P. A., and Lind, T. (1985). The effects of oral iron supplementation on zinc and magnesium levels during pregnancy. *Brit. J. Obstet. Gynaecol.* 92:892-898.

Siimes, A. S. I., and Siimes, M. A. (1986). Changes in the concentration of ferritin in the serum during fetal life in singletons and twins. *Early Human Develop.* 13:47-52.

Solomons, N. W., and Jacob, R. A. (1981). Studies on the bioavailability of zinc in humans: Effects of heme and nonheme iron on the absorption of zinc. *Amer. J. Clin. Nutr.* 34:475-482.

Taylor, D. J., and Lind, T. (1979). Red cell mass during and after normal pregnancy. *Brit. J. Obstet. Gynaecol.* 86:464-470.

Ulmer, H. U., and Goepel, E. (1988). Anemia, ferritin and preterm labor. *J. Perinat. Med.* 16:459-465.

VanNagell, J. Koepke, J., and Dilts. Jr., P. V. (1971). Preventable anemia and pregnancy. *Obstet. Gynecol. Sur.* 26:551-563.

Van Eijk, H. G., Kroos, M. J., Hoogendoorn, G. A., and Wallenburg, C. S. (1978). Serum ferritin and iron stores during pregnancy. *Clinca Chimica Acta* 83:81-91.

Wapnir, R. A. (1990). *Protein Nutrition and Mineral Absorption.* CRC Press, Boca Raton, FL. (see pages 1-9, Mechanisms of Protein Absorption.)

White, H. S. (1970). Iron deficiency in young women. *Amer. J. Pub. Health* 60:659-665.

Whittaker P. G., Lind, T., and Williams, J. G. (1991). Iron absorption during normal human pregnancy: A study using stable isotopes. *Brit. J. Nutr.* 65:457-463.

Wong, C. T., and Saha, N. (1990). Inter-relationships of storage iron in the mother, the placenta and the newborn. *Acta Obstet. Gynecol. Scand.* 69:613-616.

World Health Organization. (1970). *Requirements of Ascorbic Acid, Vitamin D, Vitamin B12, Folate and Iron.* WHO Tech. Rep. Ser., Rep. No. 452. Geneva, Switzerland.

Yepez, R., Calle, A., Galan, P., Estevez, E., Davila, M., Estrella, R., Masse-Raimbault, A. M., and Hercberg, S. (1987). Iron status in Ecuadorian pregnant women living at 2800 m altitude: Relationahip with infant iron status. *Intern. J. Vit. Nutr. Res.* 57:327-332.

Zhang, D., Hendricks, D. G., and Mahoney, A. W. (1989). Bioavailability of total iron from meat, spinace (*Spinacea oleracea L.*) and meat-spinach mixtures by anaemic and nonanaemic rats. *Brit. J. Nutr.* 61:331-343.

Zhang, D., Hendricks, D. G., Mahoney, A. W., and Cornforth, D. P. (1985). Bioavailability of iron in green peas, spinach, bran cereal and cornmean fed to anemic rats. *J. Food Sci.* 50:426-428.

Zhang, D., Hendricks, D. G., Mahoney, A. W., Yu, Y., Thannoun, A. M., and Sisson, D. V. (1991). Bioavailability of total iron from beef and soy protein isolate, alone or combined, in anemic and healthy rats. *Cereal Chem.* 68: 194-200.

Zhang, D., and Mahoney, A. W. (1989). Bioavailability of iron-milk-protein complexes and fortified Cheddar cheese. *J. Dairy Sci.* 72:2845-2855.

Zhang, D., and Mahoney, A. W. (1990). Effect of iron fortification on quality of Chedder cheese. 2. Effects of aging and fluorescent light on pilot scale cheeses. *J. Dairy Sci.* 73:2252-2258.

Chapter 5

Embryonic Nutrition and Yolk Sac Function

**M. R. Juchau, J.Creech-Kraft, Q. P. Lee
H. L. Yang, M. J. Namkung**

From the results of experimental teratology as well as from clinical observations, it is widely accepted that the mammalian embryo is maximally susceptible to the induction of congenital malformations in the period immediately after the onset of organogenesis. Prior to this point, it is believed that teratogenic agents would kill the embryo but, ordinarily, not leave it permanently malformed, presumably because the conceptal cells have not yet lost their developmental plasticity. Susceptibility to chemical insults that produce permanent or semi-permanent malformational changes is rapid in onset and then declines slowly over the remainder of the period of gestation. For most mammals, the period of early organogenesis follows shortly after implantation of the blastocyst. There is no true allantoic placenta at this time, as might be expected, since a considerable degree of organ differentiation is required for development of a functioning circulatory system in the embryo. During the early postimplantation period, the yolk sac serves as the principal membrane for placental exchange and, in rats, the embryo is wholly dependent on the visceral yolk sac for nutrition and oxygen before gestational day 12 (Freeman & Brown, 1986; Jollie, 1986; Eto & Takakubo, 1985; Beckman, *et al.*, 1991b; Thomas, *et al.*, 1990).

In terms of its function in the histiotrophic nutrition of the embryo prior to development of the transfer functions of the chorioallantoic placenta, the critical importance of the visceral yolk sac to the development of the organogenesis-stage embryo is well recognized and appreciated (Jollie, 1986; Mossman, 1986; Sobis, *et al.*, 1986; Thiriot-Hebert, 1987;

Freeman & Lloyd, 1983a). In addition, a large number of past and ongoing studies have documented the hematopoietic functions of the visceral yolk sac (Sasaki & Kendall, 1985; Migliaccio, *et al.*, 1986; Sasaki & Matsumara, 1986; Ohsaki, *et al.*, 1987). A recent update of these and other important functions of the mammalian yolk sac was presented at a symposium sponsored by the Teratology Society and published in *Teratology* (Brent, 1990; Jollie, 1990; Lloyd, 1990; Beckman, *et al.*, 1990; Brent, *et al.*, 1990). Other recognized functions of mammalian yolk sacs include, (a) production of primordial germ cells, (b) exchange/elimination of a large number of endogenous substances via active transport, (c) facillitated diffusion and cytosis, (d) protein digestion via lysosomal proteases, and (e) protein synthesis. The function of the yolk sac in the nutrition of the embryo during early organogenesis is one of the best recognized and most important. Investigators who experiment with whole embryo culture systems are acutely aware of the importance of an intact and functioning visceral yolk sac to the development of the cultured embryo.

The capacity of drugs and other foreign chemicals to disrupt the nutritive functions of the mammalian yolk sac has been studied but not extensively. It is known that damage to the visceral yolk sac can result in embryonic dysmorphogenesis, growth retardation and, if severe, loss of viability. This has been demonstrated with the use of antibodies directed against yolk sac proteins (Freeman, *et al.*, 1982; Freeman & Brown, 1986; Sahali, *et al.*, 1988, Brent, *et al.*, 1990; Beckman, *et al.*, 1991a), with inhibition of yolk sac proteolysis (Freeman & Lloyd, 1983b), and at least one chemical (trypan blue) is believed to produce secondary embryotoxicity via primary damage to the yolk sac (Beck, *et al.*, 1967; Davis & Gunberg, 1968). Examples of other implicated chemicals (including ethanol) can also be cited (Schmid, *et al.*, 1985; Steventon & Williams, 1987; Hunter, *et al.*, 1991).

The purpose of this short treatise is to examine the available information concerning the expression of functional xenobiotic-biotransforming/bioactivating enzymes in tissues of the mammalian yolk sac placenta. Focus is on P450 cytochromes of the visceral yolk sac and their capacity to catalyze bioactivation reactions resulting in the generation of reactive intermediates having the potential to damage the yolk sac and thereby compromise its nutritive functions.

Historical Perspectives

In the late 1950s, publications appeared in the literature indicating that prenantal organisms were deficient in their capacity to biotransform certain drug biotransformation reactions (Jondorf, et al., 1958; Fouts & Adamson, 1959). Since that time, it has been virtually dogmatic in the textbook literature that prenatal biotransformation of xenobiotic chemicals is negligible to non-existent and very unlikely to play a role as a determinant of either beneficial or toxic effects of chemicals to which the conceptus might be exposed. In terms of the fetal period in humans (from approximately day 60 of gestation until term), it is now recognized that this generalization does not fully apply (Juchau, et al., 1980; Pelkonen, et al., 1987; Juchau & Harris, 1990; Krauer & Dayer, 1991), but very little work applicable to xenobiotic biotransformation/bioactivation during the period of human organogenesis (approximately day 18 until day 60 of gestation) has appeared in the open literature as of this writing. However, beginnings have been made (Lee, et al., 1991a). For rodents, lagomorphs (rabbits) and other common experimental animals, the view is still widely held that conceptal biotransformation/ bioactivation of xenobiotics is extremely low to negligible during all except the very latest stages of prenatal existence. Recent results strongly indicate that even this view is outmoded (Juchau & Stark, 1988; Juchau, 1989; Juchau, et al., 1992).

Nevertheless, the possibility that metabolic conversions of foreign organic chemicals of low molecular weight (xenobiotics) might be responsible for the embryotoxic/dysmorphogenic effects producible by certain of such chemicals has been under consideration for some time. For example,

Keberle, *et al.* (1965) felt that it was possible that thalidomide might owe its teratogenic effects to metabolic conversion of the parent thalidomide to monocarboxylic metabolites after passage of the drug into conceptal tissues. King, *et al.* (1965) and Posner, *et al.* (1967) reported evidence indicating that the teratogenic effects of chlorcyclizine and meclizine administered in large doses to pregnant rats were due to metabolic conversion of these antihistaminic agents to norchlorcyclizine, a metabolite lacking antihistaminic properties. For these latter chemicals, the maternal organism was presumed to be responsible for the biotransformation reactions. Several studies have also indicated that maternal biotransformation of cyclophosphamide is requisite for the embryotoxic/dysmorphogenic effects of this widely used cancer chemotherapeutic agent (see Juchau, 1989 and references therein for reviews).

Because of the extremely short half-lives of the majority of reactive intermediates, investigators logically have become more interested in the generation of such intermediates within the target cells themselves — in this case in the cells of the developing conceptus during organogenesis. Studies by Nebert, *et al.* (Shum, *et al.*, 1979; Legraverend, *et al.*, 1984) and by Manson, *et al.* (York & Manson, 1984; York, *et al.*, 1984) suggested that genetic variability in the capacity of murine embryos to respond to inducers of cytochromes P4501a1 and P4501a2, monooxygenases, for which benzo(a)pyrene is a good substrate, was a determinant of the susceptibility of the embryos to benzo(a)pyrene-elicited embryotoxicity. These investigations pointed to the possibility that P450-dependent embryonic bioactivation could play a significant role in chemical teratogenesis. A series of more recent investigations with 2-acetylaminofluorene and cultured whole embryos has greatly reinforced this concept (Faustman-Watts, *et al.*, 1983, 1985, 1986; Juchau, *et al.*, 1985a,b). We discovered that day-10 rat embryos contained enzymes that would catalyze the N- and ring-hydroxylation of 2-acetylaminoflorene, a compound previously demonstrated to act as a proembryotoxin in culture in the presence of an added, exogenous P450-dependent bioactivating system prepared from the livers of adult male rats induced with polychlorinated biphenyls. The latter investigations showed definitively that embryos preinduced in utero and subsequently explanted in the whole embryo culture system contained more than adequate cytochrome P450 to catalyze the bioconversion of 2-acetylaminofluorene to reactive intermediates in quantities amply sufficient to produce profound, grossly observable abnormalities in the selfsame embryos. The implications of these results are enormous because they demonstrate that extremely low levels of monooxygenase activity in the target cells of the conceptus are sufficient to elicit major malformations. The entire subject of embryonic bioactivation of xenobiotic chemicals has been reviewed recently (Juchau, *et al.*, 1992), and the implications for chemical dysmorphogenesis and embryotoxicity are discussed extensively. In nearly all of the studies reported to date, it is impressive that the visceral yolk sac has exhibited higher levels of xenobiotic biotransforming enzymes and their corresponding activities than any of the other conceptal tissues examined. The implications of these observations for the nutritional functions of the visceral yolk sac and for the nutrition of the developing embryo are discussed below.

Current State of Knowledge

Initial investigations of conceptal biotransformation during the period of organogenesis did not distinguish among the relative capacities of the various conceptal tissues and organs to express the pertinent enzymes or to catalyze the corresponding reactions associated with such enzymes. As judged from published material, specific interest in the yolk sac *per se* as a xenobiotic biotransforming/bioactivating organ appears to have developed only in very recent years and the current data base is very limited. As of this writing, no published information directly pertaining to the capacity of human yolk sac tissues to effect xenobiotic biotransformations has appeared in the open literature, insofar as we are able to ascertain. To date, it appears that data pertinent to this topic are available only for rats, mice and chicks. Approximate periods of organogenesis for these three species respectively are days 9.5-16.5, 8-15 and (post egg-laying for chicks) 1-8 (Juchau, *et al.*, 1992). The rat has been studied by far the most intensively.

An early indication that tissues of the yolk sac *per se* contain a measurable complement of xenobiotic biotransforming enzymes was provided by Shiverick, *et al.* (1986). Using ethoxyresorufin as substrate, these investigators showed that fetal membranes (consisting of the unseparated visceral yolk sac and amniotic membranes) of noncultured rat conceptuses contained enzymes capable of catalyzing O-deethylation of the substrate at day 15 of gestation. The activity was barely detectable in the membranes of untreated rats but was markedly increased (8- to 20-fold) after pretreatment *in utero* with β-naphthoflavone or 3-methylcholanthrene, inducers of cytochrome P450 isoforms of the 1A subfamily. Marked inhibition of the activity by α-naphthoflavone also indicated participation of P450 isoforms of the 1A subfamily. It is noteworthy that, at this stage of gestation and after induction with 3-methylcholanthrene, enzymic activities were greatest in homogenates of placental labyrinth tissues followed by fetal membranes (visceral yolk sac plus amnion), fetus *per se*, decidual tissues and basal zone tissues in that order.

With a series of phenoxazone ethers (also commonly referred to as resorufin ethers) as substrate probes, Yang, *et al.* (1988) showed that several rat conceptal tissues, including the isolated visceral yolk sac, contain enzymes capable of catalyzing the O-debenzylation of benzyloxyphenoxazone, the O-depentylation of pentoxyphenoxazone and the O-deethylation of ethoxyphenoxazone at day 11 of gestation. Interestingly, the O-demethylation of methoxyphenoxazone, a preferential substrate for P4501A2 (Namkung, *et al.*, 1988), could not be detected, even after induction with 3-methylcholanthrene. The O-deethylation of ethoxyphenoxazone was only marginally detectable in conceptal tissue homogenates of noninduced conceptuses but, similar to the observations of Shiverick, *et al.* (1986), was markedly increased after treatment of conceptuses in utero with 3-methylcholanthrene. Again, the O-deethylation reaction appeared to be catalyzed by a conceptal cytochrome P450 isoform(s) of the 1A subfamily. Absence of detectability of methoxyphenoxazone O-demethylation suggsted that P4501A2 was not a significant participant in the reaction and also that it is probably not expressed significantly in the studied tissues. For each of the three detected reactions, activities were much higher in preparations of visceral yolk sac tissues than in analogous preparations of tissues of the embryo *per se* or of the ectoplacental cone. With tissue preparations of isolated yolk sacs, O-deethylation of ethoxyphenoxazone was readily measurable without induction by 3-methylcholanthrene. An analysis of the data obtained with the four probe substrates strongly suggested the presence of at least four separate, functional P450 isoforms in the visceral yolk sac at this comparatively early stage of gestation: a 3-methylcholanthrene-inducible isoform and three separate constitutive isoforms.

In later investigations along these lines (Yang, *et al.*, 1989), it was shown that the visceral yolk sac contained higher constitutive levels of P450 isoforms for catalysis of O-deethylation of ethoxyphenoxazone, O-depentylation of pentoxyphenoxazone and O-debenzylation of benzyloxyphenoxazone than the embryo proper or ectoplacental cone at days 10-14 of gestation. Response of the deethylation reaction to the inducing activity of 3-methylcholanthrene was also highest in the visceral yolk sac. Importantly, it was shown that a 3-methylcholanthrene-induced isoform(s) (presumably the same isoform) was capable of catalyzing the oxidative biotransformation of two promutagen/procarcinogens, *i.e.*, benzo(a)pyrene and 2-acetylaminofluorene. The experiments performed thus documented the capacity of the visceral yolk sac to convert bioactivatable substrates to their respective metabolic products. Expression of P4501A1 in yolk sac tissues may therefore be an important determinant of the capacity of certain chemicals (those that are substrates for

P4501A1) to disrupt the nutritive functions of the visceral yolk sac.

Subsequent studies have provided still further evidence for the identity of the isoform inducible by 3-methylcholanthrene and responsible for the catalysis of the monooxygenation of ethoxyphenoxazone, benzo(a)pyrene and 2-acetylaminofluorene (Yang, *et al.*, 1991). The visceral yolk sac, ectoplacental cone and embryo proper each were investigated on day 12 of gestation with and without prior exposure *in utero* to 3-methylcholanthrene as inducing agent. With two sets of discriminating oligonucleotide primers, definitive, reproducible signals were detectable only in tissues from 3-methylcholanthrene-exposed conceptuses. Signals of highest intensity were observed with visceral yolk sac tissues and signals of lowest intensity were observed with tissues of the embryos *per se.* Specificities of the amplified cDNAs were verified using Southern blotting with hybridization to an internal oligonucleotide probe. The results corroborated previous suggestions that the isoform in question is either P4501A1 or a very closely related isoform(s).

Evidence that the above-described observations pertaining to yolk sac P4501A1 need not be restricted to rats has been provided by Dey, *et al.* (1989) who showed with *in situ* hybridization studies that the murine visceral yolk sac likewise responds well to methylcholanthrene-type inducing agents and expresses higher levels of CYP1A1 mRNA than other conceptal tissues in the species of mouse investigated. These investigators detected a hybridization signal for P450 1A1 mRNA in the murine visceral yolk sac at day 8.5 of gestation and in liver and lung (but not other embryonic mouse tissues) at days 12.5 and 14.5 of gestation. The question as to whether or not functional P4501A1 was translated from the mRNA responsible for the detected signals, however, appears not to have been answered. In harmony with our own observations on rat conceptuses at days 10-14 of gestation with the P4501A2-selective substrate, methoxyphenoxazone, Dey, *et al.* (1989) were unable to detect a hybridization signal for P4501A2 mRNA in murine conceptal tissues between days 5.3 and 14.5 of gestation. Thus, currently available data permit the following tentative conclusions with respect to the presence in visceral yolk sacs of the two known members (1A1 and 1A2) of the P4501A subfamily: (1) Neither isoform appears to be expressed constitutively in the visceral yolk sacs of rats or mice during the period of organogenesis (for rats and mice, the period of organogenesis extends approximately from day 9 to 16 and from day 8 to 15 of gestation respectively); and (2) The 1A1, but not the 1A2 isoform, appears to be strongly inducible in rodent visceral yolk sacs following exposure to chemicals with inducing properties similar to those of 3-methylcholanthrene (these include the planar polyhalogenated biphenyls, dioxins, naphthoflavones, methylxanthines and polynuclear aromatic hydrocarbons and are commonly referred to as "MC-type" inducing agents). This is of importance because of the very large number of toxic organic chemicals known to undergo bioactivation catalyzed by P4501A1. The extent to which bioactivatable P4501A1 substrates are capable of disrupting the nutritional (or other) functions of rodent visceral yolk sacs, however, has not yet been investigated.

A number of investigations have also suggested, but not definitively shown, that P4501A1 may be present and functional in organogenesis-stage conceptal tissues (including the yolk sac) of the chick (Hamilton, et al., 1983; Heinrich-Hirsch, et al., 1990; Denison, et al., 1986; Brunstroem & Lund, 1988). In view of the known species and tissue distribution of P4501A1, it would, in fact, be surprising if this were not the case.

In addition to P450s 1A1 and 1A2, only one other rat isoform is currently known to be inducible by "MC-type" inducing agents. This isoform is P4502A1, but the likelihood that 2A1 represents the catalyst for the above described reactions seems very low because of considerations of substrate/inhibitor specificity, immunologic cross-reactivity and nucleic acid hybridization (Yang, et al., 1988, 1989, 1991). Nevertheless, final confirmation of the expression of functional P4501A1 in rodent yolk sac tissues remains to be achieved with the necessary sequence information.

It has been of considerable interest to us that the rat visceral yolk sac contains an enzyme(s) that will catalyze an easily measurable conversion of pentoxyphenoxazone to resorufin via P450-dependent O-depentylation (Yang, *et al.*, 1988, 1989). Pentoxyphenoxazone is a widely utilized probe substrate and its O-depentylation in tissue preparations is frequently regarded as indicative of the presence of functional P450s of the 2B subfamily (Burke et al., 1985; Lubet, *et al.*, 1985, 1990). For adult rat hepatic preparations, rates of pentoxyphenoxazone O-depentylation are proportional to quantities of P450s 2B1 and 2B2 and the reaction is regarded as a marker for these particular isoforms. We have observed that the rat visceral yolk sac, parietal yolk sac, ectoplacental cone, decidua and embryo proper each contain a P450 isoform(s) that catalyzes easily measurable depentylation and debenzylation reactions at days 10-14 of gestation. Of these tissues, the visceral yolk sac exhibited the highest activities for both reactions and initially suggested to us that functional P450s 2B1 and/or 2B2 might be expressed in cells of the rat visceral yolk sac. However, even though carbon monoxide was a very effective inhibitor of these reactions, no or minimal inhibition of the reactions was achieved with inhibitory 2B1/2B2 antibodies or with metyrapone or orphenadrine, all selective inhibitors of the monooxygenase activities of cytochromes P4502B1 and 2B2 (Lee, *et al.*, 1991b; Lee & Juchau, 1990, 1992). Failure of treatment of embryos *in utero* with phenobarbital to increase conceptal O-depentylase activities was also regarded as evidence that these two P4502B isoforms were not acting as catalysts for the reaction since, in adult rat livers, both isoforms are phenobarbital-inducible.

In addition, exposure of cultured rat conceptuses to dibutyryl cAMP or various nonselective phosphodiesterase inhibitors resulted in significant increases in conceptal O-depentylase activities (Lee, *et al.*, 1991b; Lee & Juchau, 1990, 1992). These results were somewhat surprising because it is well known that exposure of adult hepatic tissues/cells to increased levels of cAMP results in marked decreases in hepatic O-depentylase activity (Oesch-Bartlomowicz & Oesch, 1990; Eliasson, et al., 1990; Jansson, et al., 1990). The decreases represent a "short-term" regulatory mechanism and appear to be due primarily to a direct phosphorylation of P4502B cytochromes, resulting in the labilization and subsequent degradation of these as well as other xenobiotic-biotransforming P450 hemoproteins. The conceptal O-depentylase appeared to behave more analogously to certain extrahepatic (adrenal gland, ovary, testis, placenta) P450 isoforms that are known to catalyze the biosynthesis of several steroid hormones. These steroid-synthesizing P450s are upregulated following increases in cellular cAMP levels via a "long-term" regulatory mechanism(s) not involving direct P450 phosphorylation. From the perspective of this review, it is of importance to note that the visceral yolk sac not only exhibited higher O-depentylase activities than any of the other conceptal tissues studied, but also appeared to be the only tissue to respond to the increases in activities elicited by cAMP.

In summary, studies of the O-depentylation of pentoxyphenoxazone as a probe substrate are indicative of the expression of yet another (in this case, constitutive) P450 isoform in tisssues of the visceral yolk sac. However, the identity of the conceptal isoform(s) that catalyzes the O-depentylation reaction remains a mystery and a formidable challenge for future research. It does appear to be distinct from at least two other constitutive P450 isoforms present in yolk sac tissues. However, the importance of this unidentified isoform to the nutritive functions of the visceral yolk sac (or disruption thereof) is solely the subject of speculation at present.

Aside from the phenoxazone ethers discussed above, several additional substrates have been reported to undergo monooxygenation (presumably P450-catalyzed) in yolk sac tissues. Included is the ring hydroxylation of 2-acetylaminofluorene for which 5- and 7-hydroxy-2-acetylaminofluorene are the major metabolites (Juchau, et al., 1985a,b, 1991; Faustman-Watts, et al., 1986; Harris et al., 1989; Stark, et al.,

1989). Presumably, the ring hydroxylation is catalyzed by conceptal P4501A1. Importantly, the studies showed that 7-hydroxy-2-acetylaminofluorene acts as a proximate dysmorphogen. In this series of investigations it was shown that 7-hydroxy-2-acetylaminofluorene was itself a substrate for conceptal enzymes and can be further converted to the corresponding catechol that is (based on the acetaminophen model discussed below) a more proximate dysmorphogen. The identity of the conceptal enzyme(s) that catalyzes the conversion of 7-hydroxy-2-acetylaminofluorene to the catechol remains to be elucidated.

Acetaminophen, an hepatotoxic/nephrotoxic chemical that also elicits neural tube abnormalities similar to those produced by 7-hydroxy-2-acetylaminofluorene (in cultured rat embryos) is likewise a substrate for conceptal P450s. These two structurally-similar chemicals both undergo conversion to the corresponding catechol metabolites — 3-hydroxyacetaminophen in the case of the former. It was shown that 3-hydroxyacetaminophen was approximately 5 times more active than acetaminophen when added to the culture medium and approximately 100 times more active after microinjection into the amniotic cavity in direct contact with the embryo proper (Stark, et al., 1990). The studies demonstrated that the visceral yolk sac was the most active tissue in converting not only 7-hydroxy-2-acetylaminofluo-rene to its corresponding catechol (discussed above) but also in converting acetaminophen to 3-hydroxyacetaminophen as well as to N-acetyl-p-quinoneimine. The latter metabolite is commonly regarded as a proximate hepatotoxin and was also shown to exhibit embryotoxic effects in the above-cited studies. Interestingly, 7-hydroxy-2-acetylaminofluorene and acetaminophen were both virtually inactive as dysmorphogens when microinjected into the amniotic cavity but were both very active when placed in the culture medium or micro- injected into the exocoelomic fluid. These observations suggested that visceral yolk sac bioactivation was requisite for elicitation of the xenobiotic-produced neural tube abnormalities. As of yet, none of the enzymes responsible for catalyzing these reactions have been identified. It seems probable that they would be P450 isoforms.

Other chemicals shown to be converted to oxidized metabolites in yolk sac tissues include benzo(a)pyrene (discussed above), aldrin and 7-ethoxycoumarin in chick conceptuses (Heinrich-Hirsch, et al., 1990) and QA-208-199, an experimental lipoxygenase inhibitor (Bechter & Terlouw, 1990; Bechter, et al., 1992, Terlouw & Bechter, 1992). For benzo(a)pyrene, catalysis of the reaction is currently presumed to be by P4501A1, although it is now known that several other P450 isoforms will catalyze benzo(a)pyrene oxidation. For the other three substrates, the identities of the catalyzing enzymes are currently unknown. A number of other xenobiotic chemicals have been reported to undergo oxidative biotransformation in organogenesis-stage conceptal tissues (see review by Juchau, et al., 1992), but the extent to which these reactions may be localized in the visceral yolk sac remains to be determined. The chemicals include a number of synthetic steroidal and nonsteroidal estrogens, propranolol, valproic acid and diphenylhydantoin. For estrogens, propranolol and valproic acid, the oxidations are presumably P450-dependent; for diphenylhydantoin, a peroxidase-catalyzed reaction appeared to be involved (Wells, et al., 1989a,b).

Several P450-independent reactions also have been reported to be catalyzed in organogenesis-stage conceptal tissues (Juchau, et al., 1992). Again, it is presently unknown if any of these reactions occur principally in yolk sac tissues. Some studies have suggested that glutathione conjugation in the visceral yolk sac may be a significant determinant of embryotoxicity (Harris, et al., 1986, 1987). In a series of recent investigations involving the microinjections of retinoic acids and their metabolites into the amniotic and exocoelomic fluids of cultured whole rat conceptuses, the results provided evidence for a significant participation of the visceral yolk sac in determining the extent to which all-trans-retinoic acid elicited dysmorphogenic effects (Lee, et al., 1991; Creech-Kraft, et al., 1992a,b,c). Of particular interest to us in these investigations was the apparent capacity of the visceral yolk sac to effect glucuronidation of retinoids. It must be emphasized, however, that direct, systematic investigations of the visceral yolk sac in terms of its capacity to catalyze retinoid biotransformation or glutathione conjugation have not yet been undertaken. In view of the above discussion, it seems likely that significant biotransformation of retinoids would occur in yolk sac tissues. This appears to be an interesting and important area for future research.

Research Needs

It is now very well established that the visceral yolk sac subserves a highly critical function in the nutrition of the developing conceptus during organogenesis. Likewise, it is also established that the stage of organogenesis is the most sensitive stage of gestation in terms of the capacity of foreign organic chemicals of low molecular weight (xenobiotics) to elicit dysmorphogenesis/teratogenesis. This report reviews the data that indicate that the visceral yolk sacs of rodents and chicks also exhibit the capacity to express functional xenobiotic biotransforming/bioactivating enzymes throughout organogenesis, including during the earlier, highly sensitive phases. This newly-discovered yolk sac function clearly has implications for the capacity of drugs and other environmental xenobiotics to interfere with the established nutritional functions of the visceral yolk sac and thereby elicit dysmorphogenic and/or other embryotoxic effects. Bioactivation of xenobiotic chemicals in yolk sac cells results in the generation of cytotoxic reactive intermediates capable of disrupting the nutritive functions of the bioactivating cells. Thus, future research should be directed toward the following major goals:

(1) Systematic investigations of the expression and regulation of xenobiotic bioactivating enzymes in tissues of the visceral yolk sac *per se*, and of the substrate specificities of such enzymes.

(2) Ascertainment of the extent to which the nutritive functions of the visceral yolk sac are compromised in

situations for which such bioactivation reactions are occurring or have occurred.

(3) Evaluation of the qualitative and quantitative relationships between bioactivatable xenobiotic-compromised nutritive functions of the visceral yolk sac and embryonic abnormalities.

(4) Ascertainment of information pertaining both to the nutritive functions as well as the bioactivation capacity of the human yolk sac placenta during the critical stage of organogenesis.

Conclusions

From the foregoing, it can be concluded that cellular elements of the visceral yolk sacs of rodents and chicks will express significant quantities of several (at least four) catalytically functional P450 isoforms capable of catalyzing the bioactivation of xenobiotic chemicals. One of these isoforms has been identified tentatively as P4501A1, a 3-methylcholanthrene-inducible P450. Other enzymes have not yet been identified. Because these isoforms can control the rates of generation of detrimental reactive intermediates via bioactivating reactions, they have the potential to act as critical determinants of the capacity of xenobiotics to interfere with the highly important nutritive functions of the yolk sac placenta. At present, no published data pertaining to the capacity of bioactivation reactions or reactive intermediates to interfere with yolk sac nutritive functions are available. This represents an area of research that should receive immediate attention.

Summary

Recent research in our own as well as other laboratories has demonstrated that the visceral yolk sac of rat conceptuses possesses a complement of functional xenobiotic biotransforming enzymes. Focus has been largely on the highly important and interesting superfamily of cytochrome P450s. As a general rule, levels and activities of such enzymes in the visceral yolk sac appear to exceed those measured in tissues of the embryo *per se*, ectoplacental cone, parietal yolk sac or decidual elements. Reactions catalyzed include P450-dependent bioactivations of promutagens, procarcinogens, procytotoxins and prodysmorphogens. Although levels appear to be very low relative to those known to exist in adult hepatic tissues, they are adequately high to effect generation of quantites of reactive intermediates sufficient to elicit easily detectable, gross anatomic malformations in embryos cultured in vitro. This raises the distinct possibility that such bioactivation reactions could also effect significant damage to the visceral yolk sac to the extent that the highly crucial nutritional functions of this important organ could be seriously compromised. In turn, secondary maldevelopment of the growing embryo would be a logical, expected consequence. This area of research has received only very limited attention to date and now seems ripe for a major investigative effort.

Acknowledgments

Original research reported herein was supported by NIEHS grants ES-04041 and ES-07032.

References

Bechter R., and Terlouw, G. D. C. (1990). Xenobiotic metabolism in the isolated conceptus. *Toxicol. in vitro* 4/5: 480-492.

Bechter, R., Terlouw, G. D. C., Lee, Q. P., and Juchau, M. R. (1991). Effects of QA 208-199 and its metabolite 209-668 on embryonic development *in vitro* after microinjection into the exocoelomic space or into the amniotic cavity of cultured rat embryos. *Teratog. Mutag. Carcinog.* 11:185-194.

Beck, F., Lloyd, J. B., and Griffiths, A. (1967). Lysosomal enzyme inhibition by trypan blue: A theory of teratogenesis. *Science* 157:1180-1182.

Beckman, D. A., Koszalka, T. R., Jensen, M., and Brent, R.

L. (1990). Experimental manipulation of the rodent visceral yolk sac. *Teratology* 41:395-404.

Beckman, D. A., Ornoy, A., Jensen, M. Arnon, J., and Brent, R. L. (1991a). Ultrastructure and function of the rat yolk sac: Damage caused by teratogenic anti-VYS serum and recovery. *Teratology* 44:181-192.

Beckman, D. A., Pugarelli, J. E., Koszalka, T. R., Brent, R. L., and Lloyd, J. B. (1991b). Sources of amino acids for protein synthesis during early organogenesis in the rat. 2. Exchange with amino acid and protein pools in embryo and yolk sac. *Placenta* 12:37-46.

Brent, R. L. (1990). Introduction to the yolk sac symposium. *Teratology* 41:359.

Brent, R. L., Beckman, D. A., Jensen, M., and Koszalka, T.R. (1990). Experimental yolk sac dysfunction as a model for studying nutritional disturbances in the embryo during early organogenesis. *Teratology* 41:405-413.

Brunstroem, B. and Lund, J. (1988). Differences between chick and turkey embryos in sensitivity to 3,3',4,4'-tetrachlorobiphenyl and in concentration/affinity of the hepatic receptor for 2,3,7,8-tetrachlorodibenzo-p-dioxin. *Comp. Biochem. Physiol.* 91C:507-512.

Burke, M. D., Thompson, S., Elcombe, S. R., Halpert, J., Haaparanta, T. and Mayer, R. T. (1985). Ethoxy, pentoxy and benzyloxyphenoxazones and homologues: A series of substrates to distinguish between different induced cytochromes P450. *Biochem. Pharmacol.* 34:3337-3345.

Creech-Kraft, J., and Juchau, M. R. (1992a). Correlations between conceptal concentrations of all-*trans*-retinoic acid and dysmorphogenesis after microinjections of all-*trans*-retinoic acid, 13-*cis*-retinoic acid, all-*trans*-retinoyl-o-glucuronide or retinol in cultured whole rat embryos. *Drug Metab. Dispos.* 20:218-226.

Creech-Kraft, J., Bui, T., and Juchau, M. R. (1992b). Elevated levels of all-*trans*-retinoic acid in cultured rat embryos 1-5 hours after intraamniotic microinjections with 13-*cis*-retinoic acid or retinol and correlations with dysmorphogenesis. *Biochem. Pharmacol.* 42:R21-R25.

Creech-Kraft, J., Lee, Q. P., Bechter, R., and Juchau, M. R. (1992c). Microinjections of cultured rat embryos: Studies with 4-oxo-all-*trans*-retinoic acid, 4-oxo-13-*cis*-retinoic acid and all-*trans*-retinoyl-o-glucuronide. *Teratology* 45:259-271.

Davis, H. W., and Gunberg, D. L. (1968). Trypan blue in the rat embryo. *Teratology* 1:125-134.

Denison, M. S., Okey, A. B., Hamilton, J. W., Bloom, S. E., and Wilkinson, C.F. (1986). Ah receptor for 2,3,7,8-tetrachlorodibenzo-*p*-dioxin: Ontogeny in chick embryo liver. *J. Biochem. Toxicol.* 1:39-49.

Dey, A., Westphal, H., and Nebert, D. W. (1989). Cell-specific induction of mouse Cyp1A1 during development. *Proc. Natl. Acad. Sci. U.S.A.* 86:7446-7450.

Eliasson, E., Johansson, I., and Ingelman-Sundberg, M. (1990). Substrate-, hormone-, and cAMP-regulated cytochrome P450 degradation. *Proc. Natl. Acad. Sci. USA* 87:3225-3229.

Eto, K., and Takakubo, F. (1985). Role of the yolk sac in craniofacial development of cultured rat embryos. *J. Craniofac. Genet. Dev. Biol.* 5:357-361.

Faustman-Watts, E. M., Giachelli, C. M., and Juchau, M. R. (1986). Carbon monoxide inhibits embryonic monooxygenation and embryotoxic effects of proteratogens in vitro. *Toxicol. Appl. Pharmacol.* 83:590-596.

Faustman-Watts, E. M., Greenaway, J. C., Namkung, M. J., Fantel, A. G., and Juchau, M. R. (1983). Teratogenicity in vitro of 2-acetylaminofluorene: Role of biotransformation. *Teratology* 27:19-29.

Faustman-Watts, E. M., Namkung, M. J., Greenaway, J. C., and Juchau, M. R. (1985). Analyses of metabolites of 2-acetylaminofluorene generated in an embryo culture system: Relationship of biotransformation to teratogenicity in vitro. *Biochem. Pharmacol.* 34:2953-2960.

Fouts, J. R., and Adamson, R. H. (1959). Drug metabolism in the newborn rabbit. *Science* 129:897-898.

Freeman, S. J., and Brown, N. A. (1986) An *in vitro* study of teratogenicity in the rat due to antibody-induced yolk sac dysfunction. *Roux's Arch. Dev. Biol.* 195:236-242.

Freeman, S. J., and Lloyd, J. B. (1983a). Evidence that protein ingested by the rat visceral yolk sac yields amino acids for the synthesis of embryonic protein. *J. Embryol. Exp. Morphol.* 73:307-315.

Freeman, S. J., and Lloyd, J. B. (1983b). Inhibition of proteolysis in rat yolk sac as a cause of teratogenesis. Effects of leupeptin *in vitro* and *in vivo*. *J. Embryol. Exp. Morphol.* 78:183-193.

Freeman, S. J., Brent, R. L., and Lloyd, J. B. (1982). The effect of teratogenic antiserum on yolk sac function in rat embryos cultured *in vitro*. *J. Embryol. Exp. Morphol.* 71:63-74.

Hamilton, J. W., Denison, M. S., and Bloom, S. E. (1983). Development of basal and induced aryl hydrocarbon (benzo(a)pyrene) hydroxylase activity in the chick embryo in ovo. *Proc. Natl. Acad. Sci. USA* 80:3372-3376.

Harris, C., Fantel, A. G., and Juchau, M. R. (1986). Differential glutathione depletion in rat embryo vs. visceral yolk sac *in vivo* and *in vitro* by L-buthionine-S,R-sulfoximine. *Biochem. Pharmacol.* 35:4437-4442.

Harris, C., Namkung, M. J., and Juchau, M. R. (1987). Regulation of intracellular glutathione in rat embryos and visceral yolk sacs and its effect on 2-nitrosofluorene-induced malformations in the whole embryo culture system. *Toxicol. Appl. Pharmacol.* 88:141-153.

Harris, C., Stark, K. L., Luchtel, D. L., and Juchau, M. R. (1989). Abnormal neurulation induced by 7-hydroxy-2-acetylaminofluorene and acetaminophen: Evidence for catechol metabolites as proximate dysmorphogens. *Toxicol. Appl. Pharmacol.* 101:432-447.

Heinrich-Hirsch, B., Hofmann, D. Webb, J., and Neubert, D. (1990). Activity of aldrinepoxidase, 7-ethoxycoumarin-O-deethylase and 7-ethoxyresorufin O-deethylase during the development of chick embryos in ovo. *Arch. Toxicol.* 64:128-134.

Hunter III, E. S., Phillips, L. S., Goldstein, S., and Sadler, T.

W. (1991). Altered visceral yolk sac function produced by a low-molecular-weight somatomedin inhibitor. *Teratology* 43:331-340.

Jansson, I., Curti, M., Epstein, P. M., Peterson, J. A., and Schenkman, J. B. (1990). Relationship between phosphorylation and cytochrome P450 destruction. *Arch. Biochem. Biophys.* 283:285-292.

Jollie, W. P. (1986). Review article: Ultrastructural studies of protein transfer across the rodent yolk sac. *Placenta* 7: 263-281.

Jollie, W. P. (1990). Development, morphology and function of the yolk sac placenta of laboratory rodents. *Teratology* 41:361-381.

Jondorf, W. R., Maickel, R. P. and Brodie, B. B. (1958). Inability of newborn mice and guinea pigs to metabolize drugs. *Biochem. Pharmacol.* 1:352-354.

Juchau, M. R. (1989). Bioactivation in chemical teratogenesis. *Ann. Rev. Pharmacol. Toxicol.* 29:165-187.

Juchau, M. R., and Harris, C. (1990). The developing organism as a toxicological target. Pages 91-111 *in* D. B. Clayson, I. C. Munro, P. Shubik, & J. A. Swenberg, eds., *Progress in Predictive Toxicology.* Elsevier Press, New York.

Juchau, M. R., and Stark, K. L. (1988). Mechanisms in chemical teratogenesis. *ISI Atlas of Science: Pharmacology* 2:283-287.

Juchau, M. R., Bark, D. H., Shewey, L. M., and Greenaway, J. C. (1985b). Generation of reactive dysmorphogenic intermediates by rat embryos in culture: Effects of cytochrome P450 inducers. *Toxicol. Appl. Pharmacol.* 81: 533-544.

Juchau, M. R., Chao, S. T., and Omiecinski, C. J. (1980). Drug metabolism by the human fetus. *Clin. Pharmacokinet.* 5:320-339.

Juchau, M. R., Giachelli, C. M., Fantel, A. G., Greenaway, J. C., Shepard, T. H., and Faustman-Watts, E. M. (1985a). Effects of 3-methylcholanthrene and phenobarbital on the capacity of embryos to bioactivate teratogens during organogenesis. *Toxicol. Appl. Pharmacol.* 80:137-147.

Juchau, M. R., Harris, C., Stark, K. L., Lee, Q. P., Yang, H. L., Namkung, M. J., and Fantel, A. G. (1991). Cytochrome P450-dependent bioactivation of prodysmorphogens in cultured conceptuses. *Reprod. Toxicol.* 5:259-264.

Juchau, M. R., Lee, Q. P., and Fantel, A. G. (1992). Xenobiotic biotransformation/bioactivation in organogenesis-stage conceptal tissues: Implications for embryotoxicity and teratogenesis. *Drug Metab. Rev.* 24:195-238.

Keberle, H., Loustalot, P. Mallon, R. K., Faigle, J. W., and Schmid, K. (1965). Biochemical effects of drugs on the mammalian conceptus. *Ann. NY Acad. Sci.* 123:252-262.

King, C. T. G., Weaver, S. A., and Narrod, S. A. (1965). Antihistamines and teratogenicity in the rat. *J. Pharmacol. Exp. Ther.* 147:391-398.

Krauer, B., and Dayer, P. (1991). Fetal drug metabolism and its possible clinical implications. *Clin. Pharmacokinet.* 21:70-80.

Lee, Q. P., and Juchau, M. R. (1990). Regulation of conceptal P450 isoforms with cyclic nucleotides and phosphodiesterase inhibitors. *Teratology* 41:574.

Lee, Q. P., and Juchau, M. R. (1992). Glucagon and isobutyl-methyl-xanthine increase cAMP levels and rates of cytochrome P450-dependent pentoxyphenoxazone depentylation in cultured rat conceptuses. *Toxicologist* 12:484.

Lee, Q. P., Fantel, A. G., and Juchau, M. R. (1991b). Human embryonic cytochrome P450s: Phenoxazone ethers as probes for expression of functional isoforms during organogenesis. *Biochem. Pharmacol.* 42:2377-2384.

Lee, Q. P., Juchau, M. R., and Creech-Kraft, J. M. (1991). Microinjection of cultured rat embryos: Studies with retinol, 13-*cis*- and all-*trans*-retinoic acid. *Teratology* 44:313-324.

Lee, Q. P., Yang, H. L., Namkung, M. J., and Juchau, M. R. (1991a). cAMP-dependent regulation of P450-catalyzed dealkylation in rat conceptal tissues. *Reprod. Toxicol.* 5:473-481.

Legraverend, C., Guenther, T. M., and Nebert, D. W. (1984). Importance of the route of administration for genetic differences in benzo(a)pyrene-induced *in utero* toxicity and teratogenicity. *Teratology* 29:35-48.

Lloyd, J. B. (1990). Cell physiology of the rat visceral yolk sac: A study of pinocytosis and lysosome function. *Teratology* 41:383-393.

Lubet, R. A., Mayer, R.T., Cameron, J. W., Nims, R. W., Burke, M. D., Wolfe, T., and Guengerich F. P. (1985). Dealkylation of pentoxyresorufin: A rapid and sensitive assay for measuring induction of cytochrome(s) P450 by phenobarbital and other xenobiotics in the rat. *Arch. Biochem. Biophys.* 238:43-48.

Lubet, R. A., Syi, J., Nelson, J. D., and Nims, R. W. (1990). Induction of hepatic cytochrome P450-mediated alkoxyresorufin O-dealkylase activities in different species by prototype P450 inducers. *Chem-Biol. Interact.* 75:325-331.

Migliaccio, G., Migliaccio, A. R., Petti, S., Mavilio, F., Russo, G., Lazzaro, D., Testa, U., Marinucci, M., and Peschie, C. (1986). Human embryonic hemopoiesis. Kinetics of progenitors and precursors underlying the yolk sac-liver transition. *J. Clin. Invest.* 78:51-60.

Mossman, H. W. (1986). *Vertebrate Fetal Membranes. Comparative Ontogeny and Morphology; Evolution; Phylogenetic Significance; Basic Functions; Research Opportunities.* Rutgers University Press, New Brunswick, NJ. 383 pp.

Namkung, M. J., Yang, H. L., Hulla, J. E., and Juchau, M. R. (1988). On the substrate specificity of cytochrome P450 IIIA1. *Molec. Pharmacol.* 34:628-637.

Oesch-Bartlomowicz, B., and Oesch, F. (1990). Review: phosphorylation of cytochrome P450 isoenzymes in intact hepatocytes and its importance for their function in metabolic processes. *Arch. Toxicol.* 64:257-262.

Ohsaki, T., Fujimoto, E., and Miki, A. (1987). Angiogenesis

and haematopoiesis in the rat visceral yolk sac under different oxygen concentrations *in vitro*. *Kobe J. Med. Sci.* 33:125-141.

Pelkonen, O., Pasanen, M., and Vahakangas, K. (1987). Metabolic activation by the fetus and placenta. Pages 734-746 *in* D. V. Parke and R. L. Smith, eds., *Drug Metabolism: From Molecules to Man*. Taylor & Francis, London.

Posner, H. S., Graves, A., King, C. T. G., and Wilk, A. (1967). Experimental alteration of the metabolism of chlorcyclizine and the incidence of cleft palate in rats. *J. Pharmacol. Exp. Ther.* 155:494-505.

Sahali, D., Mullier N., Chatelet, F., DuPuis, R., Ronco, P., and Verroust, P. (1988). Characterization of a 280-kD protein restricted to the coated pits of the renal brush border and the epithelial cells of the yolk sac: Teratogenic effect of the specific monoclonal antibodies. *J. Exp. Med.* 167:213-218.

Sasaki, K., and Matsumara, G. (1986). Hematopoietic cells of the yolk sac and liver in the mouse embryo: Light and electron microscopy study. *J. Anat.* 148:87-97.

Sasaki, K., and Kendall, M. D. (1985). The morphology of the hemopoietic cells of the yolk sac in mice with particular reference to nucleolar changes. *J. Anat.* 140:279-295.

Schmid, B. P., Hauser, R. E., and Donatsch, P. (1985). Effects of cyproheptadine on the rat yolk sac membrane and embryonic development *in vitro*. *Xenobiotica* 15:695-699.

Shiverick, K. T., Swanson, C., Salhab, A. S., and James, M. O. (1986). Differential induction of ethoxyresorufin-O-deethylase in tissues of the rat placenta. *J. Pharmacol. Exp. Ther.* 238:1108-1113.

Shum, S., Jensen, N. M., and Nebert, D. W. (1979). The Ah locus: *In utero* toxicity and teratogenesis associated with genetic differences in benzo(a)pyrene metabolism. *Teratology* 20:365-376.

Sobis, H., Goebels, J., and Van de Putte, M. (1986). Histochemical and autoradiographic study of the cultured rat visceral yolk sac. *J. Embryol. Exp. Morphol.* 97:169-176.

Stark, K. L., Harris, C., and Juchau, M. R. (1989). Modulation of the embryotoxicity and cytotoxicity elicited by 7-hydroxy-2-acetylaminofluorene and acetaminophen via deacetylation. *Toxicol. Appl. Pharmacol.* 97:548-561.

Stark, K. L., Lee, Q. P., Namkung, M. J., Harris, C., and Juchau, M. R. (1990). Dysmorphogenesis elicited by microinjected acetaminophen analogs and metabolites in rat embryos cultured *in vitro*. *J. Pharmacol. Exp. Therap.* 255:74-83.

Steventon, G. B., and Williams, K. E. (1987). Ethanol-induced inhibition of pinocytosis and proteolysis in rat yolk sac *in vitro*. *Development* 99:247-253.

Terlouw, G. D. C., and Bechter, R. (1992). Comparison of the metabolic activity of yolk sac tissue in the whole-embryo and isolated yolk sac culture. *Reprod. Toxicol.* (in press).

Thiriot-Hebert, M. (1987). Uptake of transferrin by the rat yolk sac and its materno-fetal transfer *in vivo*. *Cell Mol. Biol.* 33:183-189.

Thomas, T., Southwell, B. R., Schreiber, G., and Jaworowski, A. (1990). Plasma protein synthesis and secretion in the visceral yolk sac of the fetal rat: Gene expression, protein synthesis and secretion. *Placenta* 11:413-430.

Wells, P. G., Nagai, M. K., and Spano Greco, G. (1989a). Inhibition of trimethadione and dimethadione teratogenicity by the cyclooxygenase inhibitor acetylsalicylic acid: A unifying hypothesis for the teratologic effects of hydantoin anticonvulsants and structurally related compounds. *Toxicol. Appl. Pharmacol.* 97:406-414.

Wells, P. G., Zubovits, J. T., Wong, S. T., Molinari, L. M., and Ali, S. (1989b). Modulation of phenytoin teratogenicity and embryonic covalent binding by acetylsalicylic acid, caffeic acid and α-phenyl-N-t-butylnitrone: Implications for bioactivation by prostaglandin synthetase. *Toxicol. Appl. Pharmacol.* 97:192-202.

Yang, H. L. Zelus, B. D., and Juchau, M. R. (1991). Organogenesis-stage cytochrome P450 isoforms: Utilization of

PCR for detection of CYP1A1 mRNA in rat conceptal tissues. *Biochem. Biophys. Res. Commun.* 178:236-241.

Yang, H. L., Namkung, M. J., and Juchau, M. R. (1988). Cytochrome P450-dependent biotransformation of a series of phenoxazone ethers in the rat conceptus during early organogenesis: Evidence for multiple P450 isoenzymes. *Molec. Pharmacol.* 34:67-73.

Yang, H. L., Namkung, M. J., and Juchau, M. R. (1989). Immunodetection, immunoinhibition, immunoquantitation and biochemical analyses of cytochrome P450IA1 in tissues of the rat conceptus during the progression of organogenesis. *Biochem. Pharmacol.* 38:4027-4036.

York, R. G., and Manson J. M. (1984). Perinatal toxicity in mice associated with the Ahb allele following *in utero* exposure to 3-methylcholanthrene. *Toxicol. Appl. Pharmacol.* 72:417-426.

York, R. G., Stemmer, K., and Manson, J. M. (1984). Lung tumorigenesis and hyperplasia in offspring associated with the Ahd allele following *in utero* exposure to 3-methylcholanthrene. *Toxicol. Appl. Pharmacol.* 72:427-439.

Chapter 6

Retinoids and Fetal Malformations

D. M. Kochhar and Michael A. Satre

Vitamin A is an essential micronutrient for humans because it is not synthesized *de novo* in the body. The normal diet provides it either as provitamin A (or carotenoids), found in plants and vegetables, or as preformed vitamin A, found in animal products (Bendich & Langseth, 1989). It was discovered almost 75 years ago by McCollum and Davis (1913) as a lipid-soluble growth factor present in certain foods. They called this substance "Fat Soluble A" to distinguish it from essential "B" nutrients that were known to be water soluble. Further studies showed that vitamin A not only maintained growth but also prevented xerophthalmia and night blindness. Vitamin A-deficient children are anemic and grow poorly, have more infections, and are more likely to die than their peers (Sommer, 1989). During pregnancy, an imbalance in vitamin A nutriture is more likely than not to result in an adverse outcome (Wallingford & Underwood, 1986). While there is only indirect evidence that deficiency compromises the ability of a pregnant female in maintaining and delivering a normal baby, there is indisputable evidence that ingestion of vitamin A-related therapeutics during pregnancy results in fetal malformations (Rosa, *et al.*, 1986; Anonymous, 1987).

Retinol, or vitamin A alcohol, is the most common form of the vitamin and is the term now used instead of vitamin A (Table 1). Retinol performs essential functions in reproduction, vision and in regulation of differentiation and proliferation of a wide variety of tissues including the epithelial tissues. Retinol yields several derivatives in the body one of which, 11-*cis* retinal, specifically functions in vision as a photolabile molecule. The most common derivative of retinol is all-*trans* retinoic acid (RA) that circulates in the blood and occurs in small quantities in a wide variety of tissues. New discoveries have singled out RA and one of its isomers, 9-*cis* retinoic acid, as natural hormones with important regulatory function in all phases of life including embryonic development (Table 1) (Packer, 1990). RA can prevent almost all symptoms of vitamin A deficiency except those in vision and the male reproductive tract.

To exploit the therapeutic value of RA, a considerable number of natural and synthetic RA analogs (termed retinoids) are under laboratory and clinical investigation (Table 1). Although the intended applications are widely based, the initial use of retinoids has been to treat diverse diseases of the skin and mucous membranes, carcinoma of the respiratory tract, and acute promyelocytic leukemia. One such retinoid, 13-*cis* retinoic acid, has been marketed since 1982 under the trade name Accutane® for treatment of disfiguring, recalcitrant cystic acne. Out of a large number of

TABLE 1. Chemical Structure of Vitamin A and
other Natural and Synthetic Retinoids

Name(s)	Structure
Retinol (vitamin A)	
All-*trans* Retinoic Acid (Tretinoin)	
13-*cis* Retinoic Acid (Isotretinoin, Accutane)	
9-*cis* Retinoic Acid	
Acitretin	
Etretinate (Tigason, Tegison)	
Ro 13-6307	
Ro 13-7410 (TTNPB)	

patients who have taken this drug were women of child-bearing age, and as of April 1990 more than 87 malformed babies and more than 40 spontaneous abortions have occurred in this group (Rosa, 1992). Etretinate (Tigason®) is another retinoid that is prescribed for treating recalcitrant psoriasis. Teratogenic outcome has also occurred with etretinate, although malformations are different from those produced by Accutane® and their frequency is difficult to ascertain.

The purpose of this presentation is to discuss the occurrence and nature of fetal malformations due to maternal ingestion of various natural and synthetic retinoids. In view of the recent discoveries of nuclear receptors that specifically bind RA and its isomers and thereby regulate expression of responsive genes, we emphasize in this chapter information on vitamin A nutrition and metabolism in the body that may serve as a starting point for understanding the molecular role of this micronutrient in normal and abnormal development. A brief review of the biochemistry and metabolism of vitamin A in nutrition during pregnancy is followed by information on the effects of its deficiency on embryonic development. The developmental role of vitamin A deficiency is complicated by the likely imposition of secondary effects in the afflicted dam. Resolution of the role of vitamin A in the embryo, therefore, has hitherto depended on information derived from teratogenic effects of retinol and retinoic acid given in excess to pregnant animals of various species of laboratory animals. This information is summarized with emphasis on the response of the embryonic tissues to variations in the chemical structure of the retinoid molecule in order to assess the risk of fetal malformations posed by vitamin A ingested as an oral supplement or taken as a therapeutic drug in the form of one of its synthetic analogs.

Vitamin A Metabolism

The following discussion of vitamin A metabolism is presented in the same sequence as illustrated in Figure 1. Thus, the metabolic reactions will be described in the context of the general systemic progression of the vitamin; from absorption in the gut, to metabolism, storage and release from the liver, transport through the circulation and finally uptake and metabolism at the target cell. Although a multitude of chemically synthesized and metabolic forms of retinoids exist, the focus here will be primarily on the major, common forms. In addition, emphasis will be placed on the metabolic route leading to the generation of "active" metabolites, with only a minimal discussion of downstream (inactivation or excretory) pathways. For more comprehensive, detailed discussions of these and other areas, readers are referred to reviews by Goodman & Blaner (1984) and Blomhoff, *et al.*, (1990).

A. Absorption

Animals are not capable of *de novo* synthesis of vitamin A active substances and must obtain their vitamin A by biosynthesis from ingested provitamin A forms from plants or from ingestion of animal products containing the preformed vitamin. Additional sources include vitamin supplements and pharmaceuticals with vitamin A activity.

Major provitamin A forms are the fat-soluble plant pigments (carotenoids), which are composed of a class of hydrocarbons (carotenes) and their oxygenated derivatives (xanthophylls). Biological activity of carotenoids with provitamin A activity results from their metabolic conversion to vitamin A by the animal. Although over 400 carotenoids have been identified, the majority possess little or no vitamin A activity (Bauernfeind, 1971; Simpson, 1983; Goodman & Blaner, 1984). Carotenoids with provitamin A activity include α-, β- and γ-carotene, citroxanthin, cryptoxanthin and various carotenals, with β-carotene the major provitamin A form (Bauernfeind, 1971; Goodman & Blaner, 1984; Underwood, 1984). Following absorption, β-carotene (and some other carotenoids) is cleaved at the central double bond by a soluble enzyme (β-carotene-15,15′-dioxygenase) into 2 molecules of retinaldehyde (retinal; RAL Figure 2). In rats, the activity of carotene-15,15′-dioxygenase has been shown to

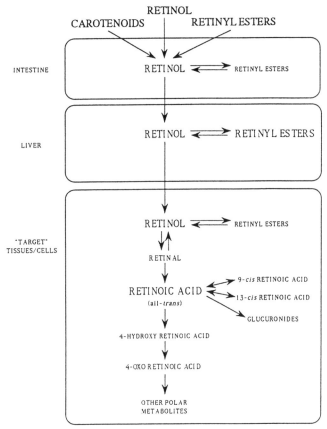

FIGURE 1. General scheme of absorption, transport, storage and release, cellular uptake and metabolism of vitamin A in the body.

increase under conditions of dietary vitamin A depletion (Villard and Bates, 1985). Other carotenoids may also be converted to RAL via excentric cleavage by additional dioxygenases (Goodman & Blaner, 1984). The majority of the RAL formed from carotenoids or other precursors is then reduced by retinal reductase to retinol (Goodman & Blaner, 1984; Lakshman, *et al.*, 1989). A recent study in the rat, however, has shown that some β-carotene may be converted directly to retinoic acid without undergoing prior conversion to RAL or retinol (Bauernfeind, 1980; Lui & Roels, 1980; Napoli & Race, 1988).

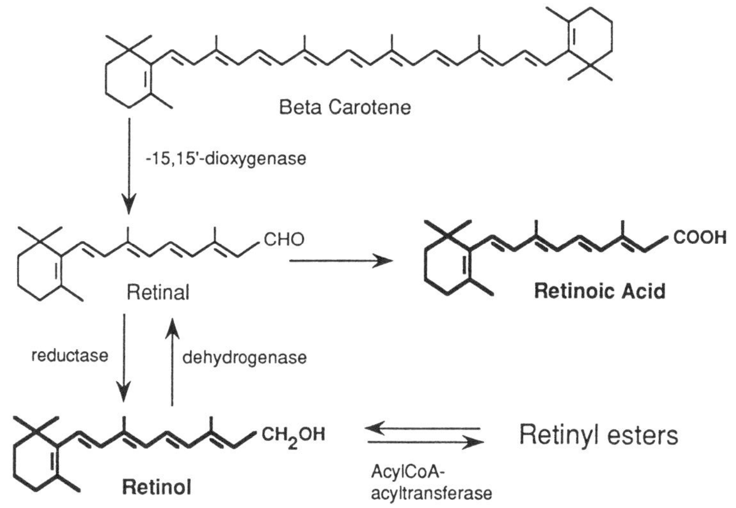

FIGURE 2. General metabolic pathways in the formation of retinol from dietary sources (carotenoids from vegetables, retinyl esters from meat products) and further oxidation of retinol to retinal and retinoic acid.

Among animal products, liver from mammals, fish and fowl are the richest sources of preformed vitamin A (retinol and retinyl esters) because of the role of this organ in uptake and storage of the vitamin. Owing to the extremely large storage capacity of the liver, acute toxicity has been documented among arctic explorers following ingestion of relatively small quantities of raw polar bear and seal livers (Underwood, 1984). Toxic symptoms have also been observed in infants fed certain fish oils (Bauernfeind, 1980) or chicken livers (Mahoney, et al., 1980).

In the intestinal lumen, virtually all retinyl esters from ingested animal products are enzymatically converted to retinol prior to absorption by intestinal cells (enterocytes). Retinyl esters are apparently hydrolyzed by the same enzymes responsible for the hydrolysis of cholesterol esters (Frolik, 1984; Goodman & Blaner, 1984).

Being lipophilic molecules, the various forms of vitamin A and carotenoids share with lipids similar requirements for dispersion and absorption. Thus, factors that affect the efficient absorption of fats also affect the fat-soluble vitamins, and especially affect absorption of carotenoids. In general, both preformed and precursor forms require solubilization into mixed-micellar solutions to facilitate efficient absorption (El-Gorab & Underwood, 1973; Hollander, 1981). Mixed micelles are formed from bile-salts and lipolytic products of ingested and endogenous fats, thus, a diet very low in fat or our interference in normal lipolysis or bile-salt availability can result in impaired intestinal absorption and uptake (Underwood, 1984).

Various distinctions exist with respect to absorption of the different forms of vitamin A. Physiological amounts of retinol are more efficiently absorbed (70->90%) than hydrocarbon carotenoids or xanthophylls (20-60%), while intact retinyl esters are absorbed relatively poorly (Olson, 1986). The absorption efficiency of retinol remains high as the amount ingested increases, whereas that of carotenoids falls markedly (to <10%) with high intake (Bauernfeind, 1971; Olson, 1972). Retinol is absorbed relatively well from a mixed micelle formed with non-ionic detergents, whereas carotenoid absorption is absolutely dependent on the presence of bile-salts (Olson, 1961; El-Gorab, et al., 1975). Finally, retinol is transported across intestinal cell membranes by a carrier-mediated process at low physiologic intakes and by diffusion from a micellar phase at higher doses. Carotenoids, on the other hand, are apparently absorbed by passive diffusion at all concentrations (El-Gorab, et al., 1975; Hollander, 1981).

The retinol formed in the intestine from either plant or animal sources is then esterified with fatty acids. Two enzymes, lecithin-retinol:acyltransferase (LRAT) (Ong, et al., 1987) and acyl-CoA-retinol:acyltransferase (ARAT) (Helgerud, et al., 1982) appear to be involved. Under conditions of normal physiologic retinol loads, retinol within the intestinal cell is bound to cellular retinol-binding protein, type II (CRBP(II)) (Ong, 1984), abundant in mature enterocytes of the adult intestine (Crow & Ong, 1985). The CRBP(II)-bound retinol can then be esterified by LRAT via a phosphatidyl choline-dependent transacylase mechanism similar to that established for the esterification of cholesterol (Ong, *et al.*, 1987; MacDonald & Ong, 1988). This esterification reaction produces predominantly retinyl palmitate and retinyl stearate in a ratio of approximately 2:1 (MacDonald & Ong, 1988) in agreement with the ratio reported in previous in vivo studies (Huang & Goodman, 1965). The retinyl ester composition appears to be essentially independent of the lipid composition of the diet (Huang & Goodman, 1965). The second esterifying enzyme, ARAT, has been characterized from rat (Helgerud, *et al.*, 1982) and human (Helgerud, *et al.*, 1983) intestinal mucosa. The activity of this enzyme is induced by large oral doses of vitamin A (Rasmussen, *et al.*, 1984). This enzyme, however, apparently does not display the appropriate fatty acyl specificity observed *in vivo*. Thus, it seems likely that retinol esterification by ARAT comes into play primarily under conditions of vitamin A excess when CRBP(II) becomes saturated.

After esterification, the retinyl esters are incorporated into the core of chylomicrons and secreted from the enterocytes into the lymph. These chylomicrons then enter the systemic blood via the lymphatic channels. The esters remain within the chylomicron particles during their catabolism in extrahepatic tissues which occurs prior to their clearance by the liver.

Although it has been clearly demonstrated that under normal physiological conditions retinol absorption occurs primarily via the lymphatic route, the existence of an alternate route of retinol absorption has been suggested. There is evidence that under abnormal conditions, such as disease or experimental closure of the thoracic duct, retinol may be absorbed via a non-lymphatic pathway in amounts sufficient to meet the nutritional needs and in a biochemical form other than chylomicron. (Lawrence, *et al.*, 1966; Herbert, *et al.*, 1983).

B. Storage

Of the four liver cell types (endothelial, Kupffer, parenchymal and stellate), only the last two appear to be of significance in hepatic vitamin A storage or metabolism. Upon reaching the liver, the chylomicron remnant is taken up by hepatic parenchymal cells (Blomhoff, *et al.*, 1983; Blomhoff, *et al.*, 1985). Chylomicron uptake appears to involve an interaction with high affinity cell-surface receptors specific for the apolipoprotein E (apoE) moiety on the chylomicron followed by receptor-mediated endocytosis (Sherill, *et al.*, 1980; Brown, *et al.*, 1981). This initial uptake into the parenchymal cells amounts to short-term storage. During the next several hours, most of the vitamin is transferred to hepatic stellate cells for long-term storage (Blomhoff, *et al.*, 1987).

Following the initial uptake into the parenchymal cells, the chylomicron remnant undergoes lysosomal degradation liberating the retinyl esters which are then hydrolyzed. Hepatic retinyl ester hydrolysis has generally been attributed to the activity of bile salt-dependent hydrolase(s) (Harrison, *et al.*, 1979; Prystowsky, *et al.*, 1981; Cooper & Olson, 1986; Cooper, *et al.*, 1987). Results from recent studies suggest that this activity is due to the same or similar enzymes as pancreatic cholesteryl ester hydrolase and/or a newly described bile salt-independent retinyl ester hydrolase (Harrison, 1988; Harrison & Gad, 1989). The activity of the later, bile salt-independent enzyme was associated with hepatic cell membranes (Harrison & Gad, 1989), suggesting that this enzyme may play a prominent role in retinyl ester hydrolysis.

Following hepatic retinyl ester hydrolysis, the liberated retinol presumably binds to CRBP and is subsequently re-esterified for storage. Hepatic retinol esterification involves two enzymes, ARAT (Ross, 1981; Rasmussen, *et al.*, 1984) and LRAT (MacDonald & Ong, 1988; Ong, *et al.*, 1988) that are the same or similar to those in the intestine. The esterification process appears to be essentially the same as that in the intestine (described previously), except that it is CRBP, not CRBP(II), that serves to bind the intracellular hepatic retinol.

In the liver ≤95% of the total vitamin A is esterified (Goodman & Blaner, 1984; Olson, 1986). Retinyl palmitate is the predominant ester present (80-90%) followed by stearate (5-10%), linoleate (1-4%), palmitoleate (1-4%), and smaller amounts of oleate, myristate, laurate and other esters

(Futterman & Andrews, 1964; Ross, 1982; Bhat & LaCroix, 1983; Tomassi & Olson, 1983; Furr, *et al.*, 1986). The composition of retinyl esters in the liver appears to be largely independent of the distribution of fatty acids in the diet (Tomassi & Olson, 1983). The ester pattern does not change appreciably with increasing liver reserves resulting from modest intakes (Batres & Olson, 1987), although it can be perturbed by very high doses (Wake, 1980).

Studies on the relative distribution of vitamin A between the parenchymal and stellate cells indicate that ≤80% of the total liver vitamin A are stored in the stellate cells, with parenchymal cells accounting for 10-20% and non-parenchymal cells <5% (Hendriks, *et al.*, 1985; Batres & Olson, 1987). This distribution of vitamin A among liver cells does not seem greatly affected over a fairly wide range of liver reserves (Batres & Olson, 1987). When very large doses of vitamin A are given, however, stellate cells clearly store a relatively larger amount (Wake, 1980), whereas in a state of severe depletion, they store very little (McKenna, *et al.*, 1983).

Both isolated parenchymal and stellate cells contain ARAT and retinyl ester hydrolase activity, with parenchymal cells accounting for >75% of the total hepatic content of these two enzyme activities. On a cell protein basis, however, both of these activities are much greater in stellate cells. Little if any enzyme activity was found in endothelial or Kupffer cells (Eriksson, *et al.*, 1984).

Based on cell protein, the concentration of CRBP in stellate cells was found to be >22-fold greater than in parenchymal cells, consistent with results from immunohistochemical studies (Eriksson, *et al.*, 1984; Kato, *et al.*, 1985b). However, because of the difference in size and number of parenchymal cells, >90% of the total hepatic CRBP is localized to parenchymal cells (Blomhoff, *et al.*, 1984).

Although initially taken up by parenchymal cells, the majority of the endocytosed retinol is transferred from these cells to the perisinusoidal stellate cells (Blomhoff, *et al.*, 1983; Blomhoff, *et al.*, 1984). A number of possible mechanisms have been proposed to account for this transfer including:

intercellular transfer mediated by retinol binding protein (RBP) (Blomhoff, *et al.*, 1984; Gjoen, *et al.*, 1987; Blomhoff, *et al.*, 1988); transfer mediated by CRBP (Nyberg, *et al.*, 1988); and transfer mediated via direct contact between parenchymal and stellate cell membranes (Fex & Johannesson, 1987). Of these, the most persuasive evidence comes from the studies by Blomhoff, *et al.* (Blomhoff, *et al.*, 1988). Using radiolabelled retinol or ester moieties, they demonstrated that while both were taken up by the parenchymal cells, only the retinol moiety was found in stellate cells. It was further noted that this transfer could be blocked by antibodies against RBP. Previous studies had shown that paranchymal cells synthesized and secreted *holo*-RBP (Rask, *et al.*, 1983; Ronne, *et al.*, 1983) and that stellate cells were capable of taking up this *holo*-RBP complex (Blomhoff, *et al.*, 1984; Gjoen, *et al.*, 1987). While stellate cells apparently contain and secrete low levels of RBP (Blomhoff, *et al.*, 1984; Blaner, *et al.*, 1985), these cells do not contain detectable quantities of RBP mRNA (Yamada, *et al.*, 1987). Thus, it appears that retinyl ester hydrolysis in parenchymal cells is very likely a prerequisite for transfer of retinol to the stellate cells. However, while the RBP-mediated transfer of retinol between parenchymal and stellate cells is plausible, the precise mechanism of this transfer remains to be definitively established.

Stellate cells (or stellate-like cells) are also found in the intestine, kidney, heart, large blood vessels, ovaries and testes, and these cells are capable of storing retinyl esters when large doses of the vitamin are consumed (Blomhoff, *et al.*, 1990). Although the liver and intestine are the primary sites of retinol esterification and hydrolysis, these reactions have recently been shown to occur in other tissues, such as the testis sertoli cells (Bishop & Griswold, 1987; Shingleton, *et al.*, 1989) and retinal pigment epithelium (Das & Gouras, 1988).

C. Transport

(1) In the Body

Under normal physiologic conditions, RBP is secreted

from the liver into the circulation in a 1:1 complex with all-*trans* retinol (*holo*-RBP) and is delivered to the body tissues as such (Goodman, 1984). The hydrophobic retinol molecule appears to be bound within a cleft in the RBP (Newcomer, *et al.*, 1984) and is thus protected from oxygen and other molecules. The size, structure and characteristics of RBP appear to be very similar among species (see Goodman, 1984 and Blaner, 1989 for complete reviews).

Within the plasma, the *holo*-RBP combines with one molecule of transthyretin (TTR); the thyroid hormone binding protein that binds one molecule of thyroxine with high affinity (Goodman, 1984). Formation of the *holo*-RBP-TTR complex significantly decreases the extent of kidney filtration (and therefore loss) compared to RBP alone. Turnover studies in humans and animals have shown that the half-life of *holo*-RBP complexed to TTR is 3-4-fold longer than uncomplexed RBP (Vahlquist, *et al.*, 1973; Peterson, *et al.*, 1974) . In addition to increasing the half-life of *holo*-RBP in the circulation, data from *in vitro* experiments has shown that binding of TTR to RBP causes a 2-fold increase in RBP avidity for retinol (Noy & Xu, 1990a) and that TTR caused a decrease in the rate of release of ^{3}H-retinol bound to RBP (Sivaprasadarao & Findlay, 1988b).

Control of circulating levels of retinol occurs primarily in the liver. If the liver stores are low, the immediate release from the parenchymal cells to the blood is more rapid and more quantitative and lower amounts of retinyl esters are transferred to the stellate cells. If, however, liver stores are adequate, most of the absorbed retinyl esters are transferred to the stellate cells and stored (McKenna *et al.*, 1983; Blomhoff, *et al.*, 1984). As yet undefined homeostatic mechanisms ensure that the plasma retinol concentration remains fairly normal despite the normal, physiological fluctuations in vitamin A intake. It is likely that saturation of CRBP and RBP along with retinoid regulation of the levels of these proteins are part of this mechanism.

During vitamin A deficiency, RBP accumulates in the liver, reaching levels 4-10-fold higher than in control livers

(Muto, *et al.*, 1972; Blaner, *et al.*, 1985). Concomitantly, plasma *holo*-RBP levels decline to very low levels while *apo*-RBP increases from <10% to the predominant circulating form (Goodman, 1984). The rate of RBP synthesis and translatable levels of liver RBP mRNA, however, remain unchanged in normal, deficient and retinol-repleted rat livers (Soprano, *et al.*, 1982; Soprano, *et al.*, 1986). Studies indicate that retinol deficiency largely prevents the movement of newly synthesized RBP from the endoplasmic reticulum to the Golgi apparatus (Rask, *et al.*, 1983; Ronne, *et al.*, 1983; Fries, *et al.*, 1984). Upon addition of vitamin A to the deficient animal, the apo-RBP within the hepatocyte quickly mobilized and *holo*-RBP increases in the plasma (Olson, 1986). Both the plasma transport of retinol and its clearance from the plasma are lower in deficiency (Donoghue, *et al.*, 1983). Interestingly, transport and clearance of retinyl esters are relatively unaffected. Turnover of plasma retinol in deficient animals is also slower (Lewis, *et al.*, 1981).

Various steroid (Yeung, 1974; Vahlquist, *et al.*, 1979; Glover, *et al.*, 1980; Borek, *et al.*, 1981; Dixon & Goodman, 1987) and adrenocortical hormones (Underwood, 1984), can modulate *holo*-RBP levels *in vivo* and *in vitro*. In addition, RA (and possibly other retinoids) can apparently cause a decrease in circulating retinol levels, presumably resulting from a decreased release of retinol from the liver, a "sparing effect"; (Keilson, *et al.*, 1979; Bhat & LaCroix, 1986). Finally, alterations in vitamin A homeostasis can result from exposure to various chemicals (*e.g.*, chlorinated and brominated biphenyls [PCBs], dioxins, and alcohols). The effects are chemical-specific and include competition/displacement of TTR from *holo*-RBP (Brouwer, *et al.*, 1985; Brouwer, *et al.*, 1988; Bank, *et al.*, 1989), inhibition of retinyl ester hydrolase activity (Powers, *et al.*, 1987), and impaired mobilization of stored vitamin A (Hakansson, *et al.*, 1988; Hakansson & Hanberg, 1989).

After the entry of retinol into the target cells, the *apo*-RBP undergoes catabolism in the kidney (Peterson, *et al.*, 1974). About 80% of the retinol bound to RBP circulating in the plasma returns to the liver (Lewis, *et al.*, 1981; Green, *et al.*, 1985). This recycling, together with the release of the vitamin as required, constitutes the homeostatic regulation of the plasma retinol level as observed over a wide range of available stores (Green, *et al.*, 1985; Olson, 1986).

(2) Cellular Uptake

At the target cell, holo-RBP may interact with a specific cell-surface receptor so that target cells take up retinol by an as yet incompletely defined mechanism, although receptor mediated endocytosis is one possibility (Olson, 1986). There is evidence for the existence of cell-surface receptors in several cell types: pigment epithelium (Heller, 1975; Pfeffer, *et al.*, 1986); intestinal mucosal cells (Rask & Peterson, 1976); testicular cells (Bhat & Cama, 1979); sertoli cells (Shingleton, *et al.*, 1989); human placenta (Torma & Vahlquist, 1986; Sivaprasadarao & Findlay, 1988a) and epithelial cells of the skin (Forsum, *et al.*, 1977). However, it is not yet clear if the cell-surface receptors are present on all cells, or if they are in fact required at all for the entry of retinol into the cell. Indeed, no cell-surface receptor has been isolated to date, and there is evidence of retinol entry into cells or membranes in the apparent absence of either a putative cell-surface receptor or RBP (Fex & Johannesson, 1988; Creek, *et al.*, 1989).

(3) Cellular Metabolism

Following uptake, many tissues/cells can metabolically convert retinol to RA. RA is a naturally occurring metabolite of vitamin A present in a variety of adult tissues following administration of physiologic doses of retinol (Emerick, *et al.*, 1967; McCormick & Napoli, 1982), retinaldehyde (Crain, *et al.*, 1967) or retinyl acetate (Ito, *et al.*, 1974; Bhat & LaCroix, 1983). Numerous *in vivo* and *in vitro* studies have demonstrated that many adult tissues and cell lines are capable of synthesizing RA (Williams, *et al.*, 1984; Napoli, 1986; Leo, *et al.*, 1987; Napoli & Race, 1987; Posch, *et al.*, 1989). Overall, however, RA is only a minor metabolite within the total spectrum of retinol metabolism, accounting for $\leq 5\%$ of the initial substrate (Napoli, 1986; Bhat, *et al.*, 1988). In the body, RA is only a minor form in tissues and circulation of animals and humans (Goodman, 1984; Olson, 1986).

Although this particular metabolic route may be minor in a quantitative sense, it is likely of significant physiologic importance given the evidence that RA may be the ultimate, "activated" metabolite of vitamin A (Roberts & Sporn, 1984; Jetten, 1986; Connor, 1988). Historically, there is abundant evidence for the role of RA in maintaining growth in otherwise vitamin A deficient animals (see Roberts & Sporn, 1984; Underwood, 1984; Olson, 1986 for reviews). More recent work has shown that this retinoid can elicit a broad spectrum of effects in target cells (Lotan, 1980; Roberts & Sporn, 1984; Jetten, 1986). In particular, RA exhibits morphogenetic activity in developing and regenerating vertebrate limbs and nervous system (Thaller & Eichele, 1987; Durston, *et al.*, 1989; Eichele, 1989).

Data from numerous studies indicate that RA can modulate the expression of genes or gene products involved in differentiation and proliferation (Chytil & Riaz-ul-Haq, 1990). This modulation occurs directly as a result of interacting of RA with nuclear receptors: RARα (Giguere, *et al.*, 1987; Petkovich, *et al.*, 1987); RARβ (Benbrook, *et al.*, 1988; Brand, *et al.*, 1988); RARγ (Krust, *et al.*, 1989; Zelent, *et al.*, 1989), for RA, and RXR (Mangelsdorf, *et al.*, 1990; Heyman, *et al.*, 1992; Levin, *et al.*, 1992), for the RA-isomer, 9-*cis* RA. These receptors function as ligand-inducible transcription factors (enhancers or suppressors). Thus, RA and its 9-*cis* isomer, can now be thought of functionally as hormones.

Classically, the metabolic generation of RA from retinol is a cytosolic reaction occurring in two sequential steps: (1) reversible dehydrogenation (oxidation) of retinol to RAL; (2) irreversible oxidation of RAL to RA. The first reaction is strongly NAD dependent and is the rate-limiting step in the conversion of retinol to RA (Napoli, 1986; Napoli & Race, 1987; Bhat, *et al.*, 1988). In the second reaction, RAL is irreversibly oxidized to RA by an aldehyde dehydrogenase (Elder & Topper, 1962; Futterman, 1962; Napoli, 1986; Leo, *et al.*, 1989). This reaction occurs 30-60 times faster than the conversion of retinol to RAL and can be stimulated by NADPH (Moffa, *et al.*, 1970; Napoli, 1986; Bhat, *et al.*, 1988). The conversion of retinol to RA may be inducible by RA pretreatment, is not inhibited by excess product, but can be inhibited by at least one synthetic retinoid (Napoli, 1986).

It is widely accepted that retinol is reversibly oxidized to RAL by a cytosolic retinol dehydrogenase (RDH) with characteristics that are identical to liver class I alcohol dehydrogenase (ADH). ADH is a well-characterized enzyme present in virtually all organisms and reversibly interconverts ethanol and acetaldehyde using NAD+/NADH as a cofactor (Branden, *et al.*, 1975). It is abundant in the liver, accounting for 2-3% of the soluble protein in adults (Lange, *et al.*, 1976; Ditlow, *et al.*, 1984). Human and rodent ADH exists as a heterogeneous group of isoenzymes that can be placed into 3 classes based on structural and functional characteristics (Strydom & Vallee, 1982; Algar, *et al.*, 1983). Human class I ADH catalyses the oxidation of a wide variety of alcohols, including ethanol and retinol (Mezey & Holt, 1971; Li, 1977). Rodent class I ADH has also been shown to function in both ethanol and retinol oxidation in the rat (Zachman & Olson, 1961; Chiao & Van Thiel, 1986; Napoli & Race, 1987) and deermouse (Leo, *et al.*, 1987; Posch, *et al.*, 1989). Examinations of retinol oxidation by human class II ADH have not been reported, but rodent class II ADH does function in retinol oxidation (Julia, *et al.*, 1986; Connor & Smit, 1987). Class III ADH is very inefficient in retinol oxidation (Beisswenger, *et al.*, 1985; Julia, *et al.*, 1987).

In humans, class I ADH is expressed in the liver where it is the most abundant class. Human class I is also produced in the intestine, kidney, stomach, lung and skin, but at levels at least an order of magnitude lower than in the liver (Smith, *et al.*, 1971; Smith, *et al.*, 1972; Smith, 1986). In rodents, class I ADH displays essentially the same expression pattern, except that it is noticeably absent from the stomach (Holmes, *et al.*, 1983; Boleda, *et al.*, 1989). Human class II ADH has only been detected in adult liver, whereas the rodent enzyme is absent from the liver but present in the stomach and sex organs of the mouse (Holmes, *et al.*, 1983), and the stomach, intestine lungs, skin and sex organs of the rat (Boleda, *et al.*, 1989). Class III ADH in both humans and rodents has been found in virtually every tissue examined (Holmes, *et al.*, 1983; Adinolfi, *et al.*, 1984; Boleda, *et al.*, 1989).

That ADH plays an important role in RA synthesis is supported by the recent experiments indicating that the expression of the human class I ADH gene (*ADH3*) is transcriptionally regulated by RA (Duester, *et al.*, 1991).

Apparent RDH activity distinct from class I ADH exists in the cytosol (Napoli & Race, 1987; Posch, *et al.*, 1989) and microsomes (Leo, *et al.*, 1987). A mutant deermouse completely lacks class I ADH activity (Leo & Leiber, 1984; Posch, *et al.*, 1989) or immunologically cross-reactive material because of a deletion of the gene (Burnett & Felder, 1978; Burnett & Felder, 1980). Compared to the wild-type, the ADH-deermouse has RA synthetic activity that is greatly reduced in the liver and kidney (Leo & Leiber, 1984), but maintains most of its RA synthetic ability in testes, lung, and intestine (Posch, *et al.*, 1989). The cytosolic RDH activity was demonstrated to be distinct from ADH based on the use of inhibitors and the observation that RAL was apparently not produced as an intermediate (Posch, *et al.*, 1989). Since the ADH-deermouse apparently reproduces and develops normally, this has been taken as evidence for specific (non-class I ADH) RDH activity that provides enough retinol oxidation to maintain RA synthesis in these animals. Recent studies, however, indicate that the ADH-deermouse does indeed have ADH species that correspond to mouse class II and III ADHs (M. Felder, pers. commun.). Since both class I and II ADH can oxidize retinol, it will be important to establish whether a unique RDH enzyme or class II ADH activity is responsible for the metabolic generation of RA in these animals.

These mutant deermice also exhibited microsomal RDH activity that accounted for virtually all of the activity observed in liver homogenates of these ADH-animals. The microsomal liver RDH activity was distinct from cytosolic RDH or cytochrome P450 (cyt.P450) retinol reductase activity that was observed in the wild-type (Leo & Leiber, 1984; Leo, et al., 1987). Since ADH II is cytosolic (Julia, et al., 1987), this microsomal activity may represent that of a specific RDH.

There is evidence that the production of RA can occur by enzyme(s) distinct from ethanol/acetaldehyde dehydrogenase or aldehyde oxidase (Napoli, 1986; Napoli & Race, 1987). Recent studies have shown that β-carotene could be converted to RA in a variety of tissues without the generation of RAL as an intermediate. Although retinol was generated in substantial amounts, it was apparently not the primary substrate for RA. This metabolic route of RA generation also differed from the classically described pathway in that it was neither NAD nor NADH dependent (Napoli & Race, 1987).

Retinol can also undergo conversion to metabolites in addition to RA. Rat liver microsomes were found to actively convert retinol to more polar metabolites (including 4-hydroxy- and 4-oxo-retinol) without generating RA as an intermediate (Leo & Leiber, 1985). Both 4-hydroxy-retinol and 4-oxo-retinol have been detected in vivo following administration of radiolabeled precursors (Barua & Olson, 1984; Williams, et al., 1984). Involvement of the cytochrome P450 system (cyt.P450) was indicated based on results using specific inhibitors and inducers, and from reconstitution experiments using purified forms of cyt.P450. This novel pathway of retinol metabolism was also documented using human liver microsomes (Leo, et al., 1989). Here the reaction was actively catalyzed by the non-inducible human cyt.P450IIC8 in both human samples and a reconstituted system. The reaction was also inhibited in the presence of a specific antibody, suggesting that retinol metabolism may be governed in part by specific cyt.P450 forms (Leo, et al., 1989).

It is now evident that retinol may undergo more complex metabolism than previously thought. In addition to the metabolic generation of RA from retinol by the traditional (ADH) route, distinct RDH enzyme(s) may in fact exist. Furthermore, retinol can be metabolized to additional products independent of the generation of RA. The extent to which these exist within a given cell or tissue and their physiologic significance remains to be determined. The RA found at or in cells is not necessarily produced there. In addition to production of RA by extrahepatic tissues, significant amounts of RA are also formed in the liver (Goodman & Blaner, 1984). Small quantities of RA are also formed in the intestine, either from the oxidation of retinol (Smith, *et al.*, 1973) or directly from β-carotene (Napoli & Race, 1988) as discussed previously. RA from these sources (or ingested as such) is transported in the plasma bound to serum albumin under physiologic conditions (Goodman & Blaner, 1984). The very little RA acquired through the diet hardly accounts for much of the systemic RA, although ingestion of pharmaceuticals containing a RA (*e.g.*, Accutane) can obviously increase the systemic load. It should be noted that unlike retinol, ingested RA is absorbed through the portal system. The balance between uptake of RA in the circulation and its generation *in situ* is regulated though imperfectly understood processes.

In the circulation and non-ocular tissues in mammals, RA is found primarily as either the all-*trans* or 13-*cis* form (Zile, *et al.*, 1967; Satre & Kochhar, 1989). All-*trans* RA is usually the predominant form and it is generally accepted that this isomeric form is responsible for the biological activity of RA (Roberts & Sporn, 1984; Connor, 1988). Both isomers are commonly observed in the plasma and tissues following physiological or pharmacological doses of either isomer alone (Creech-Kraft, *et al.*, 1987; Satre & Kochhar, 1989). Although enzymatic isomerization between all-*trans* and 11-*cis* RAL in the eye is obligatory in the visual process (Wald, 1968), no enzymatic isomerase activity has been conclusively demonstrated in non-occular tissues. While retinoids are particularly susceptible to non-enzymatic photoisomerization (Curley & Fowble, 1988) , this mechanism is not a likely to account for that observed *in vivo*. A thiol-catalyzed isomerization of all-*trans* and 13-*cis* RA has been suggested to account for both *cis* and *trans* forms of retinoids in animal tissues (Shih, *et al.*, 1986), but a definitive mechanism and the physiological significance of this isomerization remains unknown.

Within cells, RA is metabolized fairly rapidly to a variety of metabolites. It can be converted to 5,6-epoxyretinoic acid (McCormick, *et al.*, 1978; DeLuca, *et al.*, 1981; McCormick & Napoli, 1982) or conjugated to glucuronides (Sietsema & DeLuca, 1979; DeLuca, *et al.*, 1981; Miller & DeLuca, 1986). The former is not active and questions remain as to whether it is a metabolite normally formed in the body, and if so, whether it is important in the elimination pathway of RA. Retinoyl-β-glucuronide, on the other hand, is a prominent metabolite following administration of RA (Cullum & Zile, 1985) and is an endogenous component of human blood (Barua & Olson, 1986). Although it has been shown to be as active as RA in biological assays (Sietsema & DeLuca, 1982; Barua & Olson, 1987; Zile, *et al.*, 1987), it is unclear if it must first be hydrolyzed back to RA for this activity.

RA can also be metabolized to more polar, oxygenated metabolites. A major reaction is the conversion to 4-hydroxy RA and 4-oxo RA (Roberts, *et al.*, 1979a; Roberts, *et al.*, 1979b; Frolik, 1981). Both oxygenated forms have been found in the plasma and tissues following physiologic (Reitz, *et al.*, 1974; Napoli, *et al.*, 1978; Roberts, *et al.*, 1979a; Roberts, *et al.*, 1979b), or pharmacologic and teratogenic doses (Creech-Kraft, *et al.*, 1987; Satre & Kochhar, 1989). Metabolic studies indicate that the conversion of RA to its 4-oxo metabolite involves the cyt.P450 system, is unidirectional, and proceeds in two steps, generating 4-hydroxy RA as a short lived intermediate (Frolik, *et al.*, 1979; Roberts, *et al.*, 1979a; Roberts, *et al.*, 1979b; Frolik, *et al.*, 1980; Frolik, 1981). Since this metabolite was found to possess lower activity than the parent RA in the tracheal organ culture bioassay (Roberts, *et al.*, 1979a; Roberts, *et al.*, 1979b) and is one of the products found in animal urine and feces (Hanni, *et al.*, 1976; Hanni & Bigler, 1977), it has been suggested that it is a product of a detoxification pathway (Rao, 1987).

Administration of single oral doses of 4-oxo RA to pregnant animals, however, produced dose-dependent increase in the frequencies of fetal malformations of the type usually associated with RA and other active retinoids (Creech-Kraft, et al., 1989; Howard, et al., 1989; Satre, et al., 1989). This compound was as active as its parent, RA, in suppressing chondrogenesis in vitro (Satre, et al., 1989), and this activity was not due to the (re)generation of RA since the back reaction did not occur (Frolik, et al., 1979; Roberts, et al., 1979a; Roberts, et al., 1979b; Frolik, 1981).

D. Metabolism in the Embryo

Retinoid metabolism in the developing conceptus is relatively unexplored, particularly during early development and organogenesis. As discussed previously, both class I and II ADH exhibit RDH activity. Studies of human fetal livers demonstrate a 50-fold increase in the level of ADH mRNA between the 20 week fetal stage and adulthood (Bilachone et al., 1986). In humans three isoenzymes of class I ADH (α,β,γ) exist. While all three are present in the adult liver, they appear to be developmentally regulated in the embryo and fetus. Analyses of human liver extracts from several stages of development indicate that a low level of α-ADH is produced in the early fetal liver, with additional low level β-ADH occuring later, followed by the appearance of γ-ADH postnatally (Smith, et al., 1971; Smith, et al., 1972; Ikuta & Yoshida, 1986; Smith, 1986). The expression pattern for the various isozymes is different in other fetal tissues (Smith, et al., 1971; Ikuta & Yoshida, 1986; Smith, 1986). The single class I ADH form in mice and rats also appears subject to developmental regulation and increasing production during late fetal and postnatal liver development (Raiha, et al., 1967; Balak, et al., 1982; Holmes, et al., 1983). These expression patterns, however, have yet to be correlated with retinol-specific metabolic activity.

The morphogenetic activity of exogenous RA in the developing chick wing-bud is well documented (see Brickell & Tickle, 1989; Brockes, 1989; Eichele, 1989 for reviews) and the presence of an endogenous gradient of RA along the axis of the wing (Thaller & Eichele, 1987) implies that localized synthesis and/or metabolic inactivation of RA is obligatory. Recent evidence indicates that the chick wing-bud is capable of metabolically generating RA from retinol (Eichele & Thaller, 1988), although the spatial and temporal features of this reaction were not determined. *In vitro* studies indicate that supernatants from homogenates of organogenesis stage mouse embryos can also synthesize RA from retinol, and that this activity may be developmentally regulated since the activity in gestation day (GD) 10 embryos was significantly greater than in later stages (Satre, 1990). An increase in polar metabolites, indicative of increased vitamin A metabolism, has also been reported to occur during this same period in rat embryos (Rainier & McCormick, 1983).

Recently, a novel metabolite, all-*trans* 3,4-didehydro RA was identified in the chick embryo (Thaller & Eichele, 1990). Application of this retinoid to chick wing-buds demonstrated that it was as active as RA in evoking digit duplications. The 3,4-didehydroRA was generated *in situ* from retinol through a 3,4-didehydroretinol intermediate (Thaller & Eichele, 1990). The presence, metabolism, and physiologic significance of this metabolite in other species has not yet been determined.

Previous studies suggested that the chick wing bud could metabolize ^{3}H-RA to more polar compounds following administration via carrier implantation (Tickle, *et al.*, 1982; Tickle, *et al.*, 1985), however, neither the identities nor the quantities of the metabolites were conclusively determined in these studies. Supernatants from homogenized GD11 embryos were found to be capable of metabolizing RA to its 4-hydroxy- and 4-oxo- metabolites (Satre & Kochhar, unpublished observations). As noted previously, these metabolites are generated via the cytochrome P450 system (Frolik, 1981; Roberts, 1981); enzyme activities of this system are much higher in human embryonic tissues than in rodents (Nau, 1985). A rigorous characterization of RA metabolism in the embryo or embryonic tissues remains to be undertaken.

Human placental tissue displays apparent esterification and

retinyl hydrolysis activity *in vitro* (Torma & Vahlquist, 1986), and supernatants from homogenized organogenesis stage mouse placentae display retinol and RA metabolic activity (Satre & Kochhar, unpublished observations).

Vitamin A Nutrition in Pregnancy

The purpose of the following sections is to provide current thinking on the role of vitamin A in pregnancy and embryo development. To this end we will focus on three principal areas: (A) changes in maternal vitamin A homeostasis during pregnancy; (B) mechanisms of placental transport of the vitamin and its metabolites; and, (C) embryo acquisition and handling of the vitamin. In general, this discussion will be confined to the earlier part of pregnancy, particularly the period around organogenesis, since it is during this period that retinoid-induced dysmorphogenesis occurs. For further information on the role of maternal vitamin A in late pregnancy, parturition, lactation, as well as in the later stage fetus and newborn, readers are directed to comprehensive reviews by Bates (1983) and Wallingford & Underwood (1986).

A. Changes in Maternal Homeostasis

As in the adult, the mammalian embryo lacks the capability for *de novo* synthesis of vitamin A. Consequently, the developing embryo is solely dependent on the maternal circulation for its acquisition of retinoids. Although the concentration of retinol in the circulation does not reflect body stores of the vitamin (except in conditions of extreme hypo- or hypervitaminosis), circulating levels are a determinant of the amount available for immediate tissue and cellular needs.

Over the past 50 years, more than 20 studies have reported changes in maternal plasma (serum) vitamin A levels during pregnancy in humans (see Bates, 1983 and Wallingford & Underwood, 1986 for reviews). The majority of these (86%) noted a decrease in circulating levels of the vitamin. In these reports, the decrease occurred in the later part of pregnancy (2nd or 3rd trimester) with nadir values exhibiting as much as a 42% decrease compared to 1st trimester or non-pregnant levels; in women followed longitudinally the decrease was closer to 25%. In general, there is a lack of consensus among these studies with respect to the magnitude or precise temporal pattern of this change, perhaps owing to differences in methodologies and analytical techniques in addition to the natural variation in a diverse human population. Furthermore, although these results suggest changes in maternal homeostasis that may have functional consequences for the mother, it is difficult to make any correlations between this phenomenon and normal embryonic acquisition of the vitamin or abnormal developmental outcome since the decrease occurs well past the period of human embryo organogenesis (Moore, 1982).

A recent, detailed longitudinal study of maternal plasma vitamin A levels during pregnancy in the mouse revealed a significant, transient, decrease in circulating levels of retinol occurring coincident with the period of organogenesis (Satre, *et al.*, 1992). The maternal plasma retinol concentration near midgestation was about 80% lower compared to circulating levels in either the same dams at the beginning of pregnancy or in age and weight matched non-pregnant females (Figure 3). This decrease appeared specific for retinol since no changes in the plasma levels of either retinyl esters or RA were observed in these animals. Deficiency was not a factor since animals were maintained on a standard commercial (vitamin A adequate) diet and corresponding liver vitamin A values indicated ample reserves. Furthermore, fetuses allowed to go to term were apparently normal. Circulating levels of retinol at the beginning of pregnancy and in non-pregnant animals were within the range observed in other strains of mice (McPhillips, *et al.*, 1987; Brouwer, *et al.*, 1988; Creech-Kraft, *et al.*, 1989; Eckhoff, *et al.*, 1989), indicating that the phenomenon was not likely related to any particular pre-existing condition.

There is little evidence that the pregnancy-associated decrease in human maternal plasma retinol reflects inadequate vitamin A nutriture unless it is obviously exacerbated by a

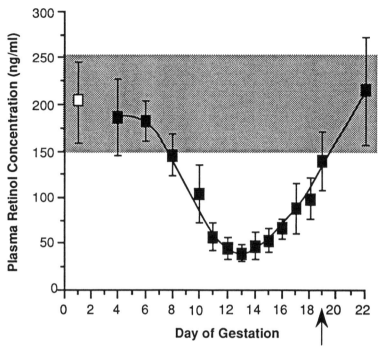

FIGURE 3. Comparison of plasma retinol concentrations in nonpregnant female (open squares; n = 23 animals) and pregnant mice (solid squares; n =≥ 7 animals per gestation day [GD]) during gestation. Values are mean ± SD. Shaded area denotes boundary of the range of values from nonpregnant animals sampled serially over the same time course. Arrow denotes day of parturition. A significant decline in retinol concentration begins on GD 10 and continues until GD 13. Thereafter, the levels gradually attain normalcy equivalent to nonpregnant females by day 19, the day of parturition (from Satre, *et al.*, 1992).

poor diet which in and of itself can result in lower circulating levels (Wallingford & Underwood, 1986) . Rather, the decrease in human maternal plasma retinol has been attributed to the hemodilution which occurs during the course of pregnancy (McGanity, *et al.*, 1954; Mattison, 1986). Relative to hematocrit, plasma vitamin A levels do not change during gestation (Dawson, *et al.*, 1969) and the 3rd trimester decrease in vitamin A and RBP appears to parallel decreases in serum albumin (Hytten & Leight, 1971) and total serum proteins (Venkatachalam, 1962). While similar hemodynamic changes may occur in other animals, the decrease observed in mice was not correlated with either a significant change in plasma protein concentration over the course of pregnancy, or with increasing body weight (Satre, *et al.*, 1992). It is worth noting that in this study the nadir concentration was followed by a steady increase over the remainder of pregnancy. Thus, levels were gradually increasing during the period most likely to exhibit hemodilution. Therefore, it is highly unlikely that the pattern of decrease observed in mice was solely due to such an alteration in hemodynamics. A similar decrease in maternal plasma retinol at mid-gestation has also been observed in the rat (Wallingford & Underwood, 1986).

The specific factors responsible for the decrease in the maternal plasma retinol are unknown. However, results from several studies indicate hormonal involvement in vitamin A homeostasis. In humans, steroids have been shown to increase maternal plasma and umbilical cord blood levels of retinol and RBP (Georgieff, *et al.*, 1988). Estrogens, either endogenous or from oral contraceptive agents, cause elevations in the circulating level of retinol, apparently as a result of an increase in circulating *holo*-RBP (Prasad, *et al.*, 1975; Yeung & Chan, 1975; Vahlquist, *et al.*, 1979; Cumming & Briggs, 1983; Olson, 1984). This estrogen mediated increase in circulating retinol may not, however, be universal among species, since rats showed no change in plasma retinol concentration in response to estrogen administration (Yeung, 1974). Studies with hepatoma cell lines and primary hepatocyte cultures indicate various degrees of hormonal modulation of RBP synthesis and secretion by other hormones (Borek, *et al.*, 1981; Dixon & Goodman, 1987). An interrelationship between hormones and vitamin A is further suggested by studies that have noted alterations in steroid hormone production in vitamin A deficiency (see Bates, 1983 for review). Further work is needed to define the role of hormones in retinoid homeostasis, particularly during pregnancy. Other factors that could contribute to the decrease in circulating retinol levels (such as increased kidney filtration of RBP, modulation of extra-hepatic RBP production and changes in systemic retinol utilization), remain to be examined.

Under certain dietary conditions, administration of RA has been shown to cause a decrease in circulating retinol levels resulting from a decreased release of retinol from the liver, (a "sparing effect" [Keilson, *et al.*, 1979; Bhat & LaCroix, 1986]). Although a decrease in maternal plasma retinol levels has also been observed in pregnant animals following administration of pharmacologic doses of RA and other retinoids (Creech-Kraft, *et al.*, 1989; Satre & Kochhar, 1989; Satre, 1990), it is unclear whether this effect in these studies is indeed the same phenomenon. It is possible that the effect observed following pharmacologic dose regimens is related directly to transport of the retinoid. Normally, RA circulates in the plasma bound to albumin, however, RA can also bind to RBP, albeit with lower affinity than retinol (Goodman, 1984). Thus, it is possible that the sudden, rapid influx resulting from a pharmacologic dose of RA (or similar retinoid) could potentially displace most, if not all of the endogenously RBP-bound retinol. An important ramification of this effect in the pregnant animal would be the delivery of a significantly high level of the retinoid to certain cells, including the relatively sensitive ones in the developing conceptus.

B. Placental Transport

The precise mechanism by which vitamin A (and other retinoids) are transferred to the developing embryo/fetus is undefined. Early studies proposed that it was β-carotene that was transferred to the fetus and subsequently converted to vitamin A (Barnes, 1951). Such a mechanism is unlikely given the relatively low circulating levels of β-carotene and the observation that embryo accumulation of vitamin A and normal developmental outcome are oberved in animals fed exclusively carotene-free diets (Takahashi, *et al.*, 1975; Ismaldi & Olson, 1982; Wallingford & Underwood, 1987). Direct transfer of retinyl esters as the primary vitamin A source is also an unlikely mechanism. As with carotenoids, retinyl esters represent only a small proportion of the vitamin A in maternal plasma (Olson, 1986; Satre, *et al.*, 1992). Recent studies indicate a relative inability of retinyl esters to enter or accumulate in the embryo. Analysis of fetal sera following maternal administration of retinyl esters revealed no significant change in fetal ester levels despite marked increases in the corresponding fraction of maternal sera (Donoghue, *et al.*, 1985; Wallingford & Underwood, 1986). Although the data suggest a relatively effective barrier to the transport of retinyl esters under conditions of normal or even moderately high intakes, pharmacologic and teratogenic doses of naturally occurring or synthetic esters can result in sustained, elevated levels of these retinoids in embryonic tissues (Reiners, *et al.*, 1988). While the possibility that these forms are an important or primary embryonic vitamin A source early in gestation has not been ruled out experimentally, it appears unlikely given the necessary metabolic capabilities required for the conversion of these substances to vitamin A active forms.

The most likely mechanism for the majority of vitamin A transfer and accumulation in the embryo involves retinol bound to RBP (*holo*RBP), with placental regulation of the transport of this complex. Indirect evidence for a role of the placenta in regulating the amount of vitamin A transferred to the embryo comes from a number of human studies comparing vitamin A and RBP levels in the maternal circulation with those in cord or fetal sera (Lewis, *et al.*, 1947; Venkatachalam, 1962; Baker, *et al.*, 1975; Ismaldi & Olson, 1975; Vahlquist, *et al.*, 1975; Baker, *et al.*, 1977; Butte & Calloway, 1982; Dostalova, 1982; Jansson & Nilsson, 1983). These studies have consistently found that the ratio favors the maternal compartment under conditions of adequate nutritional status. When the maternal serum concentration is very low, fetal concentrations often exceed those of the mother (Byrn & Eastman, 1943; McLaren & Ward, 1962; Venkatachalam, 1962; Baker, *et al.*, 1977). This inversion also occurs in rats (Takahashi, *et al.*, 1975; Wallingford & Underwood, 1986).

Pharmacokinetic studies in pregnant mice following the single dose administration of pharmacological amounts of retinol, revealed dose-dependent elevations of retinol in maternal plasma, embryo and placenta. Both the peak placental concentration and area under the concentration/time curve (AUC; reflecting exposure over time) were consistantly 2- to 3-fold greater than the corresponding values in either maternal plasma or GD 11 embryo at all dose levels (Kochhar, *et al.*, 1988; Eckhoff, *et al.*, 1989).

Previous studies in the rat provided indirect evidence for the transfer of maternal *holo*RBP to the developing conceptus and suggested that this transfer was maintained even during marginal maternal hypovitaminosis A (Takahashi, *et al.*, 1975; Takahashi, *et al.*, 1977). Studies in pregnant rhesus monkeys reported that radiolabeled RBP, TTR, and retinol were all transferred from the maternal circulation to the embryo (Vahlquist & Nilsson, 1984; Torma & Vahlquist, 1986). The specific activity of RBP in the fetus, however, reached only 13% of that in the maternal circulation, and the apparent transfer of retinol itself exceeded that of RBP, suggesting that retinol itself may be more efficiently transferred than RBP (Vahlquist & Nilsson, 1984).

Recent studies have provided direct evidence for the binding of I^{125}-*holo*RBP to specific cell-surface receptors on human placental cell membranes (Sivaprasadarao & Findlay, 1988b). Once bound, the retinol is rapidly accumulated by placental membrane vesicles while the *apo*RBP remained outside the cell (Sivaprasadarao & Findlay, 1988a). Other studies have observed that the rate of association of retinol with lipid bilayers is strongly dependent on the fatty acid acyl chain composition of the membrane lipids (Noy & Xu, 1990b). Thus, cell-specific delivery and uptake rates may be determined in part by the concentration of surface receptors as well as the cell-specific membrane lipid composition. Overall, these data suggest two distinct placental transfer mechanisms; one involving only the transport of retinol by a receptor mediated process, and another involving the uptake and transport of the intact *holo*RBP complex. The extent to which the two transfer mechanisms function simaltaneously and the existance of any gestation-associated changes in the predominant transfer mechanism remain to be determined.

Both RBP and TTR are detected in the rat placenta and visceral yolk sac around GD 14 (Soprano, *et al.*, 1986; Sklan & Ross, 1987). The first appearance of these proteins in these tissues (around GD 7) (Makover, *et al.*, 1989) preceeds their appearance in the fetal liver and other tissues (Soprano, *et al.*, 1982; Makover, *et al.*, 1989). This location and temporal expression pattern suggests that during early embryo development, the placenta (and/or visceral yolk sac) could serve as the embryonic source of these proteins. The presence of these proteins coupled with the presence of CRBP in the placenta during the same period (Kato, *et al.*, 1985a; Okuno, *et al.*, 1987) further supports the idea that the placenta plays an important role in the acquisition of vitamin A by the embryo.

In addition to the evidence presented previously for retinyl esters, results from other studies have implicated transplacental regulation of retinoids based on molecular structure. Pharmacokinetic studies in mice indicate that the all-*trans* RA is transferred to the embryo to a much greater extent than its 13-*cis* isomer. Administration of the all-*trans* form resulted in a 15-fold higher peak concentration of RA in the embryo than that following administration of an equivalent dose of 13-*cis* RA (Creech-Kraft, *et al.*, 1987; Kochhar, *et al.*, 1987). This preferential placental transfer of the all-*trans* form of the molecule has been confirmed in several mouse strains and extended to include 13-*cis*-4-oxo RA as well (Creech-Kraft, *et al.*, 1989). In these studies levels of all-*trans* RA in the embryo exceeded those of 13-*cis* RA, even when the 13-*cis* form was the administered compound. Whether these observations can be generalized to other species is not clear (Howard, *et al.*, 1989). Determination of the structural features of retinoids that influence their placental transfer will be important in understanding the developmental toxicity of these compounds.

Placental concentrations of retinol, RA, and retinyl esters remain relatively constant from GD 9 to 15 in the mouse

(Satre, *et al.*, 1992). Similarly, virtually no change in placental vitamin A concentration is observed in the rat during this developmental period or even through late gestation (Takahashi, *et al.*, 1977; Ismaldi & Olson, 1982; Wallingford & Underwood, 1986). Considering the conceptus as a developmental unit, the vitamin A content (defined as ng vitamin A per placenta or embryo) increases 5-fold from GD 9-14 (Satre, *et al.*, 1992). During early organogenesis, (GD 9-10), the placenta contains >90% of the total vitamin A content in the conceptus. Although the amount in the corresponding embryo increases rapidly, the placenta continues to contain more of the vitamin than the embryo up through GD 12. By GD 15, however, the vitamin A content of the embryo has exceeded that in the placenta by nearly 4-fold. While this pattern may be a consequence of the greater relative increase in the mass of the embryo, it could also reflect transport changes in the vitamin (and hence be indicative of changing embryonic or placental requirements).

Overall, data from a variety of studies under widely varied conditions of vitamin A nutriture suggest that, in addition to maternal plasma homeostatic mechanisms, the placenta may be capable of exerting some degree of autonomous regulation of retinol transport to the embryo.

C. Endogenous Levels in the Embryo

In studies in the mouse (Satre, *et al.*, 1992) whole embryo retinoid levels steadily increased from GD 10-16. The pattern of accumulation exhibited two phases. From GD 10-13, retinol accumulated at an apparent rate of approximately 25 ng/g/day, while the concentration of RA and retinyl esters remained essentially unchanged. A different pattern was observed between GD 13 and 16. During this period, the apparent embryo accumulation rate for both retinol and retinyl esters increased, however, the apparent rate of ester accumulation was more than 2-fold greater than that of retinol. Interestingly, the concentration of RA in the whole embryo remained relatively unchanged throughout this entire developmental period. Distinct developmental patterns of embryonic vitamin A accumulation also have been observed in the rat (Takahashi, *et al.*, 1977; Wallingford & Underwood, 1987). The earlier study described three phases of embryonic vitamin A accumulation: an early phase (GD 7-9), characterizied by a relatively large increase in retinol concentration; a second phase (GD 10-14) in which the embryonic concentration decreased; and, a third phase up until birth, of a more gradual, continued vitamin A accumulation (Takahashi, *et al.*, 1977). This general pattern was confirmed in a more recent study (Wallingford & Underwood, 1987), which further noted that the decrease in retinol concentration during mid-gestation only occurred in vitamin A sufficient animals. No decrease in mouse embryo retinol levels were observed during any period of gestation (Satre, *et al.*, 1992). This apparent difference between mice and rats may reflect a species difference. Limited evidence of species differences in vitamin A distribution and apparent placental transfer exists (Lorente & Miller, 1977). Further studies are needed to determine the reasons for this apparent difference. Apart from the transient decrease in retinol levels in the developing rat, from GD 12 on the embryonic concentrations and pattern of vitamin A accumulation are similar to those observed in the mouse.

Studies of rat (Takahashi, *et al.*, 1977; Wallingford & Underwood, 1987), mouse (Satre, *et al.*, 1992), and human fetal livers (Gebre-Medhin & Vahlquist, 1977; Montreewasuwat & Olson, 1979; Shah, *et al.*, 1987) have observed a progressive increase in the total vitamin A concentration in fetal livers beginning at midgestation and lasting through birth. Even in the early stages of its ontogeny the livers of embryonic mice and rats contain a significant proportion of the total vitamin A in the embryo. This proportion increases as gestation progresses such that near term, in the vitamin A sufficient dam, the majority of the total vitamin A in the fetus is found in the liver (Takahashi, *et al.*, 1977; Ismaldi & Olson, 1982; Wallingford & Underwood, 1987; Satre, *et al.*, 1992). In contrast, fetal livers from vitamin A deficient dams contain a much smaller proportion of the total vitamin A in the fetus, and this proportion remains essentially the same over the course of gestation (Wallingford & Underwood, 1986). In mice, GD 13 embryonic livers contained a 3-fold higher concentration of total vitamin A (retinol plus the retinyl esters), compared to the embryo as a whole. (Satre, *et al.*, 1992). The embryonic livers at this developmental age also contained a relatively higher proportion of retinyl esters (60% of the total vitamin A) compared to the GD 13 whole embryo, in which the relative proportion was only 20%. These findings suggest that the embryonic liver has developed a significant capacity for storage of vitamin A possibly as early as GD 13. This conclusion is further supported by results from radiohistochemical studies that indicated the presence of vitamin A storage cells (stellate cell) in fetal mouse livers at least as early as GD 14 (Matsumoto, *et al.*, 1984). CRBP, recently implicated in retinol esterification by rat liver microsomes (Yost, *et al.*, 1988), is also first detected in fetal rat livers around GD 11, and progressively increases over the course of gestation. The protein is initially localized only in stellate cells from GD 11-13, while after GD 14, the protein is detected in both stellate and parenchymal cells (Kato, *et al.*, 1985a). Although little is known about the development of metabolic systems during early liver organogenesis, near term fetal rat livers do exhibit the capacity for retinol esterification (Rasmussen, *et al.*, 1985).

Studies of developing rat embryos indicate a progressive increase in RBP over the course of gestation (Takahashi, *et al.*, 1977; Kato, *et al.*, 1985a). While RBP synthesis in the fetal liver is clearly evident by around GD 12-14 (Soprano, *et al.*, 1986; Sklan & Ross, 1987), mRNA for the protein has been detected in fetal rat liver primordia as early as GD 10 (Makover, *et al.*, 1989). Synthesis and secretion of the protein then progressively increase over the course of gestation (Soprano, *et al.*, 1986; Sklan & Ross, 1987; Makover, *et al.*, 1989). Altogether these studies provide strong evidence for the onset of functional development of the embryonic liver (with respect to vitamin A storage and metabolism) occurring around GD 14.

Typically, the majority of adult *holo*RBP exists in the circulation complexed with TTR with very little (3-5%) occurring in the uncomplexed form (Fex & Felding, 1984). Although early reports indicated that >95% of retinol in the fetal rat exisited in the TTR-*holo*RBP complex (Ismaldi & Olson, 1975), a number of recent studies indicate that embryonic/fetal *holo*RBP does not appear to circulate in this complex (Cullum, *et al.*, 1984; Sklan, *et al.*, 1985; Sklan & Ross, 1987). This may be attributable in part to the observation that fetal rat RBP is synthesized in a different (glycosylated) form than that in the adult (Sklan & Ross, 1987) and that the relative amounts of TTR and RBP synthesizied in the placenta, visceral yolk sac, and fetal liver are different (Sklan & Ross, 1987). Further research along these lines will certainly contribute to our knowledge of the mechanism of placental transport and mode of accumulation of retinoids in the embryo. Data from *in vitro* experiments have shown that binding of TTR to RBP causes a 2-fold increase in RBP avidity for retinol (Noy & Blaner, 1991). TTR was found to inhibit the binding of I^{125}-*holo*RBP to placental cell-surface receptors (Sivaprasadarao & Findlay, 1988b) and caused a decrease in the rate of release of ^{3}H-retinol bound to RBP (Sivaprasadarao & Findlay, 1988a).

Effects of Deficiency

The reports of Warkany and colleagues in the 1940s showed convincingly that dietary deficiencies in pregnant animals could adversely affect their developing embryos and result in malformations (see Wilson, 1977). Earlier, Hale (1933) had observed the birth of piglets without eyeballs in a vitamin A-deficient sow. Although severely deficient animals are infertile, less severe deficiency in various species (rat, pig, rabbit, monkey) produces a spectrum of fetal malformations affecting the eyes, brain, heart, and blood vessels, and the urogenital system (Palludan, 1976; Wallingford &

Underwood, 1986). In view of the paucity of definitive human studies, the results of a study on pregnant rhesus monkeys should be noted (O'Toole, *et al.*, 1974). Only four out of ten vitamin A-deficient females who mated successfully carried their pregnancies to term, and these four infants had various eye anomalies including congenital or delayed xerophthalmia, cataract, and ciliary body hyperplasia. Two of these four infants also had metaplasia of trachel/esophageal epithelia, and one had mild hydronephrosis. It is noteworthy that other gross anatomic defects seen in fetuses of deficient rats and pigs were not encountered in the monkey infants.

There is insufficient evidence to show that eye and other anomalies in human babies can occur in vitamin A-deficiency (Wallingford & Underwood, 1986). Xerophthalmic women and those suffering from night blindness, apparently due to vitamin A-deficiency, have reportedly had children afflicted with congenital xerophthalmia, anophthalmia, microphthalmia, and other eye defects. Evidence that the deficiency was the direct and the only cause of these anomalies is uncertain. Well-controlled epidemiological studies are needed to substantiate the conclusions of the isolated reports currently available in the literature. From animal studies and the recent evidence for the essential role of retinol and retinoic acid in cell differentiation and normal development (see below), the need for maintaining vitamin A-sufficiency during pregnancy cannot be overemphasized.

Wilson, *et al.* (1953) discovered that the most vulnerable period of rat gestation to vitamin A-deficiency coincided with active stages of organogenesis; supplementation with vitamin A during midgestation ameliorated maldevelopment. Pregnancy in severely deficient rats can be sustained by supplementation with RA, but animals maintained on RA alone usually resorb their conceptuses during late gestation and this is preceded by histological abnormalities in the placenta (Thompson, *et al.*, 1964; Noback & Takahashi, 1978). This indicates that retinol itself or one of its metabolites, other than RA, is indispensable for some functions in certain tissues. For additional details concerning vitamin A deficiency in pregnant animals, a recent review is recommended (Willhite, 1990).

Effects of Excess

A. *Hypervitaminosis A*

Chronic intake of vitamin A in adults invariably results in symptoms of hypervitaminosis A which can be grouped under four categories (Table 2). (Bauernfeind, 1980; Biesalski, 1989). Most of these symptoms are reversible upon cessation of intake depending on the duration and progression of the disease. Maternal hypervitaminosis A during pregnancy is teratogenic in several animal species, and evidence from several sources indicates that fetal malformations are due to the direct action of vitamin A or its derivatives on the embryo rather than the result of any of the maternal symptoms.

TABLE 2. Symptoms of Hypervitaminosis A[1]

1. CNS	increased pressure, headache, dizziness, nausea
2. LIVER	hepatomegaly, nodular cirrhosis, collagen formation
3. BONES	hyperostosis, hypercalcemia, pain, swelling
4. SKIN	dry, peeling, chelitis, brittle nails, loss of hair

[1] From Biesalski (1989)

There are several situations whereby a woman during child-bearing years may ingest excessive amounts of vitamin A: consistent consumption of vitamin A-rich foods (*e.g.*, liver), self-medication with vitamin A as nutrient supplements, and use of prescription drugs containing retinoids. Unequivocal evidence that vitamin A is teratogenic in humans comes only from the experience with 13-*cis* RA to which a large number of women became inadvertently exposed during pregnancy resulting in a fetal syndrome now known as retinoid embryopathy. This rather definitive evidence has made it possible to sort out reports from among a group of suspicious case histories numbering less than two dozen where the involvement of hypervitaminosis A in fetal malformations could be ascertained with some degree of certainty.

In this section, we discuss results of experimental studies in pregnant animals to bring out various features of retinoid-induced teratogenesis, such as comparative activities of various natural and synthetic retinoids, and particularly sensitive stages of embryonic development. This is followed by a discussion of what we know to-date about the nature of fetal malformations in human infants after maternal exposure to 13-*cis* RA and other retinoids.

(1) Laboratory Animals

Cohlan (1953; 1954) reported teratogenic effects of maternal hypervitaminosis A in pregnant rats. Healthy rats on normal diet were given orally a preparation of "natural vitamin A," presumably vitamin A esters, beginning 2-4 days after mating and ending at GD 16 (duration of gestation in the rat is 22 days). A number of exposed neonates presented such malformations as exencephaly, cleft lip and/or cleft palate, brachygnathia, and various eye defects. Giroud and colleagues (1959) extended these findings by showing that restricting dosing of rats only to a few days of gestation altered the pattern of anomalies which were stage-dependent. In addition to anencephaly, facial dysmorphia, spina bifida, syndactyly, and encephalocele, these authors also described histological abnormalities in the teeth, kidneys, and ureters of rat pups. To further refine stage-dependency of malformation, Kalter (1960) gave pregnant inbred mice a single oral dose of vitamin A palmitate, 10,000 international units (IU) per dose, on one of the GD 7-12 (birth occurs on the 19th day). A large number of embryos resorbed after treatment on GD 7 to 9. The survivors showed a specific cluster of malformations depending on the day of exposure (Kalter & Warkany, 1961). Anomalies produced affected the skin, ears, eyes, face, mouth, teeth, tongue, palate, thymus, ribs, brain, spinal cord, heart, great vessels, kidney, ureter, bladder, genital ducts, rectum, anus, tail, and limbs. Some of the defects produced were not previously recorded in rats such as supernumerary upper and lower incisors, ankyloglossia lateralis, cranio-pharyngeal duct, cervical thymus, coronary aneurysm, crossed ectopic kidney, rectovesical fistula, and absent umbilical artery.

Subsequent studies have shown that embryos of nearly all species of experimental animals are susceptible to maternal hypervitaminosis A (Geelen, 1978). In considering all natural vitamin A compounds (retinol, retinyl acetate, retiny palmitate, and all-*trans* RA) as a group, the following congenital malformations have been documented in one situation or another: exencephaly, meningocele, meningoencephalocele, spina bifida aperta or cystica, hydrocephalus, microcephaly, cyclocephaly, anophthalmia, microphthalmia, congenital cataract, coloboma, exophthalmos, hypoplastic tympanic cavity with auricular aplasia, micrognathia, median cleft mandible, mandibular ankylosis, malformed tongue and teeth, cleft palate, ventricular septal defect, overriding aorta, transposition of the great vessels, aortic stenosis, pulmonary hypoplasia, anal atresia, umbilical hernia, hydroureter, hydronephrosis, unilateral and bilateral renal or ureter agenesis, hypoplastic genital papilla, syndactyly, shortened long bones, oligodactyly, and miscellaneous skeletal malformations such as rib fusions, absent vertebrae, kyphosis, kyphoscoliosis (Kochhar & Johnson, 1965; Kochhar, 1967; Shenefelt, 1972; Geelen, 1978; Willhite, 1990).

It was later shown that all-*trans* RA was a much more potent teratogen than retinol and that the whole spectrum of congenital malformations due to maternal hypervitaminosis A was mimicked when all-*trans* RA was used alone in dosing the pregnant animals (Kochhar, 1967; Shenefelt, 1972). Since retinyl esters and retinol are capable of conversion to all-*trans* RA in the body, all-*trans* RA has been presumed to be the derivative most responsible for vitamin A-induced teratogenesis.

(2) Humans

The risk of adverse effects in the human embryo of maternal hypervitaminosis A is poorly established but is probably substantial if animal studies are taken into account. It is estimated that annually about 200 adults worldwide develop clinical symptoms of hypervitaminosis A, and certainly some of them are pregnant women. In this population, only 13 case reports are published so far describing developmental anomalies in children of exposed women. These are supplemented by a handfull of other unpublished reports (7 cases) in the FDA files (Vallet, *et al.*, 1985; Rosa, *et al.*, 1986; Rosa, 1993) for a total of 20 cases in all.

Rosa (1993) has presented a summary of congenital defects found among these 20 exposed infants and that publication should be consulted for details. A majority of women having children with congenital defects ingested 25,000 IU/day or more throughout pregnancy, a few took 2000 IU/day or less, and two ingested 150,000 IU/day during a limited period in the first trimester of pregnancy. Frequencies of organotypic defects in their children show that many organ systems were involved without any specific clustering (Table 3). Although heart and cardiovascular malformations were similar to those in children exposed to 13-*cis* RA, many of the other defects (*e.g.*, ear defects) were atypical of what later came to be characterized as the retinoid syndrome.

There are several reasons to suspect that not all of these malformations were due to hypervitaminosis A. Some of the women also took other supplements; *e.g.*, vitamin D, during pregnancy. Some of the malformations are indistinguishable from those that occur by chance in the human population; 2-3% of all newborn infants harbor anomalies. And, excepting a few instances, the syndrome is mostly unlike the retinoid syndrome due to 13-*cis* RA. In one instance, a pregnant laboratory assistant accidentally ingested a massive dose of vitamin A, estimated to contain 500,000 IU, sometime during the second month of pregnancy (Mounoud, *et al.*, 1975). The baby boy was diagnosed at 2 years of age to have Goldenhar's syndrome (hemifacial atrophy, epibulbar dermoid, micrognathia, bilateral oculomotor plasy, and unilateral preauricular tags).

Epidemiological studies undertaken to estimate the risk of birth defects due to hypervitaminosis A have been so far inconclusive, mainly because a large sample size is required

TABLE 3. Frequencies of Congenital Defects in Human Babies Exposed in utero to Vitamin A Excess or Therapeutic Retinoids[2]

(Total Cases)	Vitamin A (20)	13-cis Retinoic Acid (87)	Etretinate (12)
Heart and blood vessels	3	38	1
Craniofacial	4	26	3
Facial palsy	1	8	0
Ear, microtia	6	62	0
Eye, microphthalmia	2	3	1
Cleft lip ± cleft palate	3	0	0
Cleft palate alone	0	7	0
Brain	3	65	2
Thymus	0	7	0
Urinary	4	3	—
Gastrointestinal	2	3	0
Limb	5	1	6

[2] Adapted from Rosa (1993)

in view of the infrequent occurrence of vitamin A overdose (Vallet, *et al.*, 1985; Werler, *et al.*, 1989). Using data from the Spanish hospital-based, case-control registry, Martinez-Frias & Salvador (1990) found no statistically significant overall association between exposure to vitamin A and birth defects. The authors cautioned, however, that the data tended to suggest that some risk of teratogenic effect may exist for maternal exposure to 40,000 IU or higher.

B. Retinoic Acid

(1) Laboratory Animals

All-*trans* RA is consistently referred to in the literature as a 'potent' teratogen. The reason is that it is capable of eliciting a teratogenic response in all animal species tested so far, and this occurs at a dose which rarely produces ill-effects in the dam. Even a brief exposure during the period of organogenesis is sufficient to cause terata in virtually 100% of the fetuses of mice, rats, rabbits, and hamsters (Geelen, 1978; Willhite, 1990; Agnish & Kochhar, 1993).

Some generalizations regarding teratogenicity have emerged from a large number of experimental studies

(Shenefelt, 1972; Kochhar, 1973; Kistler, 1981; Satre & Kochhar, 1989; Agnish & Kochhar, 1993). These are:

(a) *The teratogenic response is developmental stage-dependent.* Exposure of the early postimplantation embryo (GD 8-10 in the rat) frequently results in craniofacial and overt CNS defects. Terata fails to occur if exposure occurs prior to GD 8 in the rat. Exposure occurring on GD 12-14 often is associated with limb and genitourinary defects.

(b) *The teratogenic response is dose-dependent.* Higher doses not only increase the frequency and severity of defects, they also cause embryolethality. One needs relatively low doses during early phases and higher doses during later phases of organogenesis for the teratogenic response. During the critical developmental stage of a given organ, the teratogenic response is proportional to the amount of all-trans RA localized in the embryo.

All-*trans* RA yields several metabolites in the body through isomerization and oxidation, *e.g.*, 13-*cis* RA, 11-*cis* RA, 9-*cis* RA, and 4-oxoRA; many of these are also teratogenic (Kochhar, *et al.*, 1984; Satre, *et al.*, 1989; Willhite, 1990; Kochhar & Heyman, unpublished). Since teratogenic features of 13-*cis* RA are important for comparison with its effects on the human embryo, this isomer of all-*trans* RA deserves special mention.

All therapeutic agents meant for human use are first tested for teratogenic activity in laboratory animals. In the established protocol, the dams are dosed daily during the postimplantation period so that not only the susceptibility of all aspects of organogenesis are included in the screening, but cumulative effects of the agent are also revealed. In contrast to the multiple-dose protocol, studies that aim to uncover the cellular and molecular basis of action of the teratogen prefer to employ single dose regimens. Both types of studies have shown that 13-*cis* RA produces developmental effects in embryos similar to those from all-*trans* RA, but its potency in certain species, *e.g.*, rats and mice, is lower than all-*trans*

RA. In pregnant rats, while a daily dose of up to 50 mg^{-kg} given on GD 7-15 produced no fetal effects, doses higher than 100 mg^{-kg} spared none of the exposed fetuses (Agnish & Kochhar, 1993). Cleft palate, pinna defects, exencephaly, microcephaly, spina bifida, and open eyes were the most frequently observed anomalies. Using the same protocol, a daily dose of 15 mg^{-kg} of all-*trans* RA affected all litters, and in most of the litters 65-100% of the fetuses were malformed (Agnish & Kochhar, 1993). When lowest teratogenic doses of 13-*cis* RA and all-*trans* RA under the multiple-dose regimens are compared (Table 4), it is apparent that rats and mice require much higher doses of 13-*cis* RA than all-*trans* RA for equivalent teratogenic effects. (Kistler, 1987; Hummler, *et al.*, 1990; Agnish & Kochhar, 1993; Hendrickx & Hummler, 1992).

In monkeys, however, 13-*cis* RA appears to be slightly more active as a teratogen than all-*trans* RA (Table 4). Hummler, *et al.* (1990) administered 2.5 mg^{-kg} 13-*cis* RA daily on GD 10-25 (followed by the same dose given twice daily on GD 26 and 27) to pregnant cynomolgus monkeys (*Macaca fascicularis*) and found that all fetuses (7 in number) were malformed. The lowest teratogenic dose of all-*trans* RA in the cynomolgus monkey turned out to be in the range of 5-10 mg^{-kg}, although the gestational days of exposure were not entirely the same as in the 13-*cis* RA study (Hendrickx & Hummler, 1992).

Because the maternal doses of 13-*cis* RA at which the human embryo has responded with malformations range from 0.5 to 1.5 mg^{-kg} (see later), it follows that humans are more sensitive to this retinoid than are the cynomolgus monkeys. Differences between species in bioavailability after oral doses, metabolic processing including isomerization and other pharmacokinetic parameters are among some of the explanations that have been advanced.

Some effort has been made in previous studies to address the equally puzzling phenomenon in rodents of a large disparity in teratogenic doses of the two RA isomers (Table 4). Reduced placental transfer in mice and the inability of 13-*cis*

TABLE 4. Comparison of Lowest Daily Doses (mg^{-kg}) of Retinoic Acid
Isomers Possessing Teratogenic Activity[3]

Species	13-cis RA	All-trans RA
Rat	75	0.4-2
Rabbit	5	2-10
Mouse	100	4
Cynomolgus monkey	2.5-5	5-10

[3] From Agnish & Kochhar (1993), Kistler (1987), Hendrickx & Hummler (1992), and Hummler, et al. (1990)

RA to accumulate in the embryo at concentrations requisite for teratogenesis have been reported, which explains to a great extent the reasons why higher oral doses of 13-cis RA are required (Creech-Kraft, et al., 1987; Kochhar, et al., 1987; Kochhar & Penner, 1987). There are differences between the two RA isomers in their ability to bind cellular proteins and nuclear retinoid receptors, but whether these properties impinge on their intrinsic teratogenic activities is at present an open question.

The primary targets of 13-cis RA-induced embryopathy in the cynomolgus monkey were the external ears, thymus, heart, and brain (Hummler, et al., 1990). Microtia or anotia, hypoplasia or aplasia of thymus, conotruncal defects and hypoplasia of vermis in cerebellum constituted the phenotype of the affected monkey fetuses. The monkey fetuses exposed to all-trans RA shared external ear and temporal bones defects of the 13-cis RA-treated fetuses, but showed no thymus or heart anomalies (Hendrickx & Hummler, 1992). All-trans RA-treated fetuses also had other craniofacial anomalies not seen in 13-cis RA-treated fetuses, e.g. mandibular hypoplasia and cleft palate. These differences between phenotypes may be ascribed to the small sample size inevitable in primate studies as well as to differences in the protocols followed in the two studies (Hummler, et al., 1990; Hendrickx & Hummler, 1992). However, concordance seen between the phenotypes of human babies exposed prenatally to 13-cis RA and of the cynomolgus monkeys in these and other sudies is striking (Wilson, 1974; Fantel, et al., 1977; Hendrickx, et al.,

1980). A high incidence of embryolethality in monkeys is also similar to the human experience where Lammer *et al.* (1985) reported a 20% abortion rate in women who took 13-*cis* RA within the first 10 weeks of pregnancy.

(2) Humans

13-*cis* RA was marketed under the trade name Accutane (generic name: isotretinoin) in 1982 for treatment of severe recalcitrant cystic acne, and in 1983 first cases of birth defects and instances of spontaneous abortions among drug recipients came to light (Rosa, 1993).

By April 1990, more than 40 spontaneous abortions and 87 instances of birth defect outcomes were attributable to 13-*cis* RA. The pattern of dysmorphogenesis included one or more components of malformations in the craniofacial complex, cardiovascular and central nervous systems (Table 5) (Lott, 1983; Benke, 1984; Braun, *et al.*, 1984; Cruz, 1984; Fernhoff & Lammer, 1984; Hill, 1984; Lammer, *et al.*, 1985; Lammer & Opitz, 1986; Rosa, *et al.*, 1986; Anonymous, 1991; Rizzo, *et al.*, 1991; Rosa, 1993).

The most striking feature of the syndrome is the absence or reduced size of the external ears and canals which occurred in 62 out of 87 cases (Table 3). Other craniofacial anomalies were facial asymmetry and facial palsy, micrognathia with cleft palate, and maldevelopment of the cranial bones. Thymus was reduced or absent in seven cases.

The most frequent occurrence of defects was in the CNS which included hydrocephalus, cerebellar hypoplasia, absence of vermis, and structural malformation of the cerebral cortex. Lammer & Armstrong (1991) concluded that various CNS defects arise from maldevelopment of derivatives of rhombencephalic alar plate. Preliminary findings indicate that 52% of 5-year-olds exposed during the first trimester show intellectual deficits, and these children included many (37.5%) who showed no structural CNS malformations at birth (Adams, 1990; Adams & Lammer, 1991). It is not known at present but it is probable that some neurobehavioral deficits may be encountered in children exposed to 13-*cis* RA

TABLE 5. Teratogenicity of Accutane® (13-*cis* RA) in Human Embryos[4]

0.5 to 1.5 mg/kg daily for variable period during the first 10 weeks after conception

Craniofacial defects:	Malformed external ears Midfacial and mandibular underdevelopment Wide cleft palate Absent thymus
Cardiovascular defects:	Various arch and septation anomalies
CNS:	Hydrocephalus, derivatives of rhombencephalic alar plate malformed
Limbs:	Two cases of bone dysplasia

[4] Lammer, *et al.*, 1985; Lammer & Armstrong, 1991.

during the fetal period, since the period of CNS development and maturation extends beyond the first trimester.

The cardiovascular defects occurred less frequently (38 out of 87 cases) and were less characteristic feature of the retinoid syndrome than the other defects described above. These defects could be classified as conotruncal or branchial arch tissue defects (Lammer & Opitz, 1986). Frequently observed anomalies were transposition of the great vessels, tetralogy of Fallot, truncus arteriosus communis, ventricular septal defects, interrupted aortic arch, retroesophageal right subclavian artery, and hypoplasia of the aorta (Lammer & Opitz, 1986).

Although limb defects were not encountered among the cases reported in Table 3, recently Rizzo, *et al.* (1991) described a child and a fetus who showed unusual limb reduction defects in addition to other components of the retinoid syndrome.

Lammer, *et al.* (1988) have estimated the risk for fetal malformations following maternal exposure to 13-*cis* RA during the first trimester. In that prospective study of 59 pregnancies, nine resulted in spontaneous abortions, one in a malformed stillbirth, 10 in malformed livebirths, and 37 in livebirths without apparent evidence of major malformations;

this represented a risk of 23% for fetuses that reach 20 weeks of gestation (Lammer, *et al.*, 1988).

It may be instructive to consider why so many exposures of pregnancies occurred despite warnings of teratogenic hazard of 13-*cis* RA. Cosmetic considerations allowed a more wide-spread prescription of a very effective drug intended only for recalcitrant acne. The failure of contraception device in use during treatment with 13-*cis* RA accounted for a full one-third of exposures (Lammer, *et al.*, 1985). Some other instances of exposure were preventable by various means: better communication between the dermatologist and the obstetrician, and between the physician and the patient, and knowledge of contraception methods (Rosa, 1993).

All-*trans* RA has also been used as a drug for a number of years under the trade name Retin-A® for treatment of acne, but, fortunately, it is formulated as a cream for skin application only. Its use has become more widespread since 1988 following reports suggesting its effectiveness in preventing wrinkles and ameliorating photodamage. Sporadic reports have appeared in literature of teratogenic outcome associated with the topical use of all-*trans* RA, but chance occurrences rather than causal relationships are usually indicated (Agnish & Kochhar, 1993; Camera & Pregliasco, 1992; Rosa, 1993). Experiemental studies suggest a relatively low teratogenic potential of topically applies all-*trans* RA, mainly because only limited concentrations of the drug can be externally applied from which further attenuation in the maternal circulation restricts embryonic exposure (Zbinden, 1975; Willhite, *et al.*, 1990). However, adverse outcome in human embryos resulting from topical retinoids remains a possible concern.

C. Other Retinoids

(1) Laboratory Animals

Innumerable chemical modifications have been introduced into either end of the retinol molecule and into the side-chain to generate synthetic retinoids so as to assess and compare their biological and pharmacologic properties (Table 1).

Since teratogenic effects are one of the most serious side-effects, a number of synthetic retinoids have been tested in pregnant animals (Kochhar, *et al.*, 1987; Willhite, 1990). In the teratology protocol used by us, pregnant mice are given a single oral dose on GD 11 followed by morphologic evaluation of near-term fetuses; incidences of resorption, growth retardation, palatal cleft, and limb reduction defects are consistent and reliable end-points with which to compare relative teratogenic potencies of synthetic retinoids (Kochhar, 1973; Kochhar, *et al.*, 1984; Kochhar, *et al.*, 1987). In this bioassay, 13-*cis* RA is about 4-fold less active as a teratogen than all-*trans* RA but is equal in potency to retinol (Table 6). Etretinate, an aromatic analog which has been marketed under the trade name Tigason for treatment of psoriasis, is twice as potent as all-*trans* RA. Interestingly, certain chemical modification of the molecule makes the resultant compound supremely potent teratogen; Ro 13-6307, which differs from all-*trans* RA in having an aromatic ring inserted in its side-chain next to the modified original ring, is 40-fold more active than all-*trans* RA as a teratogen (Table 6) (Kochhar & Penner, 1992). By far, the most active teratogens are benzoic and derivatives of all-*trans* RA termed arotinoids, *e.g.*, TTNPB, which is 700-fold more potent that all-*trans* RA (Zimmermann, *et al.*, 1985; Flanagan, *et al.*, 1987; Kochhar, *et al.*, 1987; Kistler, *et al.*, 1990). The chemical or biological basis for enhancement in potency is not known.

It has emerged from structure-activity correlations that an acidic end-group and a side-chain of sufficient length are necessary for a retinoid to act as a teratogen; while a ring is required at one end of the molecule for activity, the retinoid can still be an effective teratogen with changes in the ring structure that alter its lipid solubility (Willhite, 1990).

(2) Humans

Etretinate, an aromatic retinoid with an ethyl ester end group (Figure 2), marketed under the trade name Tigason (Tegison outside the United States by Sautier Laboratories, Geneva), was reported to physicians by the manufacturer in

TABLE 6. Teratogenic Potencies of Synthetic Retinoids
Relative to RA in Pregnant ICR Mice[5]

Retinoid	Structure	Tetratogenic potency
Ro 13-7410 (TTNPB)	COOH	700 X
Ro 13-6307	COOH	40 X
Etretinate (Tigason)	COOC$_2$H$_5$	2 X
13-cis RA (Isotretinoin, Accutane)	COOH	0.25 X
RA (Retinoic Acid, all-trans)	COOH	1 X
Vitamin A (Retinol)	CH$_2$OH	0.25 X

[5] Kochhar, 1973, 1987; Kochhar, et al., 1988; Kochhar & Penner, 1992.

1983 to have caused four malformed cases among patients under treatment for psoriasis. Three other cases were reported in subsequent publications (Happle, et al., 1984; Roche, 1985). Rosa (1993) concluded from a summary of a total of 12 birth outcomes ascribed to etretinate that the anomalies showed dissimilarities to the 13-cis RA syndrome (Table 3). Limb anomalies occurred more prominently (6 cases) while ear, cardiac and thymus defects were less frequent. In view of the small number of cases and the bias in reporting only the abnormal outcomes after etretinate therapy, risk estimates are not available.

Lammer (1988) reported an unusual occurrence of a malformed baby who was conceived 11 months after discontinuation of etretinate therapy where the defects resembled the retinoid syndrome. Although others have questioned if etretinate was really the causative agent in this case (Blake & Wyse, 1988), it is known that daily dosing with etretinate results in its accumulation in the body and detectable concentrations of etretinate and its metabolite acitretin have been detected in circulation in patients even at one year after cessation of treatment (Paravicini, *et al.*, 1981; Massarella, *et al.*, 1985). There are other reports of fetal malformations where conception occurred several months after cessation of etretinate therapy (Grote, *et al.*, 1985).

It is particularly disturbing that teratogenic effects occurred even when very low levels of the retinoid were detected in circulation. If these reports are confirmed, etretinate would seem to be a very potent teratogen in humans. In view of its long half-life in the body, it has been recommended that women patients contemplating pregnancy avoid the use of this drug for at least one, if not two, years prior to conception (Ward, *et al.*, 1983; Bollag, 1985). In the United States, package insert for the drug warns that "the period of time during which pregnancy must be avoided after treatment is concluded has not been determined." Because of the shorter half-life, acitretin, an analog of etretinate without the ethyl ester end group (Table 1), is currently considered a more desirable drug instead of etretinate.

Mechanisms of Teratogenesis

Research into the causation of drug-induced congenital anomalies have identified the vulnerability of a number of developmental events that may go awry; some of the events especially implicated in retinoid-induced teratogenesis are listed (Table 7). Many of the listed events are not mutually exclusive and may, in fact, be interdependent. It is not known at present if there is a primary target in the early embryo for retinoids which may lead to multiple sequelae as development

TABLE 7. Events in Teratogenesis

Growth misregulation
Failed midline fusion
Failed tissue interactions
Failed cell differentiation
Failed pattern formation
Ectopic cell death

proceeds. As the major organ systems that are components of the retinoid syndrome, *e.g.*, face, ear, brain, heart, aortic arches, and thymus, receive contributions from the neural crest cells, the latter may be a special target (Lammer, *et al.*, 1985; Anonymous, 1991). The earlist changes observed in embryos of retinoid-exposed animals were in cell cycle parameters of susceptible cell populations in neural tube, facial processes and the limb bud; this effect triggered other events including excessive cell death which disrupted the program of cell differentiation and organogenesis (Langman & Welch, 1967; Kochhar, 1968; Kochhar, 1977). Endogenous RA has been suggested to particpate in organogenetic pattern formation in normal vertebrate embryos through transcriptional control of important developmental genes such as the homeobox (*Hox*) genes, and this action is most likely mediated by its nuclear receptors (see reviews in Brockes [1989] and Tabin [1991]). This has strengthcncd the notion that an excess of RA may result in maldevelopment through an ectopic or chaotic expression of genes which disrupt pattern formation. If this turns out to be true, it is reasonable to suggest that most of cellular changes that have been observed to-date in retinoid-exposed embryos such as cell division, cell differentiation, cell interactions, migrations, and cell death could all emanate from a subtle disruption induced at the inception of organogenesis in the pattern of expression of developmental control genes.

We have hitherto relied on cells grown in culture for most of the leads on molecular role of RA in cell function or dysfunction. Many of these may not be applicable to what actually pertains to teratogenesis. Here, we summarize information from the few investigations that have been carried out in whole embryos from dams exposed to teratogenic doses of RA and other retinoids.

(A) Receptors and Binding Proteins

Discovery of nuclear RA receptors has significantly advanced our understanding of the molecular basis of RA function (Ruberte, *et al.*, 1991b). These receptors are RA-inducible transcription regulatory factors which transduce the RA signal at the level of gene expression. Three distinct receptors exist in mammalian cells: RAR-α, β and γ for which RA serves as a specific ligand (Giguere, *et al.*, 1987; Petkovich, *et al.*, 1987; Benbrook, *et al.*, 1988; Brand, *et al.*, 1988; Krust, *et al.*, 1989; Zelent, *et al.*, 1989). The genes for each of the RARs produce multiple isoforms by differential promotor usage and alternative splicing (Ruberte, *et al.*, 1991b, for review). Three additional receptors (RXR-α, β and γ) have been identified for which the favored ligand is an RA metabolite, 9-*cis* RA (Mangelsdorf, *et al.*, 1990; Heyman, *et al.*, 1992; Levin, *et al.*, 1992). In addition to the receptors, there are two other proteins which specifically bind to RA, CRABP I and II. As mentioned above, these proteins are much smaller in molecular weight than the nuclear receptors, are located in the cytoplasm, and show tissue and stage-dependent distribution in the embryo (Sani & Hill, 1976; Ong, 1985; Perez-Castro, *et al.*, 1989; Dencker, *et al.*, 1990; Maden, *et al.*, 1990; Vaessen, *et al.*, 1990; Ruberte, *et al.*, 1991a; Maden, *et al.*, 1992). Although the functions of these proteins are not entirely clear, it is believed that they serve as carrier proteins and play an important role in sequestering excess RA and thus protect against its toxicity (Balling, 1991).

(1) Distribution in the Embryo

Detailed *in situ* hybridization analyses have shown that the three RAR mRNAs are widely distributed in the developing mouse embryo (Dolle, *et al.*, 1990; Ruberte, *et al.*, 1991a; Ruberte, *et al.*, 1991b). The relative expression of each receptor type (α, β, and γ) varies from tissue to tissue and from stage to stage. While RAR-α transcripts are ubiquitously distributed, RAR-β and γ transcripts show distinct patterns of localization. In early embryos, RAR-β and γ genes are expressed in mutually exclusive domains; *e.g.*, RAR-β in the neural epithelium and RAR-γ in the underlying mesenchyme. In later development, only RAR-β shows the most restricted spatial distriubtion; its transcripts are found only in the frontonasal mesenchyme, particularly around the developing eyes, and in the lateral nasal and maxillary processes. None of the pharyngeal arches containing neural crest cells show the presence of RAR-β transcripts, while these tissues show high levels of RAR-α and γ transcripts, particularly in the neural crest-derived frontonasal mesenchyme (Dolle, *et al.*, 1990; Ruberte, *et al.*, 1991a).

In the early limb bud, RAR-α and γ transcripts are uniformly distributed throughout the mesenchyme while RAR-β is expressed only in the most proximally located mesenchyme (Dolle, *et al.*, 1990). With further development, RAR-α transcripts remain uniformly distributed while RAR-β and γ transcripts become gradually more restricted: RAR-β in the interdigital mesenchyme and in the central core region between the primordia of radius and ulna, RAR-γ in the precartilaginous condensations and later in the cartilage skeleton of the limb as well as of the whole body (Dollc, *et al.*, 1990; Ruberte, *et al.*, 1991a). These observationss implicate individual receptors as mediators of specific functions of RA in multiple tissues.

As mentioned, each of the three RAR genes are expressed in both adult and embryonic tissues as multiple isoforms which differ from each other at the 5′-end sequence, the region which presumably performs cell- and promoter-specific transcription activation function (Kastner, *et al.*, 1990; Leroy, *et al.*, 1991; Ruberte, *et al.*, 1991b; Zelent, *et al.*, 1991). The three RAR genes are expressed as eight major isoforms (α1, α2, β1-4, γ1, γ2), each of which is detectable by Northern blot analysis in the mouse embryos at various stages of gestation (Kastner, *et al.*, 1990; Leroy, *et al.*, 1991; Zelent, *et al.*, 1991; Nagpal, *et al.*, 1992). In general, a relative decrease of RAR-β2 and γ2 isoform mRNA level is observed during the course of embryogenesis with a concomitant increase in RAR-β1/β3 and γ1 mRNA (Kastner, *et al.*, 1990; Ruberte, *et al.*, 1991b; Zelent, *et al.*, 1991). This pattern suggests that some of the effects of RA may occur through isoform-specific functions (Ruberte, *et al.*, 1991b).

Only limited data are available on the presence and distribution of RXR genes (RXR-α, β, γ) in the mouse embryo, but preliminary results show that these genes are also expressed in a broad spectrum of tissues displaying unique patterns which only partially overlap with that of RARs (Mangelsdorf, et al., 1992). From the distribution pattern, it is probable that the RXR gene family is involved not only in implantation, embryogenesis and CNS differentiation, but also in aspects of adult physiology (Mangelsdorf, et al., 1992).

(2) Influence of Retinoid Treatment

The obvious developmental modulation of retinoid receptors in normal embryos has raised the question of what role(s) these receptors play in teratogenesis, and if retinoid treatment alters the expression or distribution of any receptor subtype or isoform. RA treatment of F9 and P19 embryonal carcinoma cells (EC) has been shown to increase the levels of RAR-α2 and RAR-β1, β2, β3, and β4 mRNAs while others (γ1 and γ2) are decreased (Kastner, et al., 1990; Leroy, et al., 1991; Zelent, et al., 1991; Nagpal, et al., 1992).

The expression of certain RAR isoforms has also recently been found to be altered in mouse embryos after exposure to teratogenic doses of RA, but the response is somewhat different from that of EC cells. It was found that while mRNA levels for RAR-α1, β1 and β3 were unaffected, those for RAR-α2 and β2 were elevated in embryos from mice treated with RA on day 11 of gestation (Harnish, et al., 1992; Kochhar, et al., 1993). Interestingly, RAR-β2 mRNA was specifically elevated in tissues which usually show the highest susceptibility to teratogenesis on day 11 of gestation; e.g., limb buds and craniofacial tissues. An overexpression of this isoform after RA treatment was also reported in the limb bud core mesenchyme and other tissues of transgenic mice carrying RAR-β2 promoter fused to the bacterial β-galactosidase gene (Mendelsohn, et al., 1991; Balkan, et al., 1992). These preliminary studies suggest that specific isoforms of the RARs, in particular RAR-β2, may mediate at least some of the teratogenic effects of RA.

(B) Pattern Formation

Pattern formation is defined as a process of spatial organization of cells and tissues within a developing organ so that shape and function are corrdinated in such a way that a whole, identifiable embryo emerges. The process includes both molecular and supramolecular components where, at present, only the molecular entities have been the subject of intense investigation. We believe that an understanding of the many aspects of pattern formation is crucial to resolving mechanisms of teratogenesis, since the process involves three-dimensional coordination of such events as tissue-interactions, cell growth, differentiation, cell-cell communication, and cell death (Tabin, 1991).

The first definitive evidence that the retinoids were involved in pattern formation came from an observation that endogenous RA extracted from chick limb buds, and inserted back into the anterior margin of a normal chick wing bud, induced a mirror-image duplication of the digits in the resultant limb (Eichele, 1989, for review). An analysis of the genesis of the new pattern suggested that RA had respecified information in the cells of the anterior margin so that they behaved as posterior margin cells, thus unfolding a new yet precise, mirror-image, pattern (Brickell & Tickle, 1989; Eichele, 1989; Tickle & Brickell, 1991).

The question of how RA respecified this information, called positional information, has intrigued developmental biologists for some years, and some possible clues are available. RA alters the expression pattern of a large number of genes; among them is one important class of genes called the homeobox genes which are linked intimately with pattern formation in animals from *Drosophila* to man (Akam, 1989). The mammalian genome contains 38 *Hox* genes dispersed in four clusters; a given *Hox* gene can be defined with respect to its presence within a particular cluster and with respect to its relative position within that cluster. The expression patterns of *Hox* genes during embryogenesis suggest that proteins coded by these genes could be used as positional cues in the determination of organization of cellular components within the developing organ (Akam, 1989; Izpisua-Belmonte, *et al.*, 1991).

Several reports found that RA was able to induce in EC cells *in vitro* the expression of genes in all four *Hox* clusters (Mavilio, *et al.*, 1988; Simeone, *et al.*, 1991). Also, some members of the clusters, located towards the 3'-end of group, were induced earlier and at lower RA concentrations than those located at 5'-end. In the chick embryo wing bud, introduction of RA induced individual members of *Hox*-4 cluster in the anterior tissue, thus duplicating the sequential expression of these genes that normally occurs in the posterior tissue in the absence of exogenous RA (Izpisua-Belmonte, *et al.*, 1991; Tickle & Brickell, 1991). The authors, however, considered such activation of *Hox* genes as an indirect effect requiring the presence of other factors since the ectopic expression domains were significantly smaller than normal and required a prolonged treatment interval.

Only fragmentary information is available on the role of RA-induced changes in *Hox* gene expression in teratogenesis. Using a low oral dose of RA in pregnant mice, Kessel & Gruss (1991) described a number of subtle alterations in the axial skeleton in resultant fetuses, and these alterations followed the same time-dependent, cranio-caudal sequence as changes in the expression of multiple, level-specific, *Hox* genes. From these studies, the authors (Kessel & Gruss, 1991) proposed that normal development at each vertebral level is specified by a combination of functionally active *Hox* genes, which they call a "*Hox* code." According to this concept, exogenous RA interferes with the normal establishment of *Hox* codes and thus produces stage-dependent alterations in morphogenesis. Although verification of this concept will require a concerted and labor-intensive effort, it is encouraging that the proposal is testable. It was recently reported that RA treatment of mouse embryos on GD 9 scrambled the spatio-temporal expression of two genes, *Hox-2.9* and *Krox-20*, in the hindbrain and the associated neural crest cells; the treatment resulted in the reduced size of the hindbrain and an absence of rhombomeric segmentation (Morriss-Kay, 1991; Morriss-Kay, *et al.*, 1991).

(C) Ectopic Cell Death

Although cell death is encountered in embryonic tissues after treatment with a number of unrelated teratogens, its occurrence in retinoid-treated embryos has elicited special attention (Schweichel & Merker, 1973; Scott, *et al.*, 1980; Knudsen & Kochhar, 1981; Sulik, *et al.*, 1988; Alles & Sulik, 1990). Physiological cell death is long recognized as an important component of pattern formation and organogenesis in normal embryos, yet it has been difficult to unravel molecular mechanisms associated with the process (Glucksmann, 1951; Saunders, 1966; Fallon & Saunders, 1968; Lockshin & Zakeri, 1991). In view of the morphogenetic role of endogenous RA in the embryo, the phenomenon of retinoid-induced cell death may provide a model in which one could study the cytologic and molecular correlates of cell death and further dissect the functions of the genes involved.

Certain early phases of mammalian development of the brain, neural tube derivatives, pharyngeal arches, heart, and skeletal primordia are susceptible to the action of exogenously supplied RA, and the susceptibility of each system varies with the embryonic stage of exposure (Shenefelt, 1972; Kochhar, 1973; Webster, *et al.*, 1986). As close scrutiny of the skeletal primordia of the limb bud has revealed, the effects of RA are likely to originate from a disruption of an early event in the process of cell differentiation (Kochhar, 1977). The sensitive event is likely shared by primorida of all affected organs of the RA-exposed embryo. The suggestion that the teratogenic effects of RA are not due to random episodes of cytotoxicity, previously characterized as necrosis (Kochhar, 1973; Sulik & Alles, 1991), but mediated by specific genomic activation (or suppression) is strengthened by the discovery that the RA receptors are ligand-activated transcription factors capable of activating specific genes.

Of the two distinct processes by which cells die, necrosis

and apoptosis, the cytological appearance of cells affected by RA favor apoptosis (Lockshin & Zakeri, 1990; Jiang & Kochhar, 1992). Necrosis denotes the process where acutely traumatized cells undergo rapid swelling of cytoplasmic and nuclear contents followed by lysis (Table 8) (Farber, 1985). Apoptosis defines a more active process where the affected cell controls, at least partially, its own demise; the cell shrinks and the nuclear contents condense. This is accompanied by a disintegration of the chromatin, finally resulting in fragmentation of the cell itself into dark "apoptotic" bodies and followed by phagocytosis (Wyllie & Morris, 1982; Arends & Wyllie, 1991).

TABLE 8. The Process of Cell Death

Necrosis	Apoptosis
Passive pathological process occurs due to hypoxia, ischemia, and toxins	Active morphogenetic process occurs in organogenesis, metamorphosis, tumor regression, atrophy
Affects large cell population	Affects cells within an organ field
Cells: Loss of synthetic functions Increase in cell volume Swelling of organelles Disruption of membranes	Active RNA and protein synthesis Shrinkage in volume but intact organelles Chromatin condensations Final fragmentation into dark bodies
Ca^{++} dependent activation of phospholipases	Induction of tissue transglutaminase

Recent investigations suggest that one of the proteins specifically induced during apoptosis is the peptide cross-linking enzyme tissue transglutaminase (Fesus, *et al.*, 1987). Tissue transglutaminase (tTG) is a member of a family of Ca^{++}-dependent enzymes that catalyze acyl-transfer reaction between peptide-bound glutamine residues and the ε-amino group of lysine residues of other peptide substrates (Folk, 1980). Fesus, *et al.* (1987) found an induction and activation of tTG in hepatocytes undergoing cell death during involution of the liver in response to chemically-induced hyperplasia. Piacentini, *et al.* (1991) found that tTG was expressed in cells undergoing apoptosis in two human tumor cell lines in culture. The exact function of tTG in cell death is not clear, but one could envisage its role similar to that of epidermal trans-glutaminas which cross-links epidermal proteins during terminal differentiation of the cell and formation of the epidermal envelope (Green, 1977; Folk, 1980). Such action would prevent organelles of the dying cell from dispersing into the extracellular space until the cell fragments are disposed off by phagocytosis. RA is capable of inducing tTG activity in several myeloid and tumor cell lines (Scott, *et al.*, 1982; Chiocca, *et al.*, 1988), and this has been shown to be due to activation of transcription of the gene that codes tTG (Chiocca, *et al.*, 1988).

Recently, we investigated if the maternal treatment with a teratogenic dose of RA influenced tTG activity in the embryonic limb buds at a time when cell death was also induced in the target organ (Jiang & Kochhar, 1992). We found that the limb buds experienced a rapid increase in tTG activity after RA treatment, 2-fold higher than the basal level at 1.5 h after treatment and almost 3-fold higher at 3 h. This increase was transient since by 6 h of treatment the tTG activity of the limb buds returned to the basal level. In contrast to the limb buds, maternal liver tTG activity experienced no change after RA treatment.

The increase in tTG activity effected by RA coincided in its onset with the first appearance of isolated apoptotic cells in the limb bud. The peak increase in tTG activity occurred at 3 h after treatment, a time when most of the apoptotic cells were still extracellular in location. The observation that by 6 h after treatment the tTG activity showed a return to the basal level of control limb buds indicated that the transient increase may be more important for the initial phases of cell death rather than phagocytosis which continued for several hours subsequently. The time-course of the induction and decline in tTG activity also closely follows the kinetic profile of RA concentrations in the limb bud following the teratogenic dose of RA to pregnant ICR mice (Satre & Kochhar, 1989).

Although our results only indicate that tTG activity is coincidental to apoptosis, a previous study has shown that the two events may be more intimately related (Piacentini, *et al.*,

1991). With the help of specific antibodies raised against human red blood cell soluble tTG, these authors showed that RA treatment of two human tumor cell lines not only increased tTG activity but also that the enzyme specifically accumulated in the apoptotic cells. The frequency of apoptosis was also increased after RA treatment (Piacentini, *et al.*, 1991). Several questions remain to be answered. It is important to determine if the increase in tTG activity in the limb bud occurs at the transcriptional or post-transcriptional level and if the process is mediated by the RARs. It will be necessary to define the site of action of tTG in the affected cell by first characterizing the substrates for the enzyme and then clarifying the role of tTG in apoptosis.

Summary and Conclusions

Vitamin A undergoes a series of metabolic processes during its absorption, transport, storage, and cellular uptake. One of the more important event is the formation of retinoic acid (RA) and a few other derivatives which directly interact with cellular and subcellular components including the nuclear receptors; the latter transduce the signal(s) at the level of the genome. Precise cellular site for the metabolic steps or organ-specific capability for generating RA is not fully known. Highly pleiotropic effect of RA in the body may result from a multiplicity of receptors and their isoforms which mediate these effects.

There is a high probability that oral intake of retinoids as therapeutic or nutritive supplements during pregnancy may result in fetal malformations. Retinoic acid and its synthetic congeners produce qualitatively similar fetal defects in a given animal species, but their potencies differ from one another by several orders of magnitude. While minor differences in teratogenic potency between retinoids can be reconciled on the basis of pharmacokinetic disposition in maternal and fetal compartments, major differences remain unexplained and may reside in the specificity of interaction with the receptors and/or the manner in which the activated receptor functions.

Vitamin A (retinol) in excess is likely to be teratogenic in human as it most certainly is in laboratory animals. Several lines of evidence suggest that metabolic conversion to RA and other derivatives mediates the teratogenic activity of vitamin A.

Endogenous RA has been suggested to participate in organogenetic pattern formation in normal vertebrate embryos through transcriptional control of important developmental genes such as the homeobox (*Hox*) genes, and this action is most likely mediated by its nuclear receptors. This has strengthened the notion that an excess of RA may result in maldevelopment throught an ectopic or chaotic expression of genes which disrupt pattern formation. If further evidence could be obtained to support this proposal, then one could argue that most of the cellular changes observed to-date in retinoid-exposed embryos (such as cell division, cell differentiation, cell interactions, migrations, and cell death) could all emanate from a subtle disruption induced at the inception of organogenesis in the pattern of expression of developmental control genes.

Acknowledgments

We acknowledge the assistance of John Penner for maintaining and assembling the reference data base. Reneé Anderson and Wanda Evans skillfully word-processed and assembled the manuscript. We thank Dr. Narsingh Agnish for reviewing several parts of the manuscript. Original studies reported here were funded by N.I.H. grant #HD-20925 and were aided by Reproductive Hazards in the Workplace, Home, Community, and Environment Research Grant #15-FY92-0059 from the March of Dimes Birth Defects Foundation.

References

Adams, J. (1990). High incidence of intellectual deficits in

5-year old children exposed to isotretinoin *in utero*. *Teratology* 41:614.

Adams, J., and Lammer, E. J. (1991). Relationship between dysmorphology and neuropsychological function in children exposed to isotretinoin *"in utero.*" Pages 159-168 *in* T. Fujii & G. J. Boer, eds., *Functional Neuroteratology of Short Term Exposure to Drugs*. Teikyo University Press, Tokyo.

Adinolfi, A., Adinolfi, M., and Hopkinson, D. A. (1984). Immunological and biochemical characterization of the human alcohol dehydrogenase chi-ADH isoenzyme. *Ann. Hum. Genet.*, 48:1-10.

Agnish, N. D., and Kochhar, D. M. (1993). Developmental toxicology of retinoids. Pages 47-76 *in* G. Koren, ed., *Retinoids in Clinical Practice*. Marcel Dekker, New York.

Akam, M. (1989). *Hox* and *Hom*: Homologous gene clusters in insects and vertebrates. *Cell* 57:347-349.

Algar, E. M., Seeley, T.-L., and Holmes, R. S. (1983). Purification and molecular properties of mouse alcohol dehydrogenase isoenzymes. *Eur. J. Biochem.* 137:139-147.

Alles, A. J., and Sulik, K. K. (1990). Retinoic acid-induced spina bifida: Evidence for a pathogenetic mechanism. *Development* 108:73-81.

Anonymous. (1987). Teratology Society Position Paper: Recommendations for vitamin A use during pregnancy. *Teratology* 35:269-275.

Anonymous. (1991). Recommendations for isotretinoin use in women of childbearing potential – Report from The Public Affairs Committee and the Council of the Teratology Society. *Teratology* 44:1-6.

Arends, M. J., and Wyllie, A. H. (1991). Apoptosis - mechanisms and roles in pathology. *Intern. Rev. Experim. Path.* 32:223-254.

Baker, H., Thind, I. S., Frank, O., DeAngelis, R., Caterini, H., and Louria, D. B. (1977). Vitamin levels in low-birthweight infants and their mothers. *J. Obstet. Gynecol.* 129:521-524.

Baker, H., Thompson, F. O., Langer, A. D., Munves, A.,

DeAngelis, B., and Kaminetzky, H. A. (1975). Vitamin profile of 174 mothers and newborns at parturition. *Amer. J. Clin. Nutr.* 28:59-65.

Balak, K. J., Keith, R. H., and Felder, M. R. (1982). Genetic and developmental regulation of mouse liver alcohol dehydrogenase. *J. Biol. Chem.* 257:15000-15007.

Balkan, W., Colbert, M., Bock, C., and Linney, E. (1992). Transgenic indicator mice for studying activated retinoic acid receptors during development. *Proc. Natl. Acad. Sci. USA.* 89:3347-3351.

Balling, R. (1991). CRABP and the teratogenic effects of retinoids. *Trends Gen.* 7:35-36.

Bank, P. A., Cullum, M. E., Jensen, R. K., and Zile, M. H. (1989). Effect of hexachlorobiphenyl on vitamin A homeostasis in the rat. *Biochim. Biophys. Acta.* 990:306-314.

Barnes, A. C. (1951). The placental metabolism of vitamin A. *Amer. J. Obstet. Gynecol.* 61:368-372.

Barua, A. B., and Olson, J. A. (1984). Metabolism and biological activity of all-trans 4,4-difluororetinyl acetate. *Biochim. Biophys. Acta* 199:128-134.

Barua, A. B., and Olson, J. A. (1986). Retinoyl beta-glucuronide. An endogenous compound of human blood. *Amer. J. Clin. Nutr.* 43:481-485.

Barua, A. B., and Olson, J. A. (1987). Chemical synthesis and growth-promoting activity of all-trans retinyl β-glucuronide. *Biochem. J.* 244:231-234.

Bates, C. J. (1983). Vitamin A in pregnancy and lactation. *Proc. Nutr. Soc.* 42:65-79.

Batres, R. O., and Olson, J. A. (1987). Relative amount and ester composition of vitamin A in rat hepatocytes as a function of the method of cell preparation and of total liver stores. *J. Nutr.* 117:77-82.

Bauernfeind, J. C. (1971). Carotenoid vitamin A precursors and analogs in foods and feeds. *J. Agric. Food Chem.* 20:456-473.

Bauernfeind, J. C. (1980). "The safe use of vitamin A." A report of the international vitamin A consultative group (IVACG). Nutrition Foundation, New York.

Beisswenger, T. B., Holmquist, B., and Vallee, B. L. (1985). X-ADH is the sole alcohol dehydrogenase isoenzyme of mammalian brains: Implications and inferences. *Proc. Natl. Acad. Sci. USA.* 82:8369-8373.

Benbrook, D., Lernhardt, E., and Pfahl, M. (1988). A new retinoic acid receptor identified from a hepatocellular carcinoma. *Nature* 333:669-672.

Bendich, A., and Langseth, L. (1989). Safety of vitamin A. *Amer. J. Clin. Nutr.* 49:358-371.

Benke, P. J. (1984). The isotretinoin syndrome. *J. Amer. Med. Assoc.* 251:2367-2369.

Bhat, M. K., and Cama, H. R. (1979). Gonadal cell surface receptor for plasma retinol-binding protein. *Biochem. Biophys. Res. Commun.* 587:273-281.

Bhat, P. V., and LaCroix, A. (1983). Separation and estimation of retinyl fatty acyl esters in tissues of normal rat by high-performance liquid chromatography. *J. Chromatog.* 272:269-278.

Bhat, P. V., and LaCroix, A. (1986). Effects of retinoic acid on the metabolism of vitamin A in rat liver. *Nutr. Res.* 6:429-435.

Bhat, P. V., Poissant, L., Falardeau, P., and Lacroix, A. (1988). Enzymatic oxidation of all-trans retinol to retinoic acid in rat tissues. *Biochem. Cell Biol.* 66:735-740.

Biesalski, H. K. (1989). Comparative assessment of the toxicology of vitamin A and retinoids in man. *Toxicology* 57:117-161.

Bilachone, V., Duester, G., Edwards, Y., and Smith, M. (1986). Multiple mRNAs for human alcohol dehydrogenase (ADH): Developmental and tissue-specific differences. *Nucleic Acids Res.* 14:3911-3926.

Bishop, P. D., and Griswold, M. D. (1987). Uptake and metabolism of retinol in cultured sertoli cells: Evidence for a kinetic model. *Biochemistry* 26:7511-7518.

Blake, K. O., and Wyse, R. K. H. (1988). Embryopathy in infant conceived year after termination of maternal etretinate: A reappraisal. *Lancet* 2:1254.

Blaner, W. S. (1989). Retinol-binding protein: The serum

transport protein for vitamin A. *Endocrine Rev.* 10:308-316.

Blaner, W. S., Hendriks, H. F. J., Brouwer, A., de Leeuw, A. M., Knook, D. L., and Goodman, D. S. (1985). Retinoids, retinoid binding proteins and retinyl palmitate hydrolase activities distributions in different types of rat liver cells. *J. Lipid. Res.* 26:1241-1251.

Blomhoff, R., Berg, T., and Norum, K. R. (1987). Absorption, transport and storage of retinol. *Chem. Scripta* 27: 169-177.

Blomhoff, R., Berg, T., and Norum, K. R. (1988). Transfer of retinol from parenchymal to stellate cells in liver is mediated by retinol-binding protein. *Proc. Natl. Acad. Sci. USA.* 85:3455-3458.

Blomhoff, R., Drevon, C. A., Eskild, W., Helgerud, P., Norum, K. R., and Berg, T. (1984). Clearance of acetyl low density lipoprotein by rat liver endothelial cells. *J. Biol. Chem.* 259:8898-8903.

Blomhoff, R., Green, M. H., Berg, T., and Norum, K. R. (1990). Transport and storage of vitamin A. *Science* 250: 399-404.

Blomhoff, R., Helgerud, P., Rasmussen, M., Berg, T., and Norum, K. R. (1983). *In vivo* uptake of chylomicron 3H-retinyl ester by rat liver: Evidence for retinol transfer from parenchymal to nonparenchymal cells. *Proc. Natl. Acad. Sci. USA.* 79:7326-7330.

Blomhoff, R., Norum, K. R., and Berg, T. (1985). Hepatic uptake of [3H]retinol bound to the serum retinol-binding protein involves both parencymal and perisinusoidal stellate cells. *J. Biol. Chem.* 260:13571-13575.

Boleda, M. D., Julia, P., Moreno, A., and Pares, X. (1989). Role of extrahepatic alcohol dehydrogenase in rat ethanol metabolism. *Arch. Biochem. Biophys.* 274:74-81.

Bollag, W. (1985). New retinoids with potential use in humans. Pages 274-288 *in* J. H. Saurat, ed., *Retinoids: New Trends in Research and Therapy.* Karger, Basel.

Borek, C., Smith, J. E., Soprano, D. R., and Goodman, D. S. (1981). Regulation of retinol-binding protein metabolism by glucocorticoid hormones in cultured H4II EC3 liver cells. *Endocrinology* 109:386-391.

Brand, N., Petkovich, M., Krust, A., Chambon, P., De The, H., Marchio, A., Tiollais, P., and Dejean, A. (1988). Identification of a second human retinoic acid receptor. *Nature* 332:850-853.

Branden, C.-I., Jornvall, H., Eklund, H., and Furugren, B. (1975). Alcohol dehydrogenases. Pages 103-190 *in* P. D. Boyer, ed., *The Enzymes*, Vol. XI. Academic Press, New York.

Braun, J. T., Franciosi, R. A., Mastri, A. R., Drake, R. M., and O'Neil, B. L. (1984). Isotretinoin dysmorphic syndrome. *Lancet* (8375):506-507.

Brickell, P. M., and Tickle, C. (1989). Morphogens in chick limb development. *BioEssays* 11:145-149.

Brockes, J. P. (1989). Retinoids, homeobox genes, and limb morphogenesis: specification of the limb and its axes in the chick limb bud and urodele blastema. *Neuron* 2:1285-1294.

Brouwer, A., Blaner, W. S., Kukler, A., and Van Den Berg, K. R. (1988). Study on the mechanism of interfernce of 3,4,3′,4′-tetrachlorobiphenyl with the plasma retinol-binding proteins in rodents. *Chem-Biol. Interactions* 68:203-271.

Brouwer, A., Van Den Berg, K. R., and Kukler, A. (1985). Time and dose responses of the reduction in retinoid concentrations in C57BL/Rij and DBA/2 mice induced by 3,4,3′,4′-tetrachlorobiphenyl. *Toxicol. Appl. Pharm.* 78: 180-189.

Brown, M. S., Kovanen, P. T., and Goldstein, J. L. (1981). Regulation of plasma cholesterol by lipoprotein receptors. *Science* 212:628-635.

Burnett, K. G., and Felder, M. R. (1978). *Peromyscus* alcohol dehydrogenase: Lack of cross-reacting material in enzyme-negative animals. *Biochem. Genet.* 16:1093-1105.

Burnett, K. G., and Felder, M. R. (1980). Ethanol metabolism in *Peromyscus* genetically deficient in alcohol dehydrogenase. *Biochem. Pharmacol.* 29:125-130.

Butte, N. F., and Calloway, D. H. (1982). Proteins, vitamin A, carotene, folacin, ferritin, and zinc in Navajo maternal and cord blood. *Biol. Neonat.* 41:273-278.

Byrn, J. N., and Eastman, N. J. (1943). Vitamin A levels in maternal and fetal blood plasma. *Bull. Johns Hopkins Hosp.* 73:132-137.

Camera, G., and Pregliasco, P. (1992). Ear malformation in baby born to mother using tretinoin cream. *Lancet* (339): 687.

Chiao, Y. B., and Van Thiel, D. H. (1986). Characterization of rat testicular alcohol dehydrogenase. *Alcohol alcoholism* 21:9-15.

Chiocca, E. A., Davies, P. J. A., and Stein, J. P. (1988). The molecular basis of retinoic acid action: Transcriptional regulation of tissue transglutaminase gene expression in macrophages. *J. Biol. Chem.* 263:11584-11589.

Chytil, F., and Riaz-ul-Haq (1990). Vitamin A mediated gene expression. *Crit. Rev. Euk. Gene Exp.* 1:61-73.

Cohlan, S. Q. (1953). Excessive intake of vitamin A as a cause of congenital anomalies in rat. *Science* 117:535-536.

Cohlan, S. Q. (1954). Congenital anomalies in the rat produced by excessive intake of Vitamin A during pregnancy. *Pediatrics* 13:556-567.

Connor, M. J. (1988). Oxidation of retinol to retinoic acid as a requirement for biological activity in mouse epidermis. *Canc. Res.* 48:7038-7040.

Connor, M. J., and Smit, M. H. (1987). The formation of all-trans-retinoic acid from all-trans-retinol in hairless mouse skin. *Biochem. Pharmacol.* 36:919-924.

Cooper, D. A., Furr, H. C., and Olson, J. A. (1987). Factors influencing the level and interanimal variability of retinyl ester hydrolase actrivity in rat liver. *J. Nutr.* 117: 2066-2071.

Cooper, D. A., and Olson, J. A. (1986). Properties of retinyl ester hydrolase activity in young pigs. *Biochim. Biophys. Acta* 884:251-258.

Crain, F. D., Lotspeich, F. J., and Krause, R. F. (1967).

Biosynthesis of retinoic acid by intestinal enzymes of the rat. *J. Lipid. Res.* 8:249-254.

Creech-Kraft, J., Kochhar, D. M., Scott, W. J., and Nau, H. (1987). Low teratogenicity of 13-*cis*-retinoic acid (isotretinoin) in the mouse corresponds to low embryo concentrations during organogenesis: Comparison to the all-trans isomer. *Toxicol. Appl. Pharm.* 87:474-482.

Creech-Kraft, J., Lofberg, B., Chahoud, I., Bochert, G., and Nau, H. (1989). Teratogenicity and placental transfer of all-*trans*-, 13-*cis*-, 4-oxo-all-*trans*-, and 4-oxo-13-*cis*-retinoic acid after administration of a low oral dose during organogenesis in mice. *Toxicol. Appl. Pharm.* 100:162-176.

Creek, K. E., Silverman-Jones, C. S., and DeLuca, L. M. (1989). Comparison of the uptake and metabolism of retinol delivered to primary mouse keratinocytes either free or bound to rat serum retinol-binding protein. *J. Invest. Dermatol.* 92: 283-289.

Crow, J. A., and Ong, D. E. (1985). Cell-specific immuno-histochemical localization of a cellular retinol-binding protein (type two) in the small intestine of rat. *Proc. Natl. Acad. Sci. USA.* 82:4707-4711.

Cruz, D. L. (1984). Multiple congenital malfromation associated with maternal isotretinoin therapy. *Pediatrics* 74: 428-430.

Cullum, M. E., Johnson, B. C., and Zile, M. H. (1984). Comparison of fetal and adult retinol binding proteins in bovine serum and pigment epithelium. *Intern. J. Vitam. Nutr. Res.* 54:297-305.

Cullum, M. E., and Zile, M. H. (1985). Metabolism of all-*trans*-retinoic acid and all-*trans*-retinyl acetate. Demonstration of common physiological metabolites in rat small intestinal mucosa and circulation. *J. Biol. Chem.* 260: 10590-10596.

Cumming, F. J., and Briggs, M. H. (1983). Changes in plasma vitamin A in lactating and non-lactating oral contraceptive users. *Brit. J. Obstet. Gynaecol.* 90:73-77.

Curley, R. W., and Fowble, J. W. (1988). Photoisomerization

of retinoic acid and its photoprotection in physiologic-like solutions. *Photochem. Photobiol.* 47:831-835.

Das, S. R., and Gouras, P. (1988). Retinoid metabolism in cultured human retinal pigment epithelium. *Biochem. J.* 250:459-465.

Dawson, E. B., Clark, R. R., and McGanity, W. J. (1969). Plasma vitamins and trace metal changes during teen-age pregnancy. *Amer. J. Obstet. Gynecol.* 104:953-958.

DeLuca, H. F., Zile, M., and Sietsems, W. K. (1981). The metabolism of retinoic acid to 5,6-epoxyretinoic acid, retinoyl-β-glucuronide, and other polar metabolites. *Ann. NY Acad. Sci.* 359:25-36.

Dencker, L., Annerwall, E., Busch, C., and Eriksson, U. (1990). Localization of specific retinoid-binding sites and expression of cellular retinoic-acid-binding protein (CRABP) in the early mouse embryo. *Development* 110: 343-352.

Ditlow, C. C., Holmquist, B., Morelock, M. M., and Vallee, B. L. (1984). Physical and enzymatic properties of a class II alcohol dehydrogenase isoenzyme of human liver: p-ADH. *Biochemistry* 23:6363-6368.

Dixon, J. L., and Goodman, D. S. (1987). Effects of nutritional and hormonal factors on the metabolism of retinol-binding protein by primary cultures of rat hepatocytes. *J. Cell Physiol.* 130:6-13.

Dolle, P., Ruberte, E., Leroy, P., Morriss-Kay, G., and Chambon, P. (1990). Retinoic acid receptors and cellular retinoid binding proteins. 1. A systematic study of their differential pattern of transcription during mouse organogenesis. *Development* 110:1133-1151.

Donoghue, S., Kronfeld, D. S., and Sklan, D. (1983). Retinol homeostasis in lambs fed low and high intakes of vitamin A. *Brit. J. Nutr.* 50:235-248.

Donoghue, S., Richardson, D. W., Sklan, D., and Kronfeld, D. S. (1985). Placental transport of retinol in ewes fed high intakes of vitamin A. *J. Nutr.* 115:1562-1571.

Dostalova, L. (1982). Correlation of the vitamin status between mother and newborn during delivery. *Dev. Pharmacol. Ther.*, (suppl.):45-57.

Duester, G., Shean, M. L., Mcbride, M. S., and Stewart, M. J. (1991). Retinoic acid response element in the human alcohol dehydrogenase gene ADH3 – Implications for regulation of retinoic acid synthesis. *Molec. Cell. Biol.* 11: 1638-1646.

Durston, A. J., Timmermans, J. P. M., Hage, W. J., Hendriks, H. F. J., De Vries, N. J., Heideveld, M., and Nieuwkoop, P. D. (1989). Retinoic acid causes an anteroposterior transformation in the developing central nervous system. *Nature* 340:140-144.

Eckhoff, C., Lofberg, B., Chahoud, I., Bochert, G., and Nau, H. (1989). Transplacental Pharmacokinetics and teratogenicity of a single dose of retinol (vitamin A) during organogenesis in the mouse. *Toxicol. Lett.* 48:171-184.

Eichele, G. (1989). Retinoids and vertebrate limb pattern formation. *Trends Gen.* 5:246-251.

Eichele, G., and Thaller, C. (1988). Characterization of retinoid metabolism in the developing chick limb bud. *Development* 103:473-483.

El-Gorab, M. I., and Underwood, B. A. (1973). Solubilization of β-carotene and retinol into aqueous solutions of mixed micelles. *Biochim. Biophys. Acta* 306:58-66.

El-Gorab, M. I., Underwood, B. A., and Loerch, J. D. (1975). Role of bile salts in the uptake of β-carotene and retinol by rat everted gut sacs. *Biochim. Biophys. Acta* 124:71-85.

Elder, T. D., and Topper, Y. J. (1962). The oxidation of retinene (vitamin A aldehyde) to vitamin A acid by mammalian steroid-sensitive aldehyde dehydrogenase. *Biochim. Biophys. Acta* 64:430-437.

Emerick, R. F., Zile, M., and DeLuca, H. F. (1967). Formation of retinoic acid from retinol in the rat. *Biochem. J.* 102:606-611.

Eriksson, U., Das, K., Busch, C., Norlinder, H., Rask, L., Sundelin, J., Sallstrom, J., and Peterson, P. A. (1984). Cellular retinol-binding protein: Quantitation and distribution. *J. Biol. Chem.* 259:13464-13470.

Fallon, J. F., and Saunders, J. W. (1968). *In vitro* analysis of the control of cell death in a zone of prospective necrosis from the chick wing bud. *Dev. Biol.* 18:553-570.

Fantel, A. G., Shepard, T. H., Newell-Morris, L. L., and Moffett, B. C. (1977). Teratogenic effects of retinoic acid in pigtail monkeys (*Macaca nemestrina*). I. General features. *Teratology* 15:65-72.

Farber, J. L. (1985). The biochemical pathology of toxic cell death. *Monogr. Pathol.* 26:19-31.

Fernhoff, P. M., and Lammer, E. J. (1984). Craniofacial features of isotretinoin embryopathy. *J. Pediatrics* 105: 595-597.

Fesus, L., Thomazy, V., and Falus, A. (1987). Induction and activation of tissue transglutaminase during programmed cell death. *FEBS Lett.* 224:104-108.

Fex, G., and Felding, P. (1984). Factors affecting the concentration of free holo retinol-binding protein in human plasma. *Eur. J. Clin. Invest.* 14:146-149.

Fex, G., and Johannesson, G. (1987). Studies of the spontaneous transfer of retinol from the retinol:retinol-binding protein complex to unilamellar liposomes. *Biochim. Biophys. Acta* 901:255-264.

Fex, G., and Johannesson, G. (1988). Retinol transfer across and between phospholipid bilayer membranes. *Biochim. Biophys. Acta* 944:249-255.

Flanagan, J. L., Willhite, C. C., and Ferm, V. H. (1987). Comparative teratogenic activity of cancer chemopreventive retinoidal benzoic acid congeners (arotinoids). *J Natl. Cancer Inst.* 78:533-538.

Folk, J. E. (1980). Transglutaminases. *Ann. Rev. Biochem.* 49:517-531.

Forsum, U., Rask, L., Tjernlund, U. M., and Peterson, P. A. (1977). Detection of the vitamin A carrier proteins in human epidermis. *Arch. Dermatol. Res.* 258:85-88.

Fries, E., Gustafsson, L., and Peterson, P. (1984). Four secretory proteins synthesized by hepatocytes are transported from endoplasmic reticulum to Golgi complex at different rates. *Eur. Molec. Biol. Organiz. J.* 3:147-152.

Frolik, C. A. (1981). *In vitro* and *in vivo* metabolism of all-*trans*- and 13-*cis*-retinoic acid in the hamster. *Ann. NY Acad. Sci.* 359:37-40.

Frolik, C. A. (1984). Metabolism of retinoids. Pages 177-206 *in* M. B. Sporn, A. B. Roberts and D. S. Goodman, eds., *The Retinoids*, Vol. 2. Academic Press, New York.

Frolik, C. A., Roberts, A. B., Tavela, T. E., Roller, P. P., Newton, D. L., and Sporn, M. B. (1979). Isolation and identification of 4-hydroxy- and 4-oxoretinoic acid in hamster trachea and liver. *Biochemistry* 18:2092-2097.

Frolik, C. A., Roller, P. P., Roberts, A. B., and Sporn, M. B. (1980). *In vitro* and *in vivo* metabolism of all-*trans*- and 13-*cis*-retinoic acid in hamsters: Identification of 13-*cis*-4-oxoretinoic acid. *J. Biol. Chem.* 255:8057-8062.

Furr, H. C., Cooper, D., and Olson, J. A. (1986). Separation of retinyl esters by non-aqueous reversed-phase high performance liquid chromatography. *J. Chromatog.* 378:45-53.

Futterman, S. (1962). Enzymatic oxidation of vitamin A aldehyde to vitamin A acid. *J. Biol. Chem.* 237:677-680.

Futterman, S., and Andrews, J. S. (1964). The composition of liver vitamin A ester and synthesis of vitamin A ester by liver microsomes. *J. Biol. Chem.* 239:4077-4080.

Gebre-Medhin, M., and Vahlquist, A. (1977). Vitamin A nutrition in the fetus. Pages 1-15 *in* M. Gebre-Medhin, ed., *Maternal Nutrition and Its Effect on the Offspring. Dietary, Anthropometric, Biochemical and Haematological Studies in Urban Ethiopia.* Univ. Uppsala, Uppsala, Sweden.

Geelen, J. A. G. (1978). Hypervitaminosis A induced teratogenesis. *Crit. Rev. Toxicol.* 6:351-375.

Georgieff, M. K., Chockalingam, U. M., Sasanow, S. R., Gunter, E. W., Murphy, E., and Ophoven, J. J. (1988). The effect of antenatal betamethasone on cord blood concentrations of retinol-binding protein, transthyretin, transfferin, retinol and vitamin E. *J. Pediatr. Gastroent. Nutr.* 7:713-717.

Giguere, V., Ong, E. S., Segui, P., and Evans, R. M. (1987).

Identification of a receptor for the morphogen retinoic acid. *Nature* 330:624-629.

Giroud, A., and Martinet, M. (1959). Extension ê plusiers espèces de Mammifères des malformations embryonnaires par hypervitaminose A. *Compt. Rend. Soc. Biol.* 153:201-202.

Gjoen, T., Bjerkelund, T., Blomhoff, H. K., Norum, K. R., Berg, T., and Blomhoff, R. (1987). Liver takes up retinol-binding protein from plasma. *J. Biol. Chem.* 262:10926-10930.

Glover, J., Heaf, D. J., and Large, S. (1980). Seasonal changes in plasma retinol-binding holoprotein concentration in Japanese quail (*Coturnix coturnix japonica*). *Brit. J. Nutr.* 43:357-366.

Glucksmann, A. (1951). Cell deaths in normal vertebrate ontogency. *Biol. Rev.* 26:59-86.

Goodman, D. S. (1984). Plasma retinol-binding protein. Pages 41-88 *in* M. B. Sporn, A. B. Roberts and D. S. Goodman, eds., *The Retinoids*, Vol. 2. Academic Press, New York.

Goodman, D. S., and Blaner, W. S. (1984). Biosynthesis, absorption, and hepatic metabolism of retinol. Pages 2-34 *in* M. B. Sporn, A. B. Roberts and D. S. Goodman, eds., *The Retinoids*, Vol. 2. Academic Press, New York.

Green, H. (1977). Terminal differentiation of cultured human epidermal cells. *Cell* 11:405-416.

Green, M. H., Uhl, L., and Green, J. B. (1985). A multicompartmental model of vitamin A kinetics in rats with marginal liver vitamin A stores. *J. Lipid. Res.* 26:806-818.

Grote, W., Harms, D., Janig, U., Kietzmann, H., Ravens, U., and Schwarze, I. (1985). Malformation of fetus conceived 4 months after termination of maternal etretinate treatment. *Lancet* (8440):1276.

Hakansson, H., and Hanberg, A. (1989). The distribution of [14C]-2,3,7,8-tetrachlorodibenzo-*p*-dioxin (TCDD) and its effect on the vitamin A content in parenchymal and stellate cells of rat liver. *J. Nutr.* 119:773-580.

Hakansson, H., Johansson, L., and Ahlborg, U. G. (1988).

Effects of 2,3,7,8-tetrachlorodibenzo-*p*-dioxin (TCDD) on tissue levels of vitamin A and on the distribution and excretion of the endogenous pool of vitamin A in the marginally vitamin A sufficient rat. *Chemosphere* 17:1781-1793.

Hale, F. (1933). Pigs Born Without Eyeballs. *J. Hered.* 24:105-106.

Hanni, R., and Bigler, F. (1977). Isolation and identification of three major metabolites of retinoic acid from rat feces. *Helv. Chir. Acta.* 60:881-887.

Hanni, R., Bigler, F., Meister, W., and Englert, G. (1976). Isolation and identification of three urinary metabolites of retinoic acid in the rat. *Helv. Chir. Acta* 59:2221-2227.

Happle, R., Traupe, T., Bounameaux, T., and Fisch, T. (1984). Teratogene warkung von etretinat beim menschen. *Deutsche Med. Wochencsh.* 109:1476-1480.

Harnish, D. C., Jiang, H., Soprano, K. J., Kochhar, D. M., and Soprano, D. R. (1992). Retinoic acid receptor β2 mRNA is elevated by retinoic acid *in vivo* in susceptible regions of mid-gestation mouse embryos. *Dev. Dynam.* 194:239-246.

Harrison, E. H. (1988). Role salt-dependent, neutral cholesteryl ester hydrolase of rat liver: Possible relationship with pancreatic cholesteryl ester hydrolase. *Biochim. Biophys. Acta* 963:28-34.

Harrison, E. H., and Gad, M. Z. (1989). Hydrolysis of retinyl palmitate by enzymes of rat pancreas and liver. *J. Biol. Chem.* 264:17142-17147.

Harrison, E. H., Smith, J. E., and Goodman, D. S. (1979). Unusual properties of retinyl palmitate hydrolase activity in rat liver. *J. Lipid. Res.* 20:760-771.

Helgerud, P., Petersen, L. B., and Norum, K. R. (1982). AcylCoA:retinol acyltransferase in rat small intestine: Its activity and some properties of the enzymic reaction. *J. Lipid. Res.* 23:609-618.

Helgerud, P., Petersen, L. B., and Norum, K. R. (1983). Retinol esterification by microsomes from the mucosa of human small intestine. *J. Clin. Invest.* 71:747-753.

Heller, J. (1975). Interactions of plasma retinol-binding protein with its receptor. *J. Biol. Chem.* 250:3613-3619.

Hendrickx, A. G., and Hummler, H. (1992). Teratogenicity of all-*trans* retinoic acid during early embryonic development in the cynomolgus monkey (*Macaca fascicularis*). *Teratology* 45:65-74.

Hendrickx, A. G., Silverman, S., Pellegrini, M., and Steffek, A. J. (1980). Teratological and radiocephalometric analysis of craniofacial malformations induced with retinoic acid in rhesus monkeys (*Macaca nemestrina*). *Teratology* 22:13-22.

Hendriks, H. F. J., Verhoofstad, W. A. M. M., Brouwer, A., de Leeuw, A. M., Knook, D. L., and Goodman, D. S. (1985). Perisinusoidal fat-storing cells are the main vitamin A storage sites in rat liver. *Exp. Cell Res.* 160:138-149.

Herbert, P. N., Assmann, G., Gotto, A. M., and Fredrickson, D. S. (1983). Familial lipoprotein deficiency. Pages 589-612 *in* J. B. Stanbury, J. B. Wyngaarder, D. S. Fredrickson, J. L. Goldstein and M. S. Brown, eds, *The Metabolic Basis of Inherited Disease.* McGraw-Hill, New York.

Heyman, R. A., Mangelsdorf, D. J., Dyck, J. A., Stein, R. B., Eichele, G., Evans, R. M., and Thaller, C. (1992). 9-*cis* retinoic acid is a high affinity ligand for the retinoid X receptor. *Cell* 68:397-406.

Hill, R. M. (1984). Isotretinoin teratogenicity. *Lancet* (8392):1465.

Hollander, D. (1981). Intestinal absorption of vitamin A, E, D and K. *J. Lab. Clin. Med.* 97:449-462.

Holmes, R. S., Duley, J. A., and Burnell, J. N. (1983). The alcohol dehydrogenase gene complex on chromosome 3 of the mouse. Pages 155-174 *in* M. C. Rattazzi, J. G. Scadalios and G. S. Whitt, eds., *Isoenzymes Cellular Localization, Metabolism and Physiology*, Vol. 8. Alan R. Liss, New York.

Howard, W. B., Willhite, C. C., Omaye, S. T., and Sharma, R. P. (1989). Comparative distribution, pharmacokinetics and placental permeabilities of all-*trans*-retinoic acid, 13-

cis-retinoic acid, all-*trans*-4-oxo-retinoic acid, retinyl acetate and 9-*cis*-retinal in hamsters. *Arch. Toxicol.* 63: 112-120.

Huang, H. S., and Goodman, D. S. (1965). Intestinal absorption and metabolism of ^{14}C-labelled vitamin A alcohol and β-carotene in the rat. *J. Biol. Chem.* 240:2839-2844.

Hummler, H., Korte, R., and Hendrickx, A. G. (1990). Induction of malformations in the cynomolgus monkey with 13-*cis* retinoic acid. *Teratology* 42:263-272.

Hytten, F. E., and Leight, I. (1971). *The Physiology of Human Pregnancy.* Blackwell, Oxford, UK.

Ikuta, T., and Yoshida, A. (1986). mRNA for the three human alcohol dehydrogenase subunits: Size heterogeneity and developmental changes. *Biochem. Biophys. Res. Commun.* 140:1020-1027.

Ismaldi, S. D., and Olson, J. A. (1975). Vitamin A transport in human fetal blood. *Amer. J. Clin. Nutr.* 28:967-972.

Ismaldi, S. D., and Olson, J. A. (1982). Dynamics of fetal distribution and transfer of vitamin A between fetuses and their mothers. *Intern. J. Vitam. Nutr. Res.* 52:111-118.

Ito, Y. L., Zile, M., Ahrens, H., and De Luca, H. F. (1974). Liquid-gel partition chromatography of vitamin A compounds; Formation of retinoic acid from retinyl acetate *in vivo. J. Lipid. Res.* 15:517.

Izpisua-Belmonte, J., Dolle, P., and Duboule, D. (1991). *Hox* genes and the molecular basis of vertebrate limb pattern formation. *Sem. Dev. Biol.* 2:385-391.

Jansson, L., and Nilsson, B. (1983). Serum retinol and retinol-binding protein in mothers and infants at delivery. *Biol. Neonat.* 43:269-271.

Jetten, A. M. (1986). Induction of differentiation of embryonal carcimona cells by retinoids. Pages 105-130 *in* M. I. Sherman, ed., *Retinoids and Cell Differentiation.* CRC Press, Boca Raton, FL.

Jiang, H., and Kochhar, D. M. (1992). Induction of tissue transglutaminase and apoptosis by retinoic acid in the limb bud. *Teratology* 46:333-340.

Julia, P., Boleda, M. D., Farres, J., and Pares, X. (1987).

Mammalian alcohol dehydrogenase: Characteristics of class III isoenzymes. *Alcohol Alcoholism* 34:169-173.

Julia, P., Farres, J., and Pares, X. (1986). Ocular alcohol dehydrogenasein the rat: Regional distribution and kinetics of the ADH-1 isoenzyme with retinol and retinal. *Exp. Eye Res.* 42:305-314.

Kalter, H. (1960). The teratogenic effects of hypervitaminosis A upon the face and mouth of inbred mice. *Ann. NY Acad. Sci.* 85:42-55.

Kalter, H., and Warkany, J. (1961). Experimental production of congenital malformations in strains of inbred mice by maternal treatment with hypervitaminosis A. *Amer. J. Path.* 38:1-15.

Kastner, P., Krust, A., Mendelsohn, C., Garnier, J. M., Zelent, A., Leroy, P., Staub, A., and Chambon, P. (1990). Murine isoforms of retinoic acid receptor with specific patterns of expression. *Proc. Natl. Acad. Sci. USA.* 87:2700-2704.

Kato, M., Blaner, W. S., Mertz, J. R., Das, K., Kato, K., and Goodman, D. S. (1985a). Influence of retinoid nutritional status on cellular retinol-and cellular retinoic acid-binding protein concentrations in various rat tissues. *J. Biol. Chem.* 260:4832-4838.

Kato, M., Kato, K., and Goodman, D. S. (1985b). Immunochemical studies on the localization and on the concentration of cellular retinol binding protein in rat liver during prenatal development. *Lab. Invest.* 52:475-484.

Keilson, B., Underwood, B. A., and Loerch, J. D. (1979). Effects of retinoic acid on the mobilization of vitamin A from the liver in rats. *J. Nutr.* 109:787-795.

Kessel, M., and Gruss, P. (1991). Homeotic transformations of murine vertebrae and concomitant alteration of *Hox* codes induced by retinoic acid. *Cell* 67:89-104.

Kistler, A. (1981). Teratogenesis of retinoic acid in rats: Susceptible stages and suppression of retinoic acid-induced limb malformations by cycloheximide. *Teratology* 23:25-31.

Kistler, A. (1987). Limb bud cell cultures for estimating the teratogenic potential of compounds: Validation of the test system with retinoids. *Arch. Toxicol.* 60:403-414.

Kistler, A., Galli, B., and Howard, W. B. (1990). Comparative teratogenicity of three retinoids: The arotinoids Ro 13-7410, Ro 13-6298 and Ro 15-1570. *Arch. Toxicol.* 64: 43-48.

Knudsen, T. B., and Kochhar, D. M. (1981). Limb Development in mouse embryos. III. Cellular events underlying the determination of altered skeletal patterns following treatment with 5′fluoro-2-deoxyuridine. *Teratology* 23: 241-251.

Kochhar, D. M. (1967). Teratogenic activity of retinoic acid. *Acta Path. Microbiol. Scand.* 70:393-404.

Kochhar, D. M. (1968). Studies of vitamin A-induces teratogenesis: Effects on embryonic mesenchyme and epithelium, and on incorporation of thymidine-H3. *Teratology* 1:299-310.

Kochhar, D. M. (1973). Limb development in mouse embryos. I. Analysis of teratogenic effects of retinoic acid. *Teratology* 7:289-298.

Kochhar, D. M. (1977). Cellular Basis of congenital limb deformity induced in mice by vitamin A. Pages 111-154 *in* D. Bergsma and W. Lenz, eds., *Morphogenesis and Malformation of the Limb*, Vol. 13. Alan R. Liss, New York.

Kochhar, D. M., Jiang, H., Soprano, D. R., and Harnish, D. C. (1993). Early embryonic cell response in retinoid-induced teratogenesis. Pages 383-396 *in* M. A. Livrea, ed., *Retinoids, New Trends in Research and Clinical Applications*. Marcel Dekker, New York.

Kochhar, D. M., and Johnson, E. M. (1965). Morphological and autoradiographic studies of cleft palate induced in rat embryos by maternal hypervitaminosis A. *J. Embryol. Exp. Morph.* 14:223-238.

Kochhar, D. M., Kraft, J. C., and Nau, H. (1987). Teratogenicity and disposition of various retinoids *in vivo* and *in vitro*. Pages 173-186 *in* H. Nau and W. J. Scott, eds.,

Pharmacokinetic in Teratogenesis, Vol. II. CRC Press, Boca Raton, FL.

Kochhar, D. M., and Penner, J. D. (1987). Developmental effects of isotretinoin and 4-oxo-isotretinoin: The role of metabolism in teratogenicity. *Teratology* 36:67-75.

Kochhar, D. M., and Penner, J. D. (1992). Analysis of high dysmorphogenic activity of Ro 13-6307, a tetramethylated tetralin analog of retinoic acid. *Teratology* 45:637-645.

Kochhar, D. M., Penner, J. D., and Satre, M. A. (1988). Derivation of retinoic acid and metabolites from a teratogenic dose of retinol (vitamin A) in mice. *Toxicol. & Appl. Pharm.* 96:429-441.

Kochhar, D. M., Penner, J. D., and Tellone, C. I. (1984). Comparative teratogenic activities of two retinoids: Effects on palate and limb development. *Teratogen. Carcinog. Mutagenen.* 4:377-387.

Krust, P., Kastner, P., Petkovich, M., Zelent, A., and Chambon, P. (1989). A third human retinoic acid receptor, hRARγ. *Proc. Natl. Acad. Sci. USA.* 86:5310-5314.

Lakshman, M. R., Mychkovsky, I., and Attlesey, M. (1989). Enzymatic conversion of all-*trans*-β-carotene to retinal by a cytosolic enzyme from rabbit and rat intestinal mucosa. *Proc. Natl. Acad. Sci. USA.* 86:9124-9128.

Lammer, E., and Armstrong, D. (1991). Malformations of derivatives of thombencephalic alar plate in human retinoic acid embryopathy. *8th Intern. Cong. Hum. Genet.* (Abstract).

Lammer, E. J. (1988). A phenocopy of retinoic acid embryopathy following maternal use of etretinate that ended a year before conception. *Teratology* 37:472.

Lammer, E. J., Chen, D. T., Hoar, R. M., Agnish, N. D., Benke, P. J., Braun, J. T., Curry, C. J., Fernhoff, P. M., Grix, A. W., Lott, I. T., Richard, J. M., and Sun, S. C. (1985). Retinoic acid embryopathy. *New Engl. J. Med.* 313:837-841.

Lammer, E. J., Hayes, A. M., Schunior, A., and Holmes, L. B. (1988). Unusually high risk for adverse outcomes of pregnancy following fetal isotretinoin exposure. *Amer. J. Hum. Genet.* 43:A58.

Lammer, E. J., and Opitz (1986). The Di George Anomaly as a developmental field defect. *Amer. J. Med. Genet.*, suppl 2:113-127.

Lange, L. G., Sytkowski, A. J., and Vallee, B. L. (1976). Human liver alcohol dehydrogenase: Purification, composition and catalytic features. *Biochemistry* 15:4687-4693.

Langman, J., and Welch, G. W. (1967). Excess vitamin A and development of the cerebral cortex. *J. Comp. Neurol.* 131:15-26.

Lawrence, C. W., Crain, F. D., Lotspeich, F. J., and Krause, R. F. (1966). Absorption, transport, and storage of retinyl-15-^{14}C-palmitate-9,10-^{3}H in the rat. *J. Lipid. Res.* 7:226-229.

Leo, M. A., Kim, C., and Leiber, C. S. (1987). NAD^{+}-dependent retinol dehydrogenase in liver microsomes. *Arch. Biochem. Biophys.* 259:241-249.

Leo, M. A., Lasker, J. M., Raucy, J. L., Kim, C., Black, M., and Leiber, C. S. (1989). Metabolism of retinol and retinoic acid by human liver cytochrome P450IIC8. *Arch. Biochem. Biophys.* 269:305-312.

Leo, M. A., and Leiber, C. S. (1984). Normal testicular structure and reproductive function in Deermice lacking retinol and alcohol dehydrogenase activity. *J. Clin. Invest.* 73:593.

Leo, M. A., and Leiber, C. S. (1985). New pathway for retinol metabolism in liver microsomes. *J. Biol. Chem.* 260: 5228-5231.

Leroy, P., Krust, A., Zelent, A., Mendelsohn, C., Garnier, J. M., Kastner, P., Dierich, A., and Chambon, P. (1991). Multiple isoforms of the mouse retinoic acid receptor α are generated by alternative splicing and differential induction by retinoic acid. *Eur. Molec. Biol. Organiz. J.* 10:59-69.

Levin, A. A., Sturzenbecker, L. J., Kazmer, S., Bosa-kowski, T., Huselton, C., Allenby, G., Speck, J., Kratzeisen, C., Rosenberger, M., Lovey, A., and Grippo, J. F. (1992).

9-*cis* retinoic acid stereoisomer binds and activates the nuclear receptor RXRα. *Nature* 355:359-361.

Lewis, J. M., Bodansky, O., Lillenfeld, M. C. C., and Schneider, H. (1947). Supplements of vitamin A and carotene during pregnancy. Their effect on the levels of vitamin A and carotene in the blood of mother and newborn infant. *Amer. J. Dis. Child.* 73:143-150.

Lewis, K. C., Green, M. H., and Underwood, B. A. (1981). Vitamin A turnover in rats as influenced by vitamin A status. *J. Nutr.* 111:1135-1144.

Li, T. K. (1977). Enzymology of human alcohol metabolism. *Adv. Enzymol.* 45:427-483.

Lockshin, R. A., and Zakeri, Z. F. (1990). Minireview – Programmed cell death: New thouughts and relevance to aging. *J. Gern.* 45:B135-B140.

Lockshin, R. A., and Zakeri, Z. F. (1991). Programmed cell death and apoptosis. Pages 47-60 *in* L. D. Tomei and F. O. Cope , eds., *Apoptosis: The Molecular Basis of Cell Death.* Cold Spring Harbor Laboratory Press.

Lorente, C. A., and Miller, S. A. (1977). Fetal and maternal vitamin A levels in tissues of hypervitaminotic A rats. *J. Nutr.* 107:1816-1821.

Lotan, R. (1980). Effects of vitamin A and its analogs (retinoids) on normal and neoplastic cells. *Biochim. Biophys. Acta* 605:33-91.

Lott, I. T. (1983). Fetal hydrocephalus and ear anomalies associated with maternal use of isotretinoin. *J. Pediatrics* 105:597-600.

Lui, N. S. T., and Roels, O. A. (1980). Vitamin A and carotene. Pages 142-159 *in* R. S. Goodhart and R. S. Shils, eds., *Modern Nutrition in Health and Disease.* Lea and Febiger, Philadelphia, PA.

MacDonald, P. N., and Ong, D. E. (1988). Evidence for lecithin-retinol acyltransferase activity in the rat small intestine. *J. Biol. Chem.* 263:12478-12482.

Maden, M., Horton, C., Graham, A., Leonard, L., Pizzey, J., Siegenthaler, G., Lumsden, A., and Eriksson, U. (1992). Domains of cellular retinoic acid-binding protein-I

(CRABP-I) expression in the hindbrain and neural crest of the mouse embryo. *Mech. Develop.* 37:13-23.

Maden, M., Ong, D. E., and Chytil, F. (1990). Retinoid-binding protein distribution in the developing mammalian nervous system. *Development* 109:75-80.

Mahoney, C. P., Margolis, M. T., Knauss, T. A., and Labbe, R. F. (1980). Chronic vitamin A intoxication in infants fed chiken liver. *Pediatrics* 65:893-896.

Makover, A., Soprano, D. R., Wyatt, M. L., and Goodman, D. S. (1989). An *in situ*-hybridization study of the localization of retinol-binding protein and transthyretin Messenger RNAs during fetal development in the rat. *Differentiation* 40:17-25.

Mangelsdorf, D. J., Borgmeyer, W., Heyman, R. A., Zhou, J. Y., Ong, E. S., Oro, A. E., Kakizuka, A., and Evans, R. M. (1992). Characterization of three RXR genes that mediate the action of 9-*cis* retinoic acid. *Gene Develop.* 6:329-344.

Mangelsdorf, D. J., Ong, E. S., Dyck, J. A., and Evans, R. M. (1990). Nuclear receptor that identifies a novel retinoic acid response pathway. *Nature* 345:224-229.

Martinez-Frias, M. L., and Salvador, J. (1990). Epidemiological aspects of prenatal exposure to high doses of vitamin A in Spain. *Eur. J. Epidemiol.* 6:118-123.

Massarella, J., Vane, F., Bugge, C., Rodriguez, L., Cunningham, W. J., Franz, T., and Colburn, W. (1985). Etretinate kinetics during chronic dosing in severe psoriasis. *Clin. Pharmacol. Ther.* 37:439-446.

Matsumoto, E., Kazushige, H., Kouiche, A., and Naka, S. (1984). Development of the vitamin A – storing cell in the mouse liver during late fetal and neonatal periods. *Anat. Embryol.* 169:249-254.

Mattison, D. R. (1986). Physiologic variations in pharmacokinetics during pregnancy. Pages 37-102 *in* S. Fabro and A. R. Scialli, eds., *Drug and Chemical Action in Pregnancy.* Marcel Dekker, New York.

Mavilio, F., Simeone, A., Boncinelli, E., and Andrews, P. W. (1988). Activation of four homeobox gene clusters in human embryonal carcinoma cells induces to differentiate by retinoic acid. *Differentiation* 37:73-79.

McCollum, E. V., and Davis, M. (1913). The necessity of certain lipins in the diet during growth. *J. Biol. Chem.* 15: 167-175.

McCormick, A. M., and Napoli, J. L. (1982). Identification of 5,6-epoxyretinoic acid as an endogenous retinol metabolite. *J. Biol. Chem.* 257:1730-1735.

McCormick, A. M., Napoli, J. L., Schnoes, H. K., and DeLuca, H. F. (1978). Isolation and identification of 5,6-epoxyretinoic acid: A biologically active metabolite of retinoic acid. *Biochemistry* 17:4085-4090.

McGanity, W. J., Cannon, R. O., Bridgforth, E. B., Martin, M. P., Densen, P. M., Newbill, J. A., McClennan, G. S., Christie, A., Peterson, J. C., and Darby, W. J. (1954). The Vanderbilt cooperative study of maternal and infant nutrition. IV. Relationship of obstetric performance to nutrition. *Amer. J. Obstet. Gynecol.* 67:501-527.

McKenna, M. C., Robinson, W. G., and Bieri, J. R. (1983). Cellular localization of vitamin A in rats given total perenteral nutrition (TPN) solutions intravenously or orally. *J. Nutr.* 113:1176.

McLaren, D. S., and Ward, P. G. (1962). Malarial infection of the placenta and foetal nutrition. *East Afr. Med. J.* 39: 182-189.

McPhillips, D. M., Kalin, J. R., and Hill, D. L. (1987). The pharmacokinetics of all-*trans*-retinoic acid and N-(2-Hydroxyethyl)retinamide in mice as determined with a sensitive and convenient procedure. *Drug Metab. Dispos.* 15: 207-211.

Mendelsohn, C., Ruberte, E., LeMeur, M., Morriss-Kay, G., and Chambon, P. (1991). Developmental analysis of the retinoic acid-inducible RAR-2 promoter in transgenic animals. *Development* 113:723-734.

Mezey, E., and Holt, P. R. (1971). The inhibitory effect of alcohol on retinol oxidation by human liver and cattle retina. *Exp. Molec. Pathol.* 15:148-156.

Miller, D. A., and DeLuca, H. F. (1986). Biosynthesis of

retinoyl-β-glucuronide, a biologically active metabolite of all-*trans*-retinoic acid. *Arch. Biochem. Biophys.* 244:179.

Moffa, D. J., Lotspeich, F. J., and Krause, R. F. (1970). Preparation and properties of retinal-oxidizing enzyme from rat intestinal mucosa. *J. Biol. Chem.* 245:439-447.

Montreewasuwat, N., and Olson, J. A. (1979). Serum and liver concentrations of vitamin A in Thai fetuses as a function of gestational age. *Amer. J. Clin. Nutr.* 26:601-606.

Moore, K. L. (1982). *The Developing Human.* W. B. Saunders Co., Philadelphia, PA.

Morriss-Kay, G. (1991). Retinoic acid, neural crest and craniofacial development. *Sem. in Dev. Biol.* 2:211-218.

Morriss-Kay, G. M., Murphy, P., Hill, R. E., and Davidson, D. R. (1991). Effects of retinoic acid excess on expression of *Hox*-2.9 and Krox-20 and on morphological segmentation in the hindbrain of mouse embryos. *Eur. Molec. Biol. Organiz. J.* 10:2985-2995.

Mounoud, R. L., Klein, D., and Weber, F. (1975). À propos d'un cas de syndrome de Goldenhar: Intoxication aigue à la vitamine A chez la mère pendant la grossesse. *J. Genet.* 23:135-154.

Muto, Y., Smith, J. E., Milch, P. O., and Goodman, D. S. (1972). Regulation of retinol-binding protein metabolism by vitamin A status in the rat. *J. Biol. Chem.* 247:2542-2550.

Nagpal, S., Zelent, A., and Chambon, P. (1992). RAR-β4, a retinoic acid receptor isoform is generated from RAR-beta2 by alternative splicing and usage of a CUG initiator codon. *Proc. Natl. Acad. Sci. USA.* 89:2718-2722.

Napoli, J. L. (1986). Retinol metabolism in LLC-PK1 cells. *J. Biol. Chem.* 261:13592-13597.

Napoli, J. L., McCormick, A. M., Schnoes, H. K., and DeLuca, H. (1978). Identification of 5,8-epoxyretinoic acid isolated from small intestine of vitamin A-deficient rats dosed with retinoic acid. *Proc. Natl. Acad. Sci. USA.* 75:2603-2605.

Napoli, J. L., and Race, K. R. (1987). The Biosynthesis of

Retinoic Acid from Retinol by Rat Tissues *in vitro*. *Arch. Biochem. Biophys.* 255:95-101.

Napoli, J. L., and Race, K. R. (1988). Biogenesis of retinoic acid from β-carotene: Differences between the metabolism of β-carotene and retinal. *J. Biol. Chem.* 263: 17372-17377.

Nau, H. (1985). Improvement of testing for teratogenicity by pharmacokinetics. *Concepts Toxicol.* 3:130-137.

Newcomer, M. E., Jones, T. A., Aqvist, J., Sundelin, J., Eriksson, U., Rask, L., and Peterson, P. A. (1984). The three-dimensional structure of retinol-binding protein. *Eur. Molec. Biol. Organiz. J.* 3:1451-1454.

Noback, C. R., and Takahashi, Y. I. (1978). Micromorphology of the placenta of rats reared on marginal vitamin A deficient diets. *Acta Anat.* 102:195-202.

Noy, N., and Blaner, W. S. (1991). Interactions of retinol with binding proteins – studies with rat cellular retinol-binding protein and with rat retinol-binding protein. *Biochemistry* 30:6380-6386.

Noy, N., and Xu, Z.-J. (1990a). Interactions of retinol with binding proteins: implications for the mechanism of uptake by cells. *Biochemistry* 255:3878-3888.

Noy, N., and Xu, Z.-J. (1990b). Thermodynamic parameters of the binding of retinol to binding proteins and to membranes. *Biochemistry* 29:3888-3892.

Nyberg, A., Berne, B., Nordliner, H., Bush, C., Eriksson, U., Loof, L., and Vahlquist, A. (1988). Impaired release of vitamin A from liver in primary biliary cirrhosis. *Hepatology* 8:136-141.

O'Toole, B. A., Fradkin, R., Warkany, J., Wilson, J. G., and Mann, G. V. (1974). Vitamin A deficiency and reproduction in rhesus monkeys. *J. Nutr.* 104:1513-1524.

Okuno, M., Kato, M., Moriwaki, H., Kanai, M., and Muto, Y. (1987). Purification and partial characterization of cellular retinoic acid-binding protein from human placenta. *Biochim. Biophys. Acta* 923:116-124.

Olson, J. A. (1961). The absorption of β-carotene and its conversion into vitamin A. *Amer. J. Clin. Nutr.* 9:1-11.

Olson, J. A. (1972). The prevention of childhood blindness by the administration of massive doses of vitamin A. *Israel J. Med. Sci.* 8:1199-1206.

Olson, J. A. (1984). Serum levels of vitamin A and carotenoids as reflectors of nutritional status. *J. Natl. Cancer Inst.* 73:1439-1444.

Olson, J. A. (1986). Physiologic and metabolic basis of major signs of vitamin A deficiency. Pages 19-67 *in* J. C. Baurenfeind, ed., *Vitamin A Deficiency and its Control.* Academic Press, New York.

Olson, J. A. (1987). The storage and metabolism of vitamin A. *Chem. Scripta* 27:179

Ong, D. E. (1984). A novel retinol-binding protein from rat: purification and partial characterization. *J. Biol. Chem.* 259:1476-1482.

Ong, D. E. (1985). Vitamin A-binding proteins. *Nutr. Rev.* 43:225-232.

Ong, D. E., Kakkad, B., and MacDonald, P. N. (1987). Acyl-CoA-independent esterification of retinol bound to cellular retinol-binding protein (type II) by microsomes from rat small intestine. *J. Biol. Chem.* 262:2729.

Ong, D. E., MacDonald, P. N., and Gubitosi, A. M. (1988). Esterification of retinol in rat liver. *J. Biol. Chem.* 263: 5789-5796.

Packer, L., ed. (1990). *Methods in Enzymology*, Vol. 190. *Retinoids.* Academic Press, Orlando, FL.

Palludan, B. (1976). The influence of vitamin A deficiency on fetal development in pigs with special reference to organogenesis. *Intern. J. Vitam. Nutr. Res.* 46:223-225.

Paravicini, U., Stockel, K., McNamara, P. J., Hanni, R., and Busslinger, A. (1981). On the metabolism and pharmacokinetics of an aromatic retinoid. *Ann. NY Acad. Sci.* 359: 54-67.

Perez-Castro, A. V., Toth-Rogler, L. E., Wei, L., and Nguyen-Huu, M. C. (1989). Spatial and temporal pattern of expression of the cellular retinoic acid-binding protein and the cellular retinol-binding protein during mouse embryogenesis. *Proc. Natl. Acad. Sci. USA.* 86: 8813-8817.

Peterson, P. A., Nilsson, S. F., Ostberg, L., Rask, L., and Vahlquist, A. (1974). Aspects of the metabolism of retinol-binding protein and retinol. *Vitamin Horm.* 32:181-214.

Petkovich, M., Brand, N. J., Krust, A., and Chambon, P. (1987). A human retinoic acid receptor which belongs to the family of nuclear receptors. *Nature* 330:444-450.

Pfeffer, B. A., Clark, V. M., Flannery, J. G., and Bok, D. (1986). Membrane receptors for retinol-binding protein in cultured human retinal pigment epithelium. *Invest. Ophthalmol. Vis. Sci.* 27:1031-1040.

Piacentini, M., Fesus, L., Farrace, M. G., Ghibelli, L., Piredda, L., and Melino, G. (1991). The expression of "Tissue" transglutaminase in two human cancer cell lines is related with the programmed cell death (apoptosis). *Eur. J. Cell Biol.* 54:246-254.

Posch, K. C., Enright, W. J., and Napoli, J. L. (1989). Retinoic acid synthesis by cytosol from alcohol dehydrogenase negative deermouse. *Arch. Biochem. Biophys.* 274: 171-178.

Powers, R. H., Gilbert, L. C., and Aust, S. D. (1987). The effect of 3,4,3′,4′-tetrachlorobiphenyl on plasma retinol and hepatic retinyl palmitate hydrolase activity in female Sprague-Dawley rats. *Toxicol. & Appl. Pharm.* 89:370-377.

Prasad, A. S., Lei, K. Y., Oberleas, D., Moghissi, K. S., and Stryker, J. C. (1975). Effects of oral contraceptive agents on nutrients: II. Vitamins. *Amer. J. Clin. Nutr.* 28: 385-391.

Prystowsky, J. H., Smith, J. E., and Goodman, D. S. (1981). Retinyl ester hydrolase activity in normal rat liver. *J. Biol. Chem.* 256:4498-4503.

Raiha, N. C. R., Koskinen, M., and Pikkarainen, P. H. (1967). Developmental changes in alcohol dehydrogenase activity in rat and guinea pig liver. *Biochem. J.* 103:623-626.

Rainier, S., and McCormick, A. M. (1983). *In vivo* metabolism of retinol during fetal rat development. *Fed. Amer. Soc. Exp. Biol.* 42:810.

Rao, B. (1987). Transport and metabolism of vitamin A. *J. Sci. Indust. Res.* 46:297-306.

Rask, L., and Peterson, P. A. (1976). *In vitro* uptake of vitamin A from the retinol-binding plasma protein to mucosal epithelial cells from the monkey's small intestine. *J. Biol. Chem.* 252:6360-6366.

Rask, L., Valtersson, C., Anudi, H., Kvist, S., Eriksson, U., Dallner, G., and Peterson, P. A. (1983). Subcellular localization in normal and vitamin A-deficient rat liver of vitamin A serum transport proteins, albumin, ceruloplasmin and class I major histocompatability antigens. *Exp. Cell Res.* 143:91-102.

Rasmussen, M., Petersen, L. B., and Norum, K. R. (1984). The activity of acyl CoA:retinol acyltransferase in the rat: Variation with vitamin A status. *Brit. J. Nutr.* 51:245-253.

Rasmussen, M., Petersen, L. B., and Norum, K. R. (1985). Liver retinoids and retinol esterification in fetal and pregnant rats at term. *Scand. J. Gastroent.* 20:696-700.

Reiners, J., Loefberg, B., Kraft, J. C., Kochhar, D. M., and Nau, H. (1988). Transplacental pharmacokinetics of teratogenic doses of etretinate and other aromatic retinoids in mice. *Reprod. Toxicol.* 2:19-29.

Reitz, P., Wiss, O., and Weber, F. (1974). Metabolism of vitamin A and the determination of the vitamin A status. *Vitam. Horm.* 32:237-249.

Rizzo, R., Lammer, E. J., Parano, E., Pavone, L., and Argyle, J. C. (1991). Limb reduction defects in humans associated with prenatal isotretinoin exposure. *Teratology* 44:599-604.

Roberts, A. B. (1981). Microsomal oxidation of retinoic acid in hamster liver, intestine and testis. *Ann. NY Acad. Sci.* 359:45-48.

Roberts, A. B., Frolik, C. A., Nichols, M. D., and Sporn, M. B. (1979a). Retinoid-dependent induction of *in vivo* and *in vitro* metabolism fo retinoic acid in tissues of the vitamin A-deficient hamster. *J. Biol. Chem.* 254:6303-6309.

Roberts, A. B., Nichols, M. D., Newton, D. L., and Sporn, M. B. (1979b). *In vitro* metabolism of retinoic acid in hamster intestine and liver. *J. Biol. Chem.* 254:6296-6302.

Roberts, A. B., and Sporn, M. B. (1984). Cellular biology and biochemistry of the retinoids. Pages 210-286 *in* M. B. Sporn, A. B. Roberts, & D. S. Goodman, eds., *The Retinoids*, Vol. 2. Academic Press, New York.

Roche Laboratories (1985). June 1985 presentation to FDA advisory committee and public hearing on etretinate safety.

Ronne, H., Ocklind, C., Wiman, K., Rask, L., Obrink, B., and Peterson, P. (1983). Ligand-dependent regulation of intracellular protein transport: Effect of vitamin A on the secretion of the retinol-binding protein. *J. Cell Biol.* 96: 907-910.

Rosa, F. W. (1993). Retinoid embryopathy in humans. Pages 77-109 *in* G. Koren, ed., *Retinoids in Clinical Practice*. Marcel Dekker, Inc., New York.

Rosa, F. W., Wilk, A. L., and Kelsey, F. O. (1986). Teratogen update: Vitamin A congeners. *Teratology* 33:355-364.

Ross, A. C. (1981). Separation of long chain fatty acid esters of retinol by high-performance liquid chromatography. *Analyt. Biochem.* 115:324-330.

Ross, A. C. (1982). Retinol esterification by rat liver microsomes. *J. Biol. Chem.* 257:2453-2459.

Ruberte, E., Dolle, P., Chambon, P., and Morriss-Kay, G. (1991a). Retinoic acid receptors and cellular retinoid binding proteins. 2. Their differential pattern of transcription during early morphogenesis in mouse embryos. *Development* 111:45-60.

Ruberte, E., Kastner, P., Dolle, P., Krust, A., Leroy, P., Mendelsohn, C., Zelent, A., and Chambon, P. (1991b). Retinoic acid receptors in the embryo. *Sem. Dev. Biol.* 2: 153-159.

Sani, B. P., and Hill, D. L. (1976). A retinoic acid-binding protein from chick embryo skin. *Canc. Res.* 36:409-413.

Satre, M. A. (1990). Maternal-fetal distribution of retinol (vitamin A) and its metabolite retinoic acid in pregnant mice. Ph.D. Thesis. Thomas Jefferson University, Philadelphia, PA.

Satre, M. A., and Kochhar, D. M. (1989). Elevations in the endogenous levels of the putative morphogen retinoic acid in embryonic mouse limb-buds associated with limb dysmorphogenesis. *Dev. Biol.* 133:529-536.

Satre, M. A., Penner, J. D., and Kochhar, D. M. (1989). Pharmacokinetic assessment of teratologically effective concentrations of an endogenous retinoic acid metabolite. *Teratology* 39:341-348.

Satre, M. A., Ugen, K. E., and Kochhar, D. M. (1992). Developmental changes in endogenous retinoids during pregnancy and embryogenesis in the mouse. *Biol. Reprod.* 46:802-810.

Saunders, J. W. (1966). Death in embryonic systems. *Science* 154:604-612.

Schweichel, J. U., and Merker, H. J. (1973). The morphology of various types of cell death in prenatal tissues. *Teratology* 7:253-266.

Scott, K. F. F., Meyskens, F. L., and Haddock-Russell, D. (1982). Retinoids increase transglutaminase activity and inhibit ornithine decarboxylase activity in Chinese hamster ovary cells and in melanoma cells stimulated to differentiate. *Proc. Natl. Acad. Sci. USA.* 79:4093-4097.

Scott, W. J., Ritter, E. J., and Wilson, J. G. (1980). Ectodermal and mesodermal cell death patterns in 6-mercaptopurine riboside-induced digital deformities. *Teratology* 21: 271-279.

Shah, R. S., Rajalakshmi, R., Bhat, R. V., Hazra, M. N., Patel, B. C., Swamy, N. B., and Patel, P. V. (1987). Liver stores of vitamin A in human fetuses in relation to gestational age, fetal size and maternal nutritional status. *Brit. J. Nutr.* 58:181-189.

Shenefelt, R. E. (1972). Morphogenesis of malformations in hamsters caused by retinoic acid: Relation to dose and stage at treatment. *Teratology* 5:103-118.

Sherill, B. C., Innerarity, T. L., and Mahley, R. W. (1980). Rapid hepatic clearance of the canine lipoproteins containing only E apoprotein by a high affinity receptor: Identity with the chylomicron remnant transport process. *J. Biol. Chem.* 255:1804-1807.

Shih, T. W., Shealy, Y. F., Strother, D. L., and Hill, D. L. (1986). Nonenzymatic isomerization of all-*trans* and 13-*cis* retinoids catalyzed by sulfhydryl groups. *Drug. Metab. Dispos.* 14:698-702.

Shingleton, J. L., Skinner, M. K., and Ong, D. E. (1989). Characteristics of retinol accumulation from serum retinol-binding protein by cultured sertoli cells. *Biochemistry* 28:9641-9647.

Sietsema, W. K., and DeLuca, H. F. (1979). *In vitro* epoxidation of all-*trans* retinoic acid in rat tissue homogenates. *Biochem. Biophys. Res. Commun.* 90:1091-1097.

Sietsema, W. K., and DeLuca, H. F. (1982). A new vaginal smear assay for vitamin A in rats. *J. Nutr.* 112:1481-1489.

Simeone, A., Acampora, D., Nigro, V., Faiella, A., Desposito, M., Stornaiuolo, A., Mavilio, F., and Boncinelli, E. (1991). Differential regulation by retinoic acid of the homeobox genes of the four *Hox* loci in human embryonal carcinoma cells. *Mech. Develop.* 33:215-228.

Simpson, K. L. (1983). Relative value of carotenoids as precursors of vitamin A. *Proc. Nutr. Soc.* 42:7-17.

Sivaprasadarao, A., and Findlay, J. C. B. (1988a). The interaction of retinol-binding protein with its plasma membrane receptor. *Biochem. J.* 255:561-569.

Sivaprasadarao, A., and Findlay, J. C. B. (1988b). The mechanism of uptake of retinol by plasma-membrane vesicles. *Biochem. J.* 255:571-579.

Sklan, D., and Ross, A. C. (1987). Synthesis of retinol-binding protein and transthyretin in yolk sac and fetus in the rat. *J. Nutr.* 117:436-442.

Sklan, D., Shalit, I., Labesnik, N., Spirer, Z., and Weisman, Y. (1985). Retinol transport proteins and concentrations in human amniotic fluid, placenta and fetal and maternal serum. *Brit. J. Nutr.* 54:577-583.

Smith, J. E., Muto, Y., Milch, P. O., and Goodman, D. S. (1973). The effects of chylomicron vitamin A on the metabolism of retinol-binding protein in the rat. *J. Biol. Chem.* 248:1544-1549.

Smith, M. (1986). Genetics of human alcohol and aldehyde dehydrogenases. *Adv. Hum. Genet.* 15:249-290.

Smith, M., Hopkinson, D. A., and Harris, H. (1971). Developmental changes and polymorphism in human alcohol dehydrogenase. *Ann. Hum. Genet.* 34:251-271.

Smith, M., Hopkinson, D. A., and Harris, H. (1972). Alcohol dehydrogenase isoenzymes in adult stomach and liver: Evidence for activity of the ADH3 locus. *Ann. Hum. Genet.* 35:243-253.

Sommer, A. (1989). New imperatives for an old vitamin (A). *J. Nutr.* 119:96-100.

Soprano, D. R., Smith, J. E., and Goodman, D. S. (1982). Effect of retinol status on retinol-binding protein biosynthesis rate and translatable protein messenger RNA levels in rat liver. *J. Biol. Chem.* 257:7693-7697.

Soprano, D. R., Soprano, K. J., and Goodman, D. S. (1986). Retinol-binding protein messenger RNA levels in the liver and extrahepatic tissues of the rat. *J. Lipid. Res.* 27:166-171.

Strydom, D. J., and Vallee, B. L. (1982). Characterization of human alcohol dehydrogenase isoenzymes by high performance liquid chromatographic peptide mapping. *Ann. Biochem.* 123:422-429.

Sulik, K. K., and Alles, A. J. (1991). Teratogenicity of the retinoids. Pages 282-295 *in* J. H. Saurat, ed., *Retinoids: 10 Years On.* S. Karger, Basel, Switzerland.

Sulik, K. K., Cook, C. S., and Webster, W. S. (1988). Teratogens and craniofacial malformations: Relationships to cell death. *Development* 103(suppl):213-232.

Tabin, C. J. (1991). Retinoids, homeoboxes, and growth factors – toward molecular models for limb development. *Cell* 66:199-217.

Takahashi, Y. I., Smith, J. E., and Goodman, D. S. (1977). Vitamin A and retinol-binding protein metabolism during fetal development in the rat. *Amer. J. Physiol.* 233:E263-E272.

Takahashi, Y. I., Smith, J. E., Winick, M., and Goodman, D. S. (1975). Vitamin A deficiency and fetal growth and development in the rat. *J. Nutr.* 105:1299-1310.

Thaller, C., and Eichele, G. (1987). Identification and spatial distribution of retinoids in the developing chick limb bud. *Nature* 327:625-553.

Thaller, C., and Eichele, G. (1990). Isolation of 3,4-didehydroretinoic acid, a novel morphogenetic signal in the chick wing bud. *Nature* 345:815-822.

Thompson, J. N., Howell, J. M., and Pitt, G. A. J. (1964). Vitamin A and reproduction in rats. *Proc. Roy. Soc. London*, Ser. B., 159:510-535.

Tickle, C., Alberts, B., Wolpert, L., and Lee, J. (1982). Local application of retinoic acid to the limb bud mimics the action of the polarizing region. *Nature* 296:564-565.

Tickle, C., and Brickell, P. M. (1991). Retinoic acid and limb development. *Sem. Dev. Biol.* 2:189-197.

Tickle, C., Lee, J., and Eichele, G. (1985). A quantitative analysis of the effect of all-*trans* retinoic acid on the pattern of chick wing development. *Dev. Biol.* 109:82-95.

Tomassi, G., and Olson, J. A. (1983). Effect of dietary essential fatty acids in vitamin A utilization in the rat. *J. Nutr.* 113:697-703.

Torma, H., and Vahlquist, A. (1986). Uptake of vitamin A and retinol-binding protein by human placenta *in vitro*. *Placenta* 7:295-305.

Underwood, B. A. (1984). Vitamin A in animal and human nutrition. Pages 277-282 *in* M. B. Sporn, A. B. Roberts and D. S. Goodman, eds., *The Retinoids*, Vol. 1. Academic Press, New York.

Vaessen, M., Meijers, N. H., Bootsma, D., and Geurts van Kessel, A. (1990). The cellular retinoic-acid-binding protein is expressed in tissues associated with retinoic-acid-induced malformations. *Development* 110:371-378.

Vahlquist, A., Johnsson, A., and Nygren, K.-G. (1979). Vitamin A transporting proteins and female sex hormones. *Amer. J. Clin. Nutr.* 32:1433-1438.

Vahlquist, A., and Nilsson, S. (1984). Vitamin A transfer to the fetus and amniotic fluid in rhesus monkey (*Macaca mulatta*). *Ann. Nutr. Metab.* 28:321-333.

Vahlquist, A., Peterson, P. A., and Wybell, L. (1973). Metabolism of the vitamin A transporting protein complex. I. Turnover studies in normal paersons and in patients with chronic renal failure. *Eur. J. Clin. Invest.* 3:352-362.

Vahlquist, A., Rask, L., Peterson, P. A., and Berg, T. (1975). The concentrations of retinol binding protein, prealbumin, and transferrin in the sera of newly delivered mothers and children of various ages. *Scand. J. Clin. Lab. Invest.* 35:569-575.

Vallet, H. L., Stark, A. D., Costas, K., Thompson, S., Davis, R., and Teresi, N. (1985). Isotretinoin (Accutane), vitamin A, and human teratogenicity. Presentation at the Nov. 20, 1985 meeting of the American Public Health Association, Washington, D.C.

Venkatachalam, P. S. (1962). Maternal nutritional status and its effects on the newborn. *Bull. WHO* 26:193-201.

Villard, L., and Bates, C. J. (1985). Carotene dioxygenase (EC 1.13.11.21) activity in vitamin A deficiency in pregnant rats. *Proc. Nutr. Soc.* 44:15A.

Wake, K. (1980). Perisinusoidal stellate cells (fat-storing cells, interstitial cells, lipocytes), their related structure in and around the liver sinusoids, and vitamin A-storing cells in extrahepatic organs. *Intern. Rev. Cytol.* 66:303-353.

Wald, G. (1968). Molecular basis of visual excitation. *Science* 162:230-239.

Wallingford, J. C., and Underwood, B. A. (1986). Vitamin A deficiency in pregnancy, lactation, and the nursing child. Pages 101-152 *in* J. C. Bauernfeind, ed., *Vitamin A Deficiency and Its Control.* Academic Press, Orlando, FL.

Wallingford, J. C., and Underwood, B. A. (1987). Vitamin A status needed to maintain vitamin A concentrations in nonhepatic tissues of the pregnant rat. *J. Nutr.* 117:1410-1415.

Ward, A., Brogden, R. N., Heel, R. C., Speight, T. M., and Avery, G. S. (1983). Etretinate. A review of its pharmacological properties and therapeutic efficacy in psoriasis and other disorders. *Drugs* 26:9-43.

Webster, W. S., Johnston, M. C., Lammer, E. J., and Sulik, K. K. (1986). Isotretinoin embryopathy and cranial neural crest: An *in vivo* and *in vitro* study. *J. Craniofac. Genet. Dev. Biol.* 6:211-222.

Werler, M. N., Rosenberg, L., and Mitchell, A. A. (1989). First trimester vitamin A use in relation to birth defects. *Teratology* 39:489.

Willhite, C. C. (1990). Molecular correlates in retinoid pharmacology and toxicology. Pages 539-573 *in* M. I. Dawson and W. H. Okamura, eds., *Chemistry and Biology of Synthetic Retinoids.* CRC Press, Boca Raton, FL.

Willhite, C. C., Sharma, R. P., Allen, P. V., and Berry, D. L. (1990). Percutaneous retinoid absorption and embryotoxicity. *J. Invest. Dermatol.* 95:523-529.

Williams, J. B., Pramanik, B. C., and Napoli, J. L. (1984). Vitamin A metabolism: Analysis of steady-state neutral metabolites in rat tissues. *J. Lipid. Res.* 25:638-645.

Wilson, J. G. (1974). Teratologic causation in man and its evaluation in non-human primates. Pages 191-203 *in* A. G. Motulsky, ed., *Birth Defects.* American Elsevier Publishing Co., New York

Wilson, J. G. (1977). Current status of teratology. Pages 47-74 *in* J. G. Wilson and F. C. Fraser, eds., *Handbook of Teratology*, Vol. 1. Plenum Press, New York.

Wilson, J. G., Roth, C. B., and Warkany, J. (1953). An analysis of the syndrome of malformation induced by maternal vitamin A deficiency. Effects of restoration of vitamin a at various times during gestation. *Amer. J. Anat.* 92:189-217.

Wyllie, A. H., and Morris, R. G. (1982). Hormone-induced cell death. Purification and properties of thymocytes undergoing apoptosis after glucocorticoid treatment. *Amer. J. Pathol.* 109:78-87.

Yamada, M., Blaner, W. S., Soprano, D. R., Dixon, J. L., and

Goodman, D. S. (1987). Biochemical characteristics of isolated rat liver stellate cells. *Hepatology* 7:1224-1229.

Yeung, D. L. (1974). Effects of oral contraceptives on vitamin A metabolism in the human and the rat. *Amer. J. Clin. Nutr.* 27:125-129.

Yeung, D. L., and Chan, P. L. (1975). Effects of a progestogen and a sequential type oral contraceptive on plasma vitamin A, vitamin E, cholesterol and triglycerdes. *Amer. J. Clin. Nutr.* 28:686-691.

Yost, R. W., Harrison, E. H., and Ross, A. C. (1988). Esterification by rat liver microsomes of retinol bound to cellular retinol-binding protein. *J. Biol. Chem.* 263:18693-18701.

Zachman, R. D., and Olson, J. A. (1961). A comparison of retinene reductase and alcohol dehydrogenase of rat liver. *J. Biol. Chem.* 236:2309-2313.

Zbinden, G. (1975). Investigations on the toxicity of tretinoin administered systemically to animals. *Acta. Derm. Venereol.* 74(Suppl.):36-40.

Zelent, A., Krust, A., Petkovich, M., Kastner, P., and Chambon, P. (1989). Cloning of murine α and β retinoic acid receptors and a novel receptor γ predominantly expressed in skin. *Nature* 339:714-717.

Zelent, A., Mendelsohn, C., Kastner, P., Krust, A., Garnier, J. M., Ruffenach, F., Leroy, P., and Chambon, P. (1991). Differentially expressed isoforms of the mouse retinoic acid receptor-β are generated by usage of two promoters and alternative splicing. *Eur. Molec. Biol. Organiz. J.* 10:71-81.

Zile, M. H., Cullum, M. E., Simpson, R. U., Barua, A. B., and Swartz, D. A. (1987). Induction of differentiation of human promyelocytic leukemia cell line HL-60 by retinoyl glucuronide, a biologically active metabolite of vitamin A. *Proc. Natl. Acad. Sci. USA.* 84:2208-2212.

Zile, M. H., Emerick, R. J., and DeLuca, H. F. (1967). Identification of 13-*cis* retinoic acid in tissue extracts and its biological activity. *Biochim. Biophys. Acta* 141:639-641.

Zimmermann, B., Tsambaos, D., and Sturje, H. (1985). Teratogenicity of arotinoid ethyl ester (Ro 13-6298) in mice. *Teratogen. Carcinog. Mutagenen.* 5:415-431.

Chapter 7

Selenium in Pregnancy and Fetal Development

David S. Wilson

Selenium is an essential nutrient known to have teratogenic effects when ingested in excess. Avian species are particularly affected by the toxic effects of selenium. Selenium's biologic functions are mediated by proteins that are known to incorporate selenium as the amino acid seleno-cysteine. The best characterized of these is the antioxidant enzyme glutathione peroxidase, but the list of selenium's functions is increasing as more selenoproteins are discovered. A type I deiodinase and a plasma selenoprotein are among the recently characterized selenoproteins. The National Research Council (NRC) has recently established a specific Recommended Dietary Allowance (RDA) for selenium.

Both deficiency and excess intake of selenium pose health problems for humans and other species. Selenium deficiency has been related to cancer, cardiomyopathy (disease of the heart muscle), arthritis, impaired immune function and other diseases. Most evidence for these effects remains epidemiologic. Excess selenium has been shown to produce congenital malformations or developmental defects in a number of species: birds, fish, swine, cattle, sheep, rodents. These defects include encephalocoele (cranial extrusions), anophthalmia (absence of eyes), microphthalmia (small eyes), defects of limbs and beak and morphologic changes in viscera. However, no such effects have been demonstrated in primates or in humans. During human pregnancy plasma selenium levels and GSHpx activity have been shown to drop while RBC GSHpx activity remains constant. The placental transfer of selenium is thought to assure adequate supply to the developing fetus whose requirements may exceed those of the mother.

The toxicity of selenium is such that lethality may be reached before any teratogenic effects are seen. Little is known of the mechanisms of selenite teratogenicity or selenium metabolism during pregnancy. High levels of selenium have been shown to affect the integrity of the DNA structure in cells, but the developmental implications of such effects have not been thoroughly tested. One can conclude from the data currently available, especially from studies in primates, that humans are unlikely to ingest amounts of selenium sufficient to produce teratogenic effects. Such effects are found, however, in avian species with excess intake of selenium.

Role of Selenium

Since the early work of Franke noting the production of congenital anomalies in chicks (Franke, *et al.*, 1936) and the review of Smith et al on the toxicity and pathology of selenium (Smith, *et al.*, 1937), there has been a growing interest in the potential reproductive impact of an excessive or deficient intake of selenium in its varied forms. Much recent interest in the topic has been stimulated in the United States by media dramatization of congenital defects found in wild fowl at the Kesterson Reservoir in the Central Valley of California (Fan & Kizer, 1990). Both geologic and human concentrating activities in the Western United States have indeed made excessive intake of selenium in organic and inorganic forms an issue of some concern. Self-supplementation with selenium by humans may also generate problems as claims for the disease fighting potential of selenium becomes more widely publicized.

While its essentiality has been demonstrated for many species (Combs & Combs, 1986), selenium remains potentially the most toxic of nutrients in amounts not much in excess of those required for normal biologic activity. The biologic functions of selenium and the problems of deficiency and toxicity have been addressed by several excellent recent reviews (Combs & Combs, 1986; Neve, 1991; Lockitch, 1989). The toxicology of selenium has also been reviewed

(Lo & Sandi, 1980; Wilber, 1980; Barlow & Sullivan, 1982; Olson, 1986). The focus of this paper will be on the more recent literature that explores the relationship of selenium as a nutrient to pregnancy and reproductive outcome. The discussion will concern mainly studies appearing since the publication of the excellent summary of selenium nutrition by Combs and Combs in 1986.

Selenium Metabolism

The biologic functions of selenium as they are currently understood are mediated by proteins that incorporate the element as the selenoamino acid selenocysteine (Stadtman, 1990; Sunde, 1990). As many as thirteen selenoproteins have been identified in rodents and other species by analysis of radioactively-labeled proteins (Behne, et al., 1991; Davidson & McMurray, 1988). However, it is still unclear whether or not some of the lower molecular weight forms are derived from the larger proteins that may be processed to give smaller active forms of seleno-proteins.

The mechanism of insertion of the selenoamino acid into proteins, requiring cotranslational modification of a specific tRNA, has been elucidated (Leinfelder, et al., 1988; Stadtman, 1990). mRNA for the protein contains a UGA sequence that is normally a stop codon to terminate translation, but that, in this case, becomes a signal for the insertion of selenocysteine. The DNA coding for selenocysteine thus contains the corresponding TGA base codon. Nucleotide sequences beyond the TGA position are apparently required for interpretation of this stop codon as a signal for selenocysteine insertion (Berry, et al., 1991c; Bock, et al., 1991). This peculiarity of selenium genetics is found both in prokaryotes and eukaryotes.

Glutathione Peroxidase

The best defined function of selenium is its role at the active site of the enzyme glutathione peroxidase (GSHpx) where it serves as a catalyst for the reduction of hydroperoxides with concommitant production of reduced glutathione (GSSG) (Tappel, 1987). The oxidized form of glutathione is then reduced to GSH by glutathione reductase to re-initiate the cycle. Selenium is incorporated into GSHpx at the active site as selenocysteine, the main dietary form of selenium from animal foods. Essentially universal in mammalian tissues, the GSHpx system serves as a principal weapon in the body's defenses against damage by oxygen radicals. Its activity may also be useful as an index of functional selenium status although GSHpx activity in platelets has been suggested as a better measure of short-term selenium nutrition (Kiem, 1988). Activity of GSHpx is unlikely to be useful as a marker of toxicity since its activity levels off with increasing intake of selenium. Also regulation of the expression of the GSHpx gene appears to vary substantially with different species as well as with dietary intake of selenium (Toyoda, 1989). Experiments by Saedi et al determined that livers from selenium-deficient rats had 7-17% of the GSHpx mRNA found in the livers of selenium-adequate rats (Saedi, *et al.*, 1988). Use of a cDNA probe has led to discovery of loci for the GSHpx gene on human chromosomes 3, 21 and X (McBride, *et al.*, 1988).

Other Selenoproteins

Extensive recent research has added to the list of possible functions that selenoproteins may accomplish in various species. A second selenium-dependent glutathione peroxidase has been found in plasma that is immunologically and enzymatically distinct from the cellular form (Avissar, *et al.*, 1989a). It is a tetramer of 21.5 kDa subunits similar to the cellular form, but appears to be secreted as a glycoprotein by hepatocytes (Avissar, *et al.*, 1989b; Maddipati & Marnett, 1987). Its primary structure has been determined (Takahashi, 1990) and is 44% homologous with that of the cellular form.

Another eukaryotic selenoenzyme, Type I 5'-iodothyronine deiodinase has been characterized (Berry, *et al.*, 1991a). Active mainly in liver and kidney in rats (Beckett, *et al.*, 1989;

Behne, *et al.*, 1990), this enzyme catalyzes the conversion of 3,5,3′5′-tetraiodothyronine (T4) to 3,5,3′-triiodothyronine (T3), the biologically active form of the thyroid hormone (Berry, *et al.*, 1991b). Selenium deficiency inhibits the activity of this enzyme (Beckett, *et al.*, 1989). The deiodinase contains one selenium atom per subunit polypeptide incorporated as selenocysteine. mRNA for the selenoenzyme contains the UGA codon for selenocysteine found in GSHpx coding and thus the stop codon, TGA, is found in the DNA coding for the enzyme. Selenium deficiency reduces deiodinase activity in brown adipose tissue (BAT) in rats (Arthur, *et al.*, 1991), perhaps by affecting the level of uncoupling protein in BAT (Geloen, *et al.*, 1990). However, the enzyme in BAT that converts T4 to T3 is the type II 5′-deiodinase which according to recent evidence is not a selenoenzyme (Safran, *et al.*, 1991).

This list of selenoproteins must also include a mitochondrial capsule protein that is required for normal spermatogenesis (Calvin, *et al.*, 1987). Messenger RNA for this protein and its developmental expression have been studied recently, using cDNA clones (Kleene, *et al.*, 1990). These investigators conclude that selenium is not incorporated into the protein cotranslationally as it is in other eukaryotic selenoproteins. Isotope studies with 75Se have located other polypeptides in sperm and changes in labeling over time suggest that these may be precursor forms that are processed to give the 17 kDa cap protein. An 18 kDa selenoprotein that exhibits phospholipid hydroperoxide glutathione peroxidase activity has been found in cultured tumor cell lines (Maiorino, *et al.*, 1991). Unlike the "classical" GSHpx it is resistant to changes in dietary selenium intake and is active in reduction of membrane hydroperoxides. Bansal, *et al.* (1991) have also isolated two cellular selenoproteins of 56 and 14 kDa in rodent tissues using antisera raised in rabbits. The smaller one is a fatty acid-binding protein. Synthesis of these proteins is not responsive to dietary selenium levels.

Similar techniques have been used recently by Burk's group to characterize the 57 kDa plasma selenoprotein P

(Read, *et al.*, 1990). This glycoprotein is synthesized in the liver (Motsenbocker & Tappel, 1982) and contains ten selenocysteine residues per polypeptide, nine of which are located within the terminal 122 amino acids (Hill, *et al.*, 1991). Synthesis of this protein is responsive to dietary selenium intake up to about 0.5 ppm and contains most of the selenium in rat plasma. Its synthesis also takes precedence over that of GSHpx when deficient rats are resupplied with selenium. Selenoprotein P apparently binds to cells in the brain (Burk, *et al.*, 1991) and possibly other tissues (Gomez & Tappel, 1989), but no definitive function has yet been ascribed to it. One may speculate that it is the source of proteins of similar or lower molecular weight that have been isolated from various tissues.

Requirements and Selenium-Related Disease States

The essentiality of selenium for humans has recently been emphasized in the establishment of a specific adult daily Recommended Dietary Allowance set at 70 µg for males and 55 µg for females in the United States (National Research Council, 1989). This requirement is based mainly on the biochemical function of selenium at the active site of glutathione peroxidase, but the number of selenoproteins unrelated to GSHpx that have been identified suggests that it is warranted in a broader sense. Frank disease symptoms due to selenium deficiency are hard to demonstrate in humans, but it is becoming increasingly clear that selenium status is important in a number of human diseases (Zumkley, 1988). Deficiency of selenium is associated with reduced GSHpx activity in the tissues where it is found (Combs & Combs, 1986; Combs, 1990). Deficiency predisposes to the cardiomyopathy known as Keshan disease as well as to the presenile arthritis found in Kashin-Beck disease (Li, *et al.*, 1990). Prolonged total parenteral nutrition using solutions devoid of selenium may also produce selenium-responsive muscle pain and weakness and, rarely, the cardiomyopathy characteristic of Keshan disease (Lockitch, 1989). Selenium deficiency also affects the thyroid gland and is thought to impair thermogenic adaptation to cold (Watanabe & Suzuki, 1986). It is suggested that the deficiency impairs the conversion of T4 to T3 with consequent changes in energy metabolism. Thyroid weight also decreases in such a deficiency (Arthur, *et al.*, 1991).

Other biologic effects associated with selenium deficiency support the essentiality of the nutrient and the establishment of a dietary requirement. The involvement of selenium in the immune system and resistance to infection has recently been reviewed (Dhur, *et al.*, 1990; Spallholz, *et al.*, 1990). Spallholz indicates that it is important for the control of the respiratory burst generated by phagocytic cells, for the metabolism of hydroperoxides in the production of various soluble regulatory factors and that it is needed for reduction of peroxides generated by initiators of free radical reactions. Supplementation of elderly subjects with selenium increased lymphocyte proliferation in response to pokeweed mitogen stimulation (Peretz, *et al.*, 1991). Deficiency of selenium has been shown to reduce lymphocyte proliferation without, however, affecting the production of soluble mediators of the immune function (Kiremidjian, *et al.*, 1990). On the other hand, excess selenium may suppress the activity of certain immune cells (Nair & Schwartz, 1990).

The possible functions of selenium in reducing the risk of developing certain forms of cancer have also been reviewed (Ip, 1986; Ip, *et al.*, 1991; Medina & Morrison, 1988). There is considerable epidemiologic evidence that selenium status is inversely related to the risk of developing certain types of cancer (Willett & Stampfer, 1988). For the most part, where increased risk is linked to deficiency, this protective effect appears to be related to the antioxidant functions of selenium (Levander, 1991). The feasibility of clinical trials with supraphysiologic doses of selenium has generated considerable interest (Chen & Clark, 1986). Use of selenium in chemo-prevention of cancer appears to merit additional studies on the dosage and form of the element that would have the highest therapeutic index. One can surmise that selenoproteins other than glutathione peroxidase are likely to mediate some of the potential preventive effects. Selenium may achieve a preventive effect by reducing the formation of DNA adducts with carcinogens (Ejadi, *et al.*, 1989). Its anticarcinogenic activity would thus operate during the initiation phase. Selenite may also counter the effect of methylating carcinogens by reducing the availability of glutathione for the methylating reaction (Sato, *et al.*, 1991).

Associations have been made between selenium status and the incidence of amyotrophic lateral sclerosis and cystic fibrosis, but the evidence here is somewhat tenuous. Four cases of amyotrophic lateral sclerosis were found in a population of 4000 over a ten-year period in an area of South Dakota where selenium intoxication is endemic among farm animals (Kilness & Hochberg, 1977). Cystic fibrosis and Keshan disease appear to share a common primary or induced selenium deficiency occurring around 22 weeks of fetal life, during early postnatal period or during the rapid growth period of early school years (Wallach, *et al.*, 1990). It has been proposed that oxidant stress and a deficiency of micronutrient antioxidants may be common to various forms of pancreatitis and cystic fibrosis. A preliminary trial with combined doses of such antioxidants has been successful in reducing inflammation of the pancreas (Uden, *et al.*, 1990). Several studies have revealed low plasma selenium in individuals with cystic fibrosis, but no mechanistic relationship has been clearly established (Lockitch, 1989).

Selenium in Pregnancy and Fetal Development

Concern over the possible toxicity of selenium during pregnancy as well as possible changes in requirements during gestation has produced a growing body of literature. Inadequate intake may also present problems since selenium is required for normal intrauterine growth and development (Combs & Combs, 1986). Species differences in response to deficiency or excess of selenium have been widely illustrated (Barlow & Sullivan, 1982). The exact mechanisms of these differences, however, are not well understood and knowledge of selenium metabolism in pregnancy remains limited. Teratogenic effects of excess intake of selenium have not been demonstrated in primates or humans and have been inconsistent with regard to most mammalian species. Early evidence suggested an association between inhalation of selenium dust and abortion in humans (Robertson, 1970), but no link between selenium status and reproductive effects has been established subsequently in humans. Experimental work has obviously been confined to non-human species. The question of selenium teratogenicity is admittedly complicated by a variety of factors. In addition to considering the particular species involved, it is essential in the design and interpretation of experiments on the reproductive effects of selenium that one take into account the chemical form of selenium, the route of administration, developmental stage of the conceptus, nutritional status of the mother, dosage and bioavailability of the nutrient and possibly interactions with other minerals or nutrients (Combs, 1990; Parizek, 1987; Mattison, 1991).

Effects of Pregnancy on Selenium Status

Decreases in plasma selenium and in glutathione peroxidase activity during pregnancy have been frequently observed (Butler & Whanger, 1987; Levander, et al., 1987). A comparison of pregnant and non-pregnant women found both selenium content and the GSHpx activity of plasma declined progressively throughout the course of pregnancy (Table 1). No changes were found in erythrocyte selenium content or GSHpx activity (Behne & Wolters, 1979). In rats, levels of selenium from 0.05 to 0.2 µg/g of diet did not affect these changes, which suggests that they are due mainly to the physiologic events of pregnancy (Smith & Picciano, 1986). The results of Butler & Whanger (1987) have generally confirmed data from many earlier studies. Cord levels of plasma and RBC selenium and GSHpx activity were all lower than in maternal samples although neonate whole blood selenium tended to be higher than maternal at birth. Swanson, *et*

TABLE 1. Selenium Content and GSHpx Activity
in the Plasma of Pregnant Women (X ± SD)

Group	Number of Subjects	Selenium (μg/kg)	GSHpx (U/kg)	Se Bound to GSHpx (fraction)
Non-pregnant	17	88 ± 11	170 ± 28	0.015
1st trimester	2	89 ± 1	144 ± 2	0.012
2nd trimester	14	83 ± 10	130 ± 39	0.012
3rd trimester	21	74 ± 12	116 ± 35	0.012

Adapted with permission from Behne & Wolters, 1979.

al. (1983) found that pregnant women tend to have reduced urinary selenium excretion during pregnancy, especially during late pregnancy, which points to a compensating effect that parallels decreases in serum selenium.

Maternal zinc and selenium levels in normal pregnancies and in pregnancies with fetal neural tube defect (NTD) or increased levels of alpha feto-protein (AFP) have been compared by Hinks, *et al.* (1989). Plasma selenium levels declined significantly during normal pregnancy while red blood cell selenium remained essentially unchanged. In women with fetal NTD and elevated plasma AFP, significantly lower than normal white blood cell selenium levels were found (Hinks, *et al.*, 1989). Examination of cultured fibroblasts from fetuses with NTD suggests that low levels of selenium in the diet are correlated with a higher incidence of neural tube defect (Zimmerman & Lozzio, 1989). Decreases in serum selenium concentration have been repeatedly confirmed in uncomplicated pregnancy, but in pregnant women with intrauterine growth retardation or non-inflammatory disease of the liver, serum selenium has been found to rise (Peiker, 1991a).

Several studies have examined the concentrations of selenium in umbilical cord blood as an index of fetal accumulation and placental transfer. Maternal values for plasma selenium and RBC GSHpx activity were significantly higher than those of fetal blood (Rudolph & Wong, 1978). In another investigation GSHpx activities of mothers were higher than those found in the cord blood of neonates, but were similar to those of non-pregnant women (Bannon, *et al.*, 1986). Kundu, *et al.* (1985) found no changes in serum selenium during normal pregnancies in an area of high soil selenium although the subjects studied did show increases in serum copper. The population from this region in South Dakota has shown a high incidence of infant and neonatal mortality as well as increased risk of complications during pregnancy. Others have found that zinc and selenium may interact (Chmielnicka, *et al.*, 1988), which raises the possibility that investigators should control for the presence of other nutrient interactions with selenium in determining effects relating to reproductive outcome. Zinc and selenium have, for example, been shown to form complexes in neurons (Slomianka, *et al.*, 1990). Excess selenium intake may alter tissue levels of copper as well (Chen, *et al.*, 1987).

Whole blood GSHpx activity and plasma selenium levels were determined in premature infants from a low selenium area of Northern Ireland (Tubman, *et al.*, 1990). Seventy-five preterm infants followed from birth to 70 days of age showed a decline in plasma selenium, but no change in GSHpx activity from birth to age 10 weeks. At birth GSHpx activity was 2.74 U/ml; plasma selenium was 34 µg/l. These selenium levels appear lower than those found in preterm infants elsewhere (Table 2). In a study of preterm infants fed human milk, preterm formula or sodium selenite-supplemented preterm formula, the authors were led to conclude that measurement of blood selenium does not adequately reflect dietary intake of preterm infants (Smith, *et al.*, 1991). After three weeks of supplementation, no differences in plasma selenium or erythrocyte GSHpx activity were found. No evaluation of amounts excreted was offered. Healthy infants and children generally show plasma selenium levels in the range of 50-150 µg/l (Litov & Combs, 1991).

Changes in maternal and fetal selenium levels during pregnancy in tissues other than blood have not been widely studied. In experiments designed to determine the relative effects of selenite or selenomethionine on GSHpx activity in developing rats, it was found that maternal intake of the two forms of selenium or of a selenium-deficient basal diet had

TABLE 2. Plasma or Serum Concentrations (mmol/kg) in Neonates

Location	No.	Group	Mean ± SD
Verona	38	Term-cord sample	0.49 ± 0.10
Dusseldorf	12	Term-cord sample	0.63
Helsinki	200	Term-cord sample	0.51 ± 0.08
Oslo	31	Term-cord sample	0.66
	20	Preterm-cords	0.66
Antwerp	9	Term-cord sample	0.83 ± 0.18
Vancouver, Canada	20	<2.5 kg infants	0.81 ± 0.19
	20	>1.5 kg infants	0.96 ± 0.12
Vancouver, Canada	35	<1.5 kg infants	0.77 ± 0.17
	39	1.5-2.5 kg infants	0.86 ± 0.22
	56	>2.5 kg infants	1.03 ± 0.24
Hamilton, Canada	6	Preterm infants	1.13 ± 0.38
	12	Preterm infants	0.63 ± 0.38
New York	68	Preterm infants	1.10 ± 0.40
	18	Term infants	1.23 ± 0.31
Portland	9	<1.5 kg infants	1.24 ± 0.71
	9	<1.5 kg infants	1.55 ± 0.98
New York	30	<32 weeks	1.25 ± 0.13
New York	25	Term-cord sample	1.75 ± 0.38

Adapted with permission from Lockitch, 1989.

little effect on fetal GSHpx activity (Lane, *et al.*, 1991). Supplementation of the maternal diet with selenomethionine did, however, increase the activity of GSHpx in fetal eye tissue. Milk from selenomethionine-fed mothers had higher levels of selenium than did milk from those fed selenite. Lung tissue from developing rat pups born to mothers deficient in selenium during pregnancy and lactation showed a greater extent of histologic lesions when subjected to elevated oxygen tension (Kim, *et al.*, 1991). Whole blood and liver selenium concentrations have been examined in samples from 101 dairy cattle and fetuses (Van Saun, *et al.*, 1989). Fetal liver selenium and whole blood GSHpx activity were significantly higher than corresponding maternal values while serum selenium concentration was significantly lower. No differences were found between whole blood or erythrocyte selenium levels in paired fetuses and dams.

Requirements for Pregnancy and Lactation

Changes in selenium levels and GSHpx activity in blood along with estimates of selenium balance during pregnancy and lactation have been used to justify the need for increased selenium in both periods. The most recent NRC recommendation is an increase of 10 µg/day for pregnancy and an additional 20 µg/day during lactation. The latter assumes an average selenium content for human milk of 15-20 µg/l (Mannan & Picciano, 1987). Selenium is found in foods in the organic forms as selenocysteine (animal sources) and selenomethionine (plant sources) or in inorganic forms in drinking water. Selenium balance in pregnant and non-pregnant women on controlled diets has been evaluated in an often cited study (Swanson, et al., 1983). The comparison between the non-pregnant state and late pregnancy shown in Table 3 reveals a decrease in urinary excretion accompanied by an increase in absorption and retention measured over a 12 day period. Average daily retention of selenium during the full term of pregnancy was estimated to be 3.5-5.0 µg. It is possible, however, that homeostatic regulation of selenium balance by mammalian systems may make use of the balance technique inappropriate for estimation of selenium requirements (Levander & Burk, 1986). Tissue selenium and GSHpx activity in 18 day old rat pups were found to be strongly correlated with maternal selenium intake and milk concentra-

TABLE 3. Selenium Balance in Pregnant and Non-Pregnant Women[1,2]

	$NP (n=6)$[3]	$EP (n=6)$[3]	$LP (n=4)$[3]
Selenium intake (µg/day)	150 ± 2^a	154 ± 1^a	158 ± 2^a
Fecal selenium (µg/day)	28 ± 1^a	33 ± 3^a	28 ± 1^a
Urinary selenium (µg/day)	111 ± 2^a	100 ± 6^a	96 ± 2^a
Apparent retention (µg/day)	11 ± 2^a	21 ± 4^b	34 ± 2^c

[1] Data expressed as mean ± SEM. Within a row, means sharing common superscripts are not significantly different (p>0.05).

[2] Measurements made over the last 12 days of a 20-day confined metabolic study in which a constant diet was fed.

[3] NP = non-pregnant; EP = 10-20 wks of gestation; LP = 30-40 wks of gestation.

Selenium in sweat or expired air was not measured.
Adapted with permission from Swanson, et al., 1983.

tions (Smith & Picciano, 1986). In two day old pups, however, selenium levels and GSHpx activity in liver, heart and kidney did not reflect maternal selenium status. The differences between the two stages were ascribed to the selenium intake from the dams' milk. Adequate maternal selenium intake during lactation is, then, a critical component of post-natal development (Kumpulainen, 1989). Current research is investigating the fact that selenium in milk appears to be bound mainly to proteins (Ellis, *et al.*, 1990). Experimental analysis has allowed detection of 8-10 selenium-containing protein fractions in milk from cows, goats and humans (Debski, *et al.*, 1987). Utilization of selenium from selenite or selenomethionine has been studied recently (Mangels, *et al.*, 1990). Selenomethionine appeared to be better absorbed than selenite by all groups studied (lactating, non-lactating and never-pregnant women), appearing in plasma and milk in higher concentrations.

Placental Involvement

Placental transfer of selenium is a significant factor in regulating availability of selenium to the fetus. The form in which selenium is transferred is not known. In bovine species, the placenta appears to concentrate selenium. A study of placental transfer of selenium in beef cattle indicated that the element readily crosses the placenta and that fetal concentrations of blood selenium can achieve higher levels than those of the mother (Koller, *et al.*, 1984). Trials with sustained-release supplements in cows also indicated significant placental transfer of maternal selenium to the fetus (Campbell, *et al.*, 1990). Schrammel, *et al.* (1988) examined levels of selenium and heavy metal concentrations in the maternal blood and the placentae and cord blood of neonates. These authors found a positive correlation between maternal and cord blood selenium but no correlation between maternal blood selenium and that in the placenta. The mechanisms of placental transfer of selenate and selenite have been studied in vitro using brush border membrane vesicles from fresh normal term human placentae (Shennan, 1987; Shennan, 1988). Transfer of these compounds was inhibited by sulfate and anions similar in ionic stucture to selenate. Selenium appears thus in these experiments to share a transport pathway with sulfur. Offspring appear not to be affected by these decreases in maternal selenium concentrations or GSHpx activity. Placentae of women with low blood selenium from an area with low soil selenium were found to have selenium levels similar to those of the placentae of women with higher blood selenium (Korpela, *et al.*, 1984). This suggests again that the placenta may operate to assure adequate fetal availability of selenium. These more recent studies confirm results of many earlier investigations in other species showing that the placenta appears able to sequester selenium to assure adequate supplies to the fetus (Smith & Picciano, 1986).

Pregnancy-Induced Hypertension

Women with pregnancy-induced hypertension (PIH) were found to have increased levels of lipid peroxidation products (Peiker, *et al.*, 1991b). Wickens, *et al.* (1981) measured free radical oxidation products in women with PIH. They found a continuous rise of such products during pregnancy along with a progressive increase in the severity of the condition. Serum selenium was not correlated with this increase. Erythrocyte GSHpx activity was found to be significantly higher in women with severe or superimposed hypertension as compared to levels in women with a mild form (Uotila, *et al.*, 1990). The increases may be due to the large increase of peroxides generated in PIH (Kaupilla, *et al.*, 1987). Disturbed prostaglandin metabolism may also contribute. No significant differences could be found between amniotic fluid selenium levels of normal and hypertensive pregnant women (Karunanithy, *et al.*, 1989). Amniotic fluid selenium gradually decreased during the course of pregnancy in healthy women (Roy, *et al.*, 1989). It appears that while GSHpx activity may increase in PIH, the rise does not affect selenium levels in the blood.

Effects on Fetal Development

Since Robertson's suggestion that selenium may be teratogenic (Robertson, 1970), considerable effort has been devoted to investigating the teratogenic potential of the different forms of selenium. It is clear that species respond differently to excesses and deficiencies of selenium (Barlow & Sullivan, 1982; Shamberger, 1985).

Avian species have presented the most striking evidence of the teratogenic potential of high intakes of selenium. The regional accumulation of high levels of selenium and their distribution in waters, soils and the food chain has been documented since 1984 (Schuler, *et al.*, 1990). Feeding studies and field studies have demonstrated an extensive range of malformations that can be ascribed to excessive intake of selenium. Offspring of mallard ducks fed levels of selenomethionine as high as 16 ppm exhibited congenital defects of the eyes, bill, legs and feet (Heinz, *et al.*, 1989). Selenocysteine feeding did not lead to impaired reproduction. Selenium teratogenesis among populations of aquatic species at the Kesterson Reservoir in Central California has been thoroughly documented (Ohlendorf, *et al.*, 1986; Hoffman, *et al.*, 1988). Effects ranged from high levels of embryo mortality through anophthalmia, microphthalmia and limb defects to morphologic changes in heart, liver and gastric tissue (Ohlendorf, *et al.*, 1986). Selenium concentrations in food sources for these species were 12-130 times higher than those from control areas. The grasslands area nearby also showed elevated concentrations of selenium in the tissues of the species examined (Ohlendorf, *et al.*, 1987). Bioconcentration of selenium in various forms has been demonstrated in several microorganisms and in plants common to aquatic ecosystems (Brown & Schrift, 1982). Biotic concentrating activity may ultimately achieve a nearly 5000-fold increase in the concentration of selenium over surrounding water levels (Schuler, *et al.*, 1990). For the cyanobacterium *Anabaena flos-aquae*, common to this environment, bioconcentration effects increased in the order selenate, selenite and selenomethionine, suggesting that both organic and inorganic forms may achieve increased toxicity in this process (Kiffney & Knight, 1990).

Mammalian species inhabiting the region around Kesterson have also been examined. Clark found no apparent biologic effects of the high selenium intake among raccoons (Clark, *et al.*, 1989) or smaller mammals such as rodents (Clark, 1987). However, use of the Frog Embryo Teratogenesis assay to measure the developmental toxicity of sodium selenite has produced results indicating moderate teratogenic potential (DeYoung, *et al.*, 1991). Embryos in this study exhibited edema and malformations of the gut, heart and face.

In an investigation of embryotoxicity in hamsters, Ferm, *et al.* (1990) administered selenate, selenite and selenomethionine during critical periods of embryogenesis. Doses ranged from 1.8-8.7 mg/kg and were administered either orally or intravenously by injection or infusion. Again the oral routes produced the most frequent effects with the development of cranial extrusions as the most common malformation. Significant maternal toxicity was seen with single oral doses or injections. In another study with a single equimolar intravenous or oral dose of selenate or selenomethionine (4.73 mg/kg), embryonic selenium from selenate plateaued at 0.6 $\mu g/g$, but continued to increase after the dose of selenomethionine to a level of 15.7 $\mu g/g$ (Willhite, *et al.*, 1990). No teratogenic effects were found in hamsters receiving selenate and selenomethionine either orally or intravenously. These investigators suggest that maternal lethality may be reached before teratogenic effects are seen. No teratogenic effects were observed before doses reached maternal toxicity even though placental and embryonic tissue did accumulate selenium.

A mouse model has been proposed as a means for evaluation of placental and fetal development in studies on the teratogenicity of potentially toxic compounds (Hau, *et al.*, 1987). In the evaluation of this assay system, moderate doses of selenite initiated 11 days before mating did not negatively affect growth of placenta or fetuses. Large doses, however,

(330 µg/mouse/day), caused a significant rate of abortion with a reduction of weight in those animals born.

Intravenous injection of selenate and selenite in mice at different stages of pregnancy produced similar embryonic and fetal uptake of the two forms (Danielsson, *et al.*, 1990a). Uptake by specific tissues varied with gestational age. Placental transfer appeared to increase with time and dose level. During embryonic development neuro-epithelial tissue showed the greatest rate of uptake while the eye, liver and skeleton had the highest accumulations during the fetal period. Results from an in vitro assay with mesenchymal limb bud cells suggested that selenite toxicity was greater than that of selenate. In pregnant mice dosed by gavage from day 7-15 of gestation with 7 mg selenium/kg as sodium selenite, no apparent maternal or fetal effects were observed (Plasterer, *et al.*, 1985). The authors caution that the dose may have been below that required for observation of gestational toxicity, but that there is a very narrow range of dose levels where congenital effects might be seen before maternal lethality occurs.

In an important study of the developmental toxicity of selenomethionine in primates, *Macaca fascicularis,* Tarantal, *et al.* (1991) found no evidence of teratogenic effects of selenium in this form. Pregnant animals were given doses of 0, 25, 150 and 300 µg/kg body weight/day during the gestational period of organogenesis. Offspring exhibited no developmental defects that were ascribed to the treatments. The authors concluded that the non-human primate embryo is no more sensitive to this form of selenium than is the mother and that the principal effect of high doses of selenomethionine is on fertility rather than on pregnancy-related events.

Dietary selenite may in some conditions have a protective effect against compounds known to induce embryo- and fetotoxicity. Supplementation of selenite prior to and during gestation reduced embryotoxicity of infused salicylate, but did not counteract a decline in fetal growth due to the salicylate (Bergman, *et al.*, 1990). However, selenite supplementation was found to increase the incidence of fetal malformations after repeated gavage with salicylate. In those animals receiving selenite alone (3.0 or 4.5 µg/g of diet), without the salicylate, no negative impact on fetal development was observed. An unsual supplementation of pregnant mice with selenocarrageenan at about the levels of requirement found that the dose increased litter size by 53% and average litter weight by five percent (Chiachun, *et al.*, 1991). The time of administration is another complicating factor in studies relating to the developmental impact of high doses of selenium. Dose-dependent fetal death and growth retardation were observed in pregnant mice injected subcutaneously on day 12 but not on day 16 of gestation (Yonemoto, *et al.*, 1983).

Young animals injected with selenite may develop cataracts, an outcome that probably derives from the interference of high levels of selenite with normal ocular metabolism of glutathione (Bunce & Hess, 1981). The effects of selenite on epithelial tissue in the lens appear to occur before or during DNA synthesis (Cenedella, 1987; Cenedella, 1989). Poulsen, *et al.* (1989) have investigated the effects of excessive dietary selenium fed to sows giving birth for the first time and their offspring. Levels of sodium selenite as high as 16 mg/kg diet did not impair reproductive outcome. Neither maternal mortality nor the incidence of fetal anomalies was increased by these levels of supplementation. Selenium toxicosis during pregnancy has, however, produced bleeding claw lesions in piglets (Mensink, *et al.*, 1990). Localization of the lesion to the claw may be due to the fact the selenotic ration was fed during the second half of pregnancy.

Freshwater fish may also show toxic concentrations of selenium with transfer from parent to progeny (Schultz & Hermanutz, 1990). Bioaccumulation of selenium through the food chain may be responsible for reproductive failure in different species of fish. Redear sunfish in a selenium-contaminated lake showed impaired reproductive capacity in both sexes (Sorenson & Thomas, 1988). However, Ogle and Knight found no impact of high environmental levels of selenium on the growth and reproduction of fathead minnows (Ogle & Knight, 1989).

Deficiency of selenium during gestation and the early neonatal period may also present problems. The pathologic effects of selenium deficiency during gestation appear mainly in neonates and in the early and late postnatal stages of development (Bostedt & Schramel, 1990). Congenital muscular dystrophy has been seen in lambs, calves and foals. Biochemical signs of congenital nutritional muscular dystrophy have been found in fetuses from selenium-deficient ewes two weeks before parturition (Hamliri, *et al.*, 1990). Fetuses showed low blood selenium concentrations and increased plasma creatine kinase and lactate dehydrogenase activities. Maternal selenium deficiency has been reported to enhance the fetolethality of methylmercury (Nishikido, *et al.*, 1988) but not to affect the incidence or the critical gestational period for methylmercury-induced cleft palate (Nishikido, *et al.*, 1987). Mercury concentrations in maternal and fetal tissues did not correlate with selenium levels in the diet. Glutathione peroxidase activity in maternal tissues was unaffected by methylmercury administration while activity of the fetal liver enzyme was decreased and selenium concentrations in fetal liver increased. Analysis of fetal liver cytosol suggested that selenium was not in the form of selenocysteine, *i.e.*, incorporated into proteins.

Low serum selenium and GSHpx are associated with the development of a form of cretinism found in areas of endemic goitre (Goyens, *et al.*, 1987; Vanderpas, *et al.*, 1990). This disease is due to a primary thyroid deficiency that develops before or early after birth. The investigators attributed the problem to oxidative damage to the thyroid in individuals with low antioxidant system defenses. No link was made between the disease and the effects of selenium deficiency on the activity of the type I seleno-deiodinase discussed above. A connection has also been suggested between Sudden Infant Death Syndrome and selenium status during gestation and at birth (Reid, 1991).

Selenium and Nucleic Acid Metabolism

The potential genotoxicity of selenium has been discussed previously along with its effects on nucleic acids (Shamberger, 1985). Recent literature provides further insights into the possible interactions of selenium with genetic material and raises the possibility that such interactions are involved in the teratogenicity of selenium in affected species. Very little is understood about the mechanisms of such interactions. Selenite has been found to inhibit DNA synthesis in a number of studies (Frenkel & Falvey, 1988). Morrison & Medina (1989) have found that cells from the MOD mammary epithelial cell line cultured with 395 µg/l selenite exhibit reduced DNA synthesis. This effect is enhanced by the addition of methionine and serine and is also accompanied by the appearance of a 58 kDa selenoprotein (Morrison, *et al.*, 1988a; Morrison, *et al.*, 1988b).

Endogenous sulfhydryl compounds appear to be involved in the inhibiting effects of selenite on DNA synthesis. Selenotrisulfide derivatives of sulfhydryl interactions with selenite appear to inhibit both DNA and RNA polymerases (Frenkel, *et al.*, 1987). Most of these studies focus on the anticarcinogenic aspects of selenite metabolism without considering the possible teratogenic implications of such interactions between selenite and nucleic acids. Studies with cultured hepatocytes suggest that cytotoxic levels of selenite (20-30 µM) may achieve their effect through DNA fragmentation (Garberg, *et al.*, 1987). Selenite-induced redox cycles may lead to cell lysis not only through depletion of energy supplies, but through DNA damage and subsequent polymerase activation as well. Selenite may also affect mitochondrial calcium fluxes and NAD(P)H oxidation states with subsequent toxic impact (Vlessis & Mela-Riker, 1987).

Doses of sodium selenite from 63 to 231 mg/l in culture have been shown to induce DNA fragmentation, DNA-repair synthesis, chromosome aberrations and inhibition of mitosis in human fibroblasts (Lo, *et al.*, 1978). It remains difficult to separate mutagenic, teratogenic and lethal effects given the high toxicity of selenite. Similar studies in cultured leuko-cytes have confirmed the damage to chromosomes by selenite (Nakamuro, *et al.*, 1976). Tests for the mutagenicity of sele-nate and selenite in bacterial assay systems have produced base-pair substitutions (Noda, *et al.*, 1978). The compounds thus appear to be weakly mutagenic. Effects are clearly dose-dependent.

Synthetic organoselenium compounds have been shown to have cytotoxic effects. A dimer of *p*-methoxybenzeneselenol and benzylselenocyanate that has shown some promise as a chemopreventive agent also causes chromosome aberrations (deletions, rings, dicentrics) as well as sister-chromatid ex-changes and changes in the process of mitosis in the cell (Khalil & Maslat, 1990). Snyder found that incubation of human fibroblasts with 50-500 µM selenite produced damage to DNA in a dose-dependent manner (Snyder, 1987). He contends that such damage is not related to reduced ability to defend against increases in oxidative stress. Addition of re-duced glutathione to the culture medium greatly enhanced the cells' sensitivity to the selenite which supports the suggestion that the toxicity of selenite requires a glutathione-selenite conjugant for activation (Whiting, *et al.*, 1980). Pretreatment with sodium selenite has been found to enhance the increase in DNA strand breakage caused by sodium chromate (Sug-iyama, *et al.*, 1987). Such pretreatment resulted in increased cellular levels of glutathione.

It is possible that selenium deficiency with concurrent decreases in GSHpx activity might lead to oxidative damage to DNA. Investigations in cultured human cells found that selenite supplementation produced a 2-4 fold increase in GSHpx activity in P31 and HT29 cell lines (Sandstrom & Marklund, 1990). A small but significant decrease in single-strand DNA breaks in the p31 cells due to exposure to increased oxidant levels was seen with increased GSHpx activity. No differences were seen in cell survival rates with supplementation. Prior selenium status, however, had no effect on radiation-induced cell death or DNA strand break-age in cultured cells (Sandstrom, *et al.*, 1989).

Effects of Selenium on Male Reproduction

One could expect selenium deficiency to have an effect on the male contribution to reproductive function given the requirement of selenium for normal spermatogenesis. Selenium deficiency leads to changes in sperm mitochondrial capsule morphology and to reduced stability of the sperm tail. Sperm count and fertility are severely reduced as a consequence (Wallace, *et al.*, 1987). In mice fed a selenium deficient diet for five weeks, a high proportion of abnormal sperm was found compared to those of controls (Ernst & Lauritsen, 1991).

Conclusions and Research Needs

The recent literature relating to selenium nutrition during pregnancy and development confirms results from earlier work. Knowledge on the subject remains limited and much more work is needed to extend our understanding of normal and abnormal selenium metabolism during pregnancy. It is clear that maternal selenium status changes with gestation. Plasma selenium and glutathione peroxidase activity decline progressively while erythrocyte selenium normally remains constant. This decline appears to be a normal accompaniment of pregnancy. RBC GSHpx activity is not apparently impaired. Attempts to reverse the decline with moderate increases in dietary selenium have been unsuccessful. The NRC recommends an additional 10 µg of selenium per day during pregnancy. This additional intake may enhance selenium deposition in other tissues and thus prepare for the increased demand during lactation in as much as that additional selenium becomes available for transfer via milk. Levander, *et al.* (1987) found an average intake of 80 µg per day by American subjects that appears sufficient to cover the increased demand during pregnancy and lactation. Normal increases in food intake during pregnancy and lactation would make supplementation unwarranted outside of regions of endemically low intake. One must be reminded that selenium supplementation, especially during pregnancy, presents risks, however in-completely defined.

While adequate maternal selenium status is important for fetal growth and development, the ability of the placenta to make maternal selenium available may dampen the effect of maternal selenium deficiency on the fetus. Studies are needed to determine the degree to which this may be true. It is not known whether the placenta is able to reduce the teratogenic potential of high selenium intake by the mother. One may speculate that the presence of the placenta explains in part differences between avian and mammalian developmental responses to selenosis.

Species differences in response to selenosis have been accentuated by media treatment of congenital malformations found in waterfowl and deaths due to high environmental levels of selenium in California. There are, however, some resemblances between malformations found in birds and other species. Additional research needs to be done to explain these different responses. The difficulty of such efforts is compounded by the need to control for all the various factors related to selenium biochemistry. It may be that selenium exhibits a narrow range of teratogenicity before the level of lethality is reached. Moreover, it is possible that nutrient interactions with high levels of selenium may indirectly cre-ate developmental problems. Gestational deficiency or excess may also cause effects in the developing fetus that are mani-fested only some time after birth and which are not in the strict sense teratogenic. Such problems merit further experimental inquiry.

In all of these cases, the mechanisms of developmental injury related to selenium intake are poorly defined. It is not known whether selenoproteins as mediators of the biologic effects of selenium are involved in developmental events. They have not been investigated in avian species. Determin-ing their involvement in the events of pregnancy and birth outcome may be of great value. Further study of the interac-tions of selenium and nucleic acids as they affect development is also warranted. Effects appear to be both chemical and biochemical. It would be important to further distinguish between these two categories and to investigate the relationships between selenoproteins and nucleic acid metabolism. The molecular biology of selenium is an area of intense interest and certainly would help understand the potential teratogenicity of the nutrient. Data currently available, however, especially those from studies done in primates (Tarantal, *et al.*, 1991) suggest that teratogenic effects relating to high selenium intake are unlikely to occur in humans. It also appears that physiological changes in selenium metabolism in pregnant humans may operate to reduce the potential effects of excess or deficient maternal intake on the fetus.

Acknowledgment

This study was supported in part by PHS-NIH-NIEHS Grant # 1- P42 E505961-01.

References

Arthur, J. R., Nicol, F., Beckett, G. J., and Trayhurn, P. (1991). Impairment of iodothyronine 5′-deiodinase activity in brown adipose tissue and its acute stimulation by cold in selenium deficiency. *Can. J. Physiol. Pharmacol.* 69:782-785.

Avissar, N., Whitin, J. C., Allen, P. Z., Palmer, I. S., and Cohen, H. J. (1989a). Antihuman plasma glutathione peroxidase antibodies: immunologic investigations to determine plasma gluthathione peroxidase protein and selenium content in plasma. *Blood* 73:318-323.

Avissar, N., Whitin, J. C., Allen, P.Z., Wagner, D. D., Liegey, P., and Cohen, H. J. (1989b). Plasma selenium-dependent glutathione peroxidase, cell of origin and secretion. *J. Biol. Chem.* 264:15850-15855.

Bannon, M., Halliday, H. L., and McMaster, D. (1986). Glutathione peroxidase activity in cord blood: Effects of fetal sex and maternal smoking. *Biol. Neonate* 50:274-277.

Bansal, M. P., Clement, I. P., and Medina, D.(1991). Levels and 75Se-labeling of specific proteins as a consequence of dietary selenium concentration in mice and rats. *Soc. Exp. Biol. Med.* 196:147-154.

Barlow, S. M., and Sullivan, F. M., eds. (1982). Selenium and its compounds. Pages 483-500 *in* S. M. Barlow and F. M. Sullivan, eds., *Reproductive Hazards of Industrial Chemicals: An Evaluation of Animal and Human Data.* Academic Press, New York.

Beckett, G. J., MacDougall, D. A., Nicol, F., and Arthur, J. R. (1989). Inhibition of type I and type II iodothyronine deiodinase activity in rat liver, kidney and brain produced by selenium deficiency. *Biochem. J.* 259:887- 892.

Behne, D., and Wolters, W. (1979). Selenium content and glutathione peroxidase activity in the plasma and erythrocytes of non-pregnant and pregnant women. *J. Clin. Chem. Clin. Biochem.* 17:133-135.

Behne, D., Kyriakopoulos, A., Meinhold, H., and Kohrle, J.(1990). Identification of type I iodothyronine 5-deiodinase as a selenoenzyme. *Biochem. Biophy. Res. Comm.* 173:1143-1149.

Behne, D., Kyriakopoulos, A. Scheid, S., and Gessner, H. (1991). Incorporation of selenium into tissue proteins in rats. *J. Nutr.* 806-814.

Bergman, K., Cekan, E., Slanina, P., Gabrielsson, J., and Hellenas, K.-E. (1990). Effects of dietary sodium selenite supplementation on salicylate-induced embryo- and fetotoxicity in the rat. *Toxicol.* 61:135-146.

Berry, M. J., Banu, L., and Larsen, P.R. (1991a). Type I iodothyronine deiodinase is a selenocysteine-containing enzyme. *Nature* 349:438-440.

Berry, M. J., Kieffer, J. D., Harney, J. W., and Larsen, P. R. (1991b). Selenocysteine confers the biochemical properties characteristic of the type I iodothyronine deiodinase. *J. Biol. Chem.* 266:14155-14158.

Berry, M. J., Banu, L. Chen, Y. Y., Mandel, S. J.Kieffer, J. D., Harney, J. W., and Larsen, P. R. (1991c). Recognition of UGA as a selenocysteine codon in type I deiodinase requires sequences in the 3′ untranslated region. *Nature* 353:273-276.

Bock, A., Forchhammer, K., Heider, J., Leinfelder, W., Sawers, G., Veprek, B., and Zinoni, F. (1991). Selenocysteine: The 21st amino acid. *Molec. Micro.* 5:515-520.

Bostedt, H., and Schramel, P. (1990). The importance of selenium in the prenatal and postnatal development of calves and lambs. *Biol. Trace Elem. Res.* 24:163-171.

Brown, T. A., and Schrift, A. (1982). Selenium: Toxicity and tolerance in higher plants. *Biol. Rev.* 57:59-84.

Bunce, G. E., and Hess, J. L.(1981). Biochemical changes associated with selenite-induced cataract in the rat. *Exp. Eye. Res.* 33:505-514.

Burk, R. F., Hill, K. E., Read, R., and Bellew, T. (1991). Response of rat selenoprotein P to selenium administration and fate of its selenium. *Amer. J. Physiol.* 261: E26-30.

Butler, J. A., and Whanger, P. D. (1987). Dietary selenium requirements of pregnant women and their infants. Pages 688-700 *in* G. F. Combs, Jr., J. E. Spallholz, O. A. Levander and J. E. Oldfield, eds., *Selenium in Biology and Medicine*, Part B. Avi, New York.

Calvin, J. I., Grosshans, K., Musicant-Shikora, S. R., and Turner, S. I. (1987). A developmental study of rat sperm and testis selenoproteins. *J. Reprod. Fert.* 81:1-11.

Campbell, D. T., Maas, J., Weber, D. W., Hedstrom, O. R., and Norman, B. B. (1990). Safety and efficacy of two sustained-release intrareticular selenium supplements and the associated placental and colostral transfer of selenium in beef cattle. *Amer. J. Vet. Res.* 5:813-817.

Cenedella, R. J. (1987). Direct chemical measurement of DNA synthesis and net rates of differentiation of rat lens epithelial cells *in vivo*: Applied to the selenium cataract. *Exp. Eye Res.* 44:677-690.

Cenedella, R. J. (1989). Cell cycle specific effects of selenium on the lens epithelium studied *in vivo* by the direct chemical approach. *Curr. Eye Res.* 8:429-433.

Chen, J., and Clark, L. C. (1986). Proposed supplemental dosages of selenium for a phase I trial based on dietary and supplemental selenium intakes and episodes of chronic selenosis. *J. Amer. Coll. Toxicol.* 5:71-78.

Chen, S. Y., Collipp, P. J., and Hsu, J. M. The effect of selenium toxicity on tissue distribution of zinc, iron, and copper in rats. Pages 367-376 *in* G. F. Combs, Jr., J. E. Spallholz, O. A. Levander and J. E. Oldfield, eds., *Selenium in Biology and Medicine*, Part A. Avi, New York.

Chiachun, T., Hong, C., and Haifun, R. (1991). The effects of selenium on gestation, fertility, and offspring in mice. *Biol. Trace Elem. Res.* 30:227-231.

Chmielnicka, J., Zareba, G., Witasik, M., and Brzeznicka, E. (1988). Zinc-selenium interaction in the rat. *Biol. Trace Elem. Res.* 15:267-276.

Clark, D. R., Jr. (1987). Selenium accumulation in mammals exposed to contaminated California irrigation drainwater. *Sci. Total. Environ.* 66:147-168.

Clark, D. R., Jr., Ogasawara, P. A., Smith, G. J., and Ohlendorf, H. M. (1989). Selenium accumulation by raccoons exposed to irrigation drainwater at Kesterson National Wildlife Refuge, California, 1986. *Arch. Environ. Contam. Toxicol.* 18:787-794.

Combs, F. G., Jr., and Combs, S. B. (1986). *The Role of Selenium in Nutrition.* Academic Press, Orlando, FL.

Combs, G. F., Jr. (1990). Growing interest in selenium. *West J. Med.* 154:192-194.

Danielsson, B. R. G., Danielson, M., Khayat, A., and Wide, M.(1990a). Comparative embryotoxicity of selenite and selenate: Uptake in murine embryonal and fetal tissues and effects on blastocysts and embryonic cells in vitro. *Toxicology* 63:123-136.

Danielsson, B. R., Khayat, A., and Dencker. L. (1990b). Foetal and maternal distribution of inhaled mercury vapour in pregnant mice: Influence of selenite and dithiocarbamate. *Pharmacol. Toxicol.* 67:222-226.

Davidson, W. B., and McMurray, C. H. (1988). Selenium-labeled sheep plasma: The time course of changes in 75Selenium distribution. *J. Inorgan. Biochem.* 34:1-9.

Debski, B., Picciano, M. F., and Milner, J. H. (1987). Selenium content and distribution of human, cow and goat milk. *J. Nutr.* 117:1091-1097.

DeYoung, D. J., Bantle, J. A., and Fort, D. J. (1991). Assessment of the developmental toxicity of ascorbic acid, sodium selenate, coumarin, serotonin, and 13-cis retinoic acid using fetax. *Drug Chem. Toxicol.* 14:127-141.

Dhur, A., Galan, P., and Hercberg, S. (1990). Relationship between selenium, immunity and resistance against infection. *Comp. Biochem. Physiol. Chem.* 96:271-280.

Ejadi, S., Bhattacharya, I. D., Voss, K., Singletary, K., and Milner, J.A. (1989). *In vitro* and *in vivo* effects of sodium selenite on 7,12-dimethylbenz[a]anthracene – DNA adduct formation in isolated rat mammary epithelial cells. *Carcinogenesis* 10:823-826.

Ellis, L., Picciano, M. F., Smith, A. M., Hamosh, M., and Mehta, N. R. (1990). The impact of gestational length on human milk selenium concentration and glutathione peroxidase activity. *Pediatr. Res.* 27:32-50.

Ernst, E., and Lauritsen, J. G. (1991). Effect of organic and inorganic mercury on human sperm motility. *Pharmacol. Toxicol.* 68:440-444.

Fan, A. M., and Kizer, K. W. (1990). Selenium – nutritional, toxicologic and clinical aspects. *West J. Med.* 153:160-167.

Ferm, V. H., Hanlon, D. P., Willhite, C. C., Choy, W. N., and Book, S.A. (1990). Embryotoxicity and dose-response relationships of selenium in hamsters. *Repro. Toxiocl.* 4:183:190.

Franke, K. W., Moxon, A. L., Poley, W. E., and Tully, W. C.(1936). Monstrosities produced by the injection of selenium salts into hens' eggs. *Anat. Rec.* 65:15-22.

Frenkel, G. D., Walcott, A., and Middleton, C. (1987). Inhibition of RNA and DNA polymerases by the product of the reaction of selenite with sulfhydryl compounds. *Molec. Pharmacol.* 31:112-116.

Frenkel, G. D., and Falvey, D. (1988). Evidence for the involvement of sulfhydryl compounds in the inhibition of cellular DNA synthesis by selenite. *Molec. Pharmacol.* 34:573- 577.

Garberg, P., Stahl, A., Warholm, M., and Hogberg, J. (1987). Studies of the role of DNA fragmentation in selenium toxicity. *Biochem. Pharmacol.* 37:3401-3406.

Geloen, A., Arthur, J. R., Beckett, G. J., and Trayhurn, P.(1990). Effect of selenium and iodine deficiency on the level of uncoupling protein in brown adipose tissue of rats. *Biochem. Soc. Trans.* 18:1269-1270.

Gomez, B., Jr., and Tappel. A.L.(1989). Selenoprotein P receptor from rat. *Biochim. Biophy. Acta* 979:20-26.

Goyens, P., Golstein, J., Nsombola, B. Vis, H., and Dumont, J.E. (1987). Selenium deficiency as a possible factor in the pathogenesis of myxoedematous endemic cretinism. *Acta Endocrinol.* 114:497-502.

Hamliri, A., Olson, W. G., Johnson, D. W., and Kessabi, M.(1990). Evaluation of biochemical evidence of congenital nutritional myopathy in two-week prepartum fetuses from selenium-deficient ewes.*Amer. J. Vet. Res.* 51: 1112-1115.

Hau, J., Basse, A., and Wolstrup, C.(1987). A murine model for the assessment of placental and fetal development in teratogenicity studies. *Lab. Animals* 21:26-36.

Heinz, G. H., Hoffman, D. J., and Gold, L. G. (1989). Impaired reproduction of mallards fed an organic form of selenium. *J. Wildl. Manage.* 53:418-428.

Hill, K. E., Lloyd, R. S., Yang, J. G., Read, R., and Burk, R. F.(1991). The cDNA for rat selenoprotein P contains 10 TGA codons in the open reading frame. *J. Biol. Chem.* 266:10050-10053.

Hinks, L. J., Ogilvy-Stuart, A., Hambidge, K. M., and Walker, V. (1989). Maternal zinc and selenium status in pregnancies with a neural tube defect or elevated plasma alpha-fetoprotein. *Brit. J. Obstet. Gynocol.* 96:61-66.

Hoffman, D. J., Ohlendorf, H. M., and Aldrich. T. W. (1988). Selenium teratogenesis in natural populations of aquatic birds in central California. *Arch. Environ. Contam. Toxicol.* 17:519-525.

Ip, C. (1986). The chemopreventive role of selenium in carcinogenesis. *J. Amer. Coll. Toxicol.* 5:7-20.

Ip, C., Hayes, C., Budnick, R. M., and Ganther, H. E. (1991). Chemical form of selenium, critical metabolites, and cancer prevention. *Cancer Res.* 51:595-600.

Karunanithy, R., Roy, A. C., and Ratnam, S. S. (1989). Selenium status in pregnancy: Studies in amniotic fluid from normal pregnant women. *Gynecol. Obstet. Invest.* 27:148- 150.

Kauppila, A., Makila, U. M., Korpela, H., Viinikka, L., and Yrjanheikki, E. (1987). Relationship of serum selenium and lipid peroxidation in preeclampsia. Pages 996-1001 *in* G. F. Combs, Jr., J. E. Spallholz, O. A. Levander and J. E. Oldfield, eds., *Selenium in Biology and Medicine*, Part B. Avi, New York.

Khalil, A. M., and Maslat, O.(1990). Chromosome aberrations, sister-chromatid exchanges and cell-cycle kinetics in human peripheral blood lymphocytes exposed to organoselenium in vitro. *Mutat. Res.* 232:227-232.

Kiem, J. (1988). Selenium in platelets. *Biol. Trace Elem. Res.* 15:83-88.

Kiffney, P., and Knight, A. (1990). The toxicity and bioaccumulation of selenate, selenite and seleno-L-methionine in the cyanobacterium *Anabaena flos-acquae*. *Arch. Environ. Contam. Toxicol.* 19:488-494.

Kilness, A. W., and Hochberg, F. H. (1977). Amyotrophic lateral sclerosis in a high selenium environment. *J. Amer. Med. Assoc.* 237:2843-2844.

Kim, H. Y., Picciano, M. F., Wallig, M. A., and Milner, J. A. (1991). The role of selenium nutrition in the development of neonatal rat lung. *Pediatr. Res.* 29:440- 445.

Kiremidjian, L., Roy, M., Wiske, H. I., Cohen, M. W., and Stotsky, G. (1990). Selenium and immune cell functions. 1. Effect on lymphocyte proliferation and production of interleukin 1 and interleukin 2. *Proc. Soc. Exp. Biol. Med.* 193:136-42.

Kleene, K. C., Smith, J., Bozorgzadeh, A., Harris, M., Hahn, L., Karimpour, I., and Gerstel, J. (1990). Sequence and developmental expression of the mRNA encoding the seleno-protein of the sperm mitochondrial capsule in the mouse. *Dev. Biol.* 137:395-402.

Koller, L. D., Whitbeck, G. A., and South, P. J. (1984). Transplacental transfer and colostral concentrations of selenium in beef cattle. *Amer. J. Vet. Res.* 45:2507-2510.

Korpela, H. Loueniva, R. Yrjanheikki, E., and Kauppila, A. (1984). Selenium concentration in maternal and umbilical cord blood, placenta and amniotic membranes. *Intern. J. Vit. Nutr. Res.* 54:257-262.

Kumpulainen, J. (1989). Selenium: Requirement and supplementation. *Acta Paediatr. Scand.*, Suppl. 351:114- 117.

Kundu, N., Parke, P., and Petersen, L. P. (1985). Distribution of serum selenium, copper, and zinc in normal human pregnancy. *Arch. Environ. Hlth.* 40:268-273.

Lane, H. W., Strength, R., Johnson, J., and White M. (1991). Effect of chemical form of selenium on tissue glutathione peroxidase activity in developing rats. *J. Nutr.* 121:80-86.

Leinfelder, W., Zehelein, E., Mandrand-Berthelot, M., and Bock, A. (1988). Gene for a novel tRNA species that accepts L-serine and cotranslationally inserts selenocysteine. *Nature* 331:723-725.

Levander, O. A., and Burk, R. F. (1986). Report on the 1986 A.S.P.E.N. Research Workshop on Selenium in Clinical Nutrition. *J. Parenter. Enteral. Nutr.* 10:545-549.

Levander, O. A., Moser, P. B., and Morris, V. C. (1987). Dietary selenium intake and selenium concentrations of plasma, erythrocytes, and breast milk in pregnant and postpartum lactating and nonlactating women. *Amer. J. Clin. Nutr.* 46:694-698.

Li, F., Duan, Y., Yan, S., Guan, J., Zou, L., Wei, F., Mong, L., Li., L., and Li, S. (1990). Presenile (early ageing) changes in tissues of Kaschin-Beck disease and its pathogenetic significance. *Mech. Ageing Devlop.* 54:102-120.

Litov, R. E., and Combs, G. F. Jr. (1991). Selenium in pediatric nutrition. *Pediatrics* 87:339-351.

Lo, M-T., and Sandi, E. (1980). Selenium: Occurrence in

foods and its toxicological significance – A review. *J. Environ. Pathol. Toxicol.* 4:193-218.

Lo, L. W., Koropatnick, J., and Stich, H. F. (1978). The mutagenicity and cytotoxicity of selenite, "activated" selenite and selenate for normal and DNA repair-deficient human fibroblasts. *Mutat. Res.* 49:305-312.

Lockitch, G.(1989). Selenium: Clinical significance and analytical concepts. *Crit. Rev. Clin. Lab. Sci.* 27:483- 541.

Maddipati, K. R., and Marnett, L. J. (1987). Characterization of the major hydroperoxide-reducing activity of human plasma. *J. Biol. Chem.* 262:17398-17403.

Maiorino, M., Chu, F. F., Ursini, F., Davies, K. J. A., Doroshow, J. H., and Esworthy, R. S. (1991). Phospholipid hydroperoxide glutathione peroxidase is the 18-kDa selenoprotein expressed in human tumor cell lines. *J. Biol. Chem.* 12:7728-7732.

Mangels, A. R., Moser-Veillon, P. B., Patterson, K. Y., and Veillon, C. (1990). Selenium utilization during human lactation by use of stable-isotope tracers. *Amer. J. Clin. Nutr.* 52:621-627.

Mannan, S., and Picciano, M. F. (1987). Influence of maternal selenium status on human milk selenium concentration and glutathione peroxidation activity. *Amer. J. Clin. Nutr.* 98:383-389.

Mattison, D. R. (1991). An overview on biological markers in reproductive and developmental toxicology: Concepts, definitions and use in risk assessment. *Biomed. Environ. Sci.* 4:8-34.

McBride, O. W., Mitchell, A., Lee, B. J., Mullenbach, G., and Hatfield, D. (1988). Gene for selenium-dependent glutathione peroxidase maps to human chromosomes 3, 21 and X. *Biofactors* 1:285-292.

Medina, D., and Morrison, D. G. (1988). Current ideas on selenium as a chemopreventive agent. *Pathol. Immunopathol. Res.* 7:187-199.

Mensink, C. G., Koeman, J. P., Veling, J., and Gruys, E. (1990). Haemorrhagic claw lesions in newborn piglets due to selenium toxicosis during pregnancy. *Vet. Rec.* 620-622.

Morrison, D. G., Dishart, M. K., and Medina, D. (1988a). Intracellular 58-kd selenoprotein levels correlate with inhibition of DNA synthesis in mammary epithelial cells. *Carcinogenesis* 9:1801-1810.

Morrison, D. G., Dishart, M. K., and Medina, D. (1988b). Serine and methionine enhancement of selenite inhibition of DNA synthesis in a mouse mammary epithelial cell line. *Carcinogenesis* 9:1811-1815.

Morrison, D. G., and Medina, D. (1989). Time course of selenite metabolism in confluent cultures of mouse mammary epithelial cells. *Chem. Bio. Interactions* 71:177-186.

Motsenbocker, M. A., and Tappel, A. L. (1982). A selenocysteine-containing selenium-transport protein in rat plasma. *Biochem. Biophy. Acta* 719:147-153.

Nair, M. P., and Schwartz, S. A. (1990). Immunoregulation of natural and lymphokine-activated killer cells by selenium. *Immunopharmacology* 19:177-183.

Nakamuro, K., Yoshikawa, K., Sayato, Y., Kurata, H., Tonomura, M., and Tonomura, A. (1976). Studies in selenium-related compounds. V. Cytogenetic effect and reactivity with DNA. *Mutat. Res.* 40:177-184.

National Research Council. (1989). *Recommended Dietary Allowances.* National Academy Press, Washington, D.C.

Neve, J. (1991). Physiological and nutritional importance of selenium. *Experientia* 47:187-193.

Nishikido, N., Furuyashiki, K., Naganuma, A., Suzuki, T., and Imura, N. (1987). Maternal selenium deficiency enhances the fetolethal toxicity of methylmercury. *Toxicol. Appl. Pharmacol.* 88:322-328.

Nishikido, N., Satoh, Y., Naganuma, A., and Imura, N. (1988). Effect of maternal selenium deficiency on the teratogenicity of methylmercury. *Toxicol. Lett.* 40:153-157.

Noda, M., Takano, T., and Sakurai, H. (1979). Mutagenic activity of selenium compounds. *Mutat. Res.* 66:175-179.

Ogle, R. S., and Knight, A. W. (1989). Effects of elevated

foodborne selenium on growth and reproduction of the fathead minnow (*Pimephales promelas*). *Arch. Environ. Contam. Toxicol.* 18:795-803.

Ohlendorf, H. M., Hoffman, D. J. Saiki, M. K., and Aldrich, T. W. (1986). Embryonic mortality and abnormalities of aquatic birds: Apparent impacts by selenium from irrigation drainwater. *Sci. Total. Environ.* 52:49-63.

Ohlendorf, H. M., Hothem, R. L., Aldrich, T. W., and Krynitsky, A. J. (1987). Selenium contamination of the Grasslands, a major California waterfowl area. *Sci. Total. Environ.* 66:169-183.

Olson, O. E. (1986). Selenium toxicity in animals with emphasis on man. *J. Amer. Coll. Toxicol.* 5:45-70.

Parizek, J. (1987). Dose-response aspects of selenium in nutritional toxicology. Pages 66-77 *in* G. F. Combs, Jr., J. E. Spallholz, O. A. Levander, and J. E. Oldfield, eds., *Selenium in Biology and Medicine*, Part A. Avi, New York

Peiker, G., Muller, B., Dawczynski, H., and Winnefeld, K. (1991a). Das erhalten von selen im serum und erythrozyten bei frauen mit cornaler und risikoschwangerschaft (schwangerschaftsinduzierte hypertonie, fetale retardierung und hepatose). *Zentbl. Gynakol.* 113:45-48.

Peiker, G., Kretzschmar, J., Dawczynski, H., and Muller, B.(1991b). Lipidperoxidation in der pathologischen schwangerschaft: Schwangerschaftsinduzierte hypertonie. *Zentbl. Gynakol.* 113:183-188.

Peretz, A., Neve, J., Desmedt, J., Duchateau, J., Dramaix, J., and Famaey, J. P. (1991). Lymphocyte response is enhanced by supplementation of elderly subjects with selenium-enriched yeast. *Amer. J. Clin. Nutr.* 53:1323- 1328.

Plasterer, M. R., Bradshaw, W. S., Booth, G. M., and Carter, M. W. (1985). Developmental toxicity of nine selected compounds following prenatal exposure in the mouse: Naphthalene, p-nitrophenol, sodium selenite, dimethyl phthalate, ethylenethiourea, and four glycol ether derivatives. *J. Toxicol Environ. Health* 15:25-38.

Poulsen, H. D., Danielsen, V., Nielsen, T. K., and Wolstrup,

C. (1989). Excessive dietary selenium to primiparous sows and their offspring. *Acta Vet. Scand.* 30:371-378.

Read, R., Bellow, T., Yang, J., Hill, K. E., Palmer, I. S., and Burk, R. F. (1990). Selenium and amino acid composition of selenoprotein P, the major selenoprotein in rat serum. *J. Biol. Chem.* 265:17899-17905.

Reid, G. M. (1991). Sudden infant death syndrome (SIDS): A time lag factor. *Med. Hypoth.* 34:186-189.

Robertson, D. S. F. (1970). Selenium – a possible teratogen. *Lancet* (7645):518-519.

Roy, A. C., Ratnam, S. S., and Karunanithy, R. (1989). Amniotic fluid selenium status in pre-eclampsia. *Gynecol. Obstet. Invest.* 28:161-162.

Rudolph, N., and Wong. S. L. (1978). Selenium and glutathione peroxidase activity in maternal and cord plasma and red cells. *Pediat. Res.* 12:789-792.

Saedi, M. S., Smith, C. G., Frampton, J., Chambers, I., Harrison, P. R., and Sunde, R. A. (1988). Effect of selenium status on mRNA levels for glutathione peroxidase in rat liver. *Biochem. Biophys. Res. Commun.* 153:855-861.

Safran, M., Farwell, A. P., and Leonard J. L. (1991). Evidence that Type II 5'-deiodinase is not a selenoprotein. *J. Biol. Chem.* 266:13477-13480.

Sandstrom, B. E., Carlsson, J., and Marklund, S. L. (1989). Selenite-induced variation in glutathione peroxidase activity of three mammalian cell lines: No effect on radiation-induced cell killing or DNA strand breakage. *Radiat. Res.* 117:318-325.

Sandstrom, B. E., and Marklund, S. F. (1990). Effects of variation in glutathione peroxidase activity on DNA damage and cell survival in human cells exposed to hydrogen peroxide and t-butyl hydroperoxide. *Biochem. J.* 271:17-23.

Sato, M., Nunoshiba, T., Nishioka, H., Yagi, T., and Takebe, H. (1991). Protective effects of sodium selenite on killing and mutation by N-methyl-N'-nitro-N-nitrosoguanidine in *E. coli*. *Mutat. Res.* 250:73-77.

Schramel, P., Hasse, S., and Ovcar-Pavlu, J. (1988). Selenium, cadmium, lead, and mercury concentrations in human breast milk, in placenta, maternal blood, and the blood of the newborn. *Biol. Trace Elem. Res.* 15:111-124.

Schuler, C. A., Anthony, R. G., and Ohlendorf, H. M. (1990). Selenium in wetlands and waterfowl foods at Kesterson Reservoir, California, 1984. *Arch. Environ. Contam. Toxicol.* 19:845-853.

Schultz, R., and Hermanutz, R. (1990). Transfer of toxic concentrations of selenium from parent to progeny in the fathead minnow (*Pimephales promelas*). *Bull. Environ. Contam. Toxicol.* 45:568-573.

Shamberger, R. J. (1985). The genotoxicity of selenium. *Mutat. Res.* 154:29-48.

Shennan, D. B. (1987). A study of selenate efflux from human placental microvillus membrane vesicles. *Biosci. Rep.* 7: 675-680.

Shennan, D. B. (1988). Selenium (selenate) transport by human placental brush border membrane vesicles. *Brit. J. Nutr.* 59:13-19.

Slomianka, L., Danscher, G., and Frederickson, C. J. (1990). Labeling of the neurons of origin of zinc-containing pathways by intraperitoneal injections of sodium selenite. *Neurosci* 38:843-854.

Smith, A. M., and Picciano, M. F. (1986). Evidence for increased selenium requirement for the rat during pregnancy and lactation. *J. Nutr.* 116:1068-1079.

Smith, A. M., Chan, G. M., Moyer-Mileur, L. J., Johnson, C. E., and Gardner, B. R. (1991). Selenium status of preterm infants fed human milk, preterm formula, or selenium-supplemented preterm formula. *J. Pediatr.* 119:429-433.

Smith, M. I., Stohlman, E. F., and Lillie, R. D. (1937). The toxicity and pathology of selenium. *J. Pharm. Exp. Therapeu.* 60:449-471.

Snyder, R. D. (1987). Effects of sodium selenite on DNA and carcinogen induced DNA repair in human diploid fibroblasts. *Cancer Letts.* 34:73-81.

Sorensen, E. M., and Thomas, P. (1988). Selenium accumulation, reproductive status, and histopathological changes in environmentally exposed redear sunfish. *Arch. Toxicol.* 61:324-329.

Spallholz, J. E., Boylan, M., and Larsen, H. S. (1990). Advances in understanding selenium's role in the immune system. Pages 123-139 *in* G. T. Keusch, A. Cerami and F. Takaku, eds., *Micronutrients and Immune Functions.* New York Academy of Sciences, New York.

Stadtman, T. C. (1990). Selenium biochemistry. *Annu. Rev. Biochem.* 59:111-127.

Sugiyama, M., Ando, A., Furuno, A., Furlong, N. B., Hidaka, T., and Ogura, R. (1987). Effects of vitamin E, vitamin B2 and selenite on DNA single strand breaks induced by sodium chromate (VI). *Cancer Letts.* 38:1-7.

Sunde, R. A. (1990). Molecular biology of selenoproteins. *Annu. Rev. Nutr.* 10:451-474.

Swanson, C. A., Reamer, D. C., Veillon, C., King, J. C., and Levander, O. A. (1983). Quantitative and qualitative aspects of selenium utilization in pregnant and nonpregnant women: an application of stable isotope methodology. *Amer. J. Clin. Nutr.* 38:169-180.

Takahashi, K., Akasaka, M., Yamamoto, Y., Kobayashi, C., Mizoguchi, J., and Koyama, J. (1990). Primary structure of human plasma glutathione peroxidase deduced from cDNA sequences. *J. Biochem.* 108:145-148.

Tappel, A. L. (1987). Glutathione peroxidase and other selenoproteins. Pages 122-132 *in* G. F. Combs, Jr., O. A. Levander, J. E. Spallholz and J. E. Oldfield, eds., *Selenium in Biology and Medicine*, Part A. Avi, New York.

Tarantal, A. F., Willhite, C. C., Lasley, B. L., Murphy, C. J. Miller, C. J., Cukierski, M. J., Book, S. A., and Hendrickx, A. G. (1991). Developmental toxicity of L-seleno-methionine in *Macaca fascicularis. Fund. Applied Toxicol.* 16: 147-160.

Toyoda, H., Himeno, S., and Imura, N. (1989). The regulation of glutathione peroxidase gene expression relevant to species differences and the effects of dietary selenium manipulation. *Biochim. Biophy. Acta* 1008:301-308.

Tubman, T. R. J., Halliday, H. L., and McMaster, D. (1990).

Glutathione peroxidase and selenium levels in the preterm infant. *Biol. Neonate* 58:305-310.

Uden, S., Bilton, D., Guyan, P. M., Kay, P. M., and Braganza, J. M. (1990). Rationale for antioxidant therapy in pancreatitis and cystic fibrosis. *Adv. Exp. Med. Biol.* 264:555-572.

Uotila, J., Tuimala, R., and Pyykko, K. (1990). Erythrocyte glutathione peroxidase activity in hypertensive complications of pregnancy. *Gynecol. Obstet. Invest.* 29:259-262.

Vanderpas, J. B., Contempre, B., Duale, N. L., Goossens, W., Bebe, N., Thorpe, R., Ntambue, K., Dumont, J., Thilly, C. H., and Diplock, A. T. (1990). Iodine and selenium deficiency associated with cretinism in northern Zaire. *Amer. J. Clin. Nutr.* 52:1087-1093.

Van Saun, R. J., Herdt, T. H., and Stowe, H. D. (1989). Maternal and fetal selenium concentrations and their interrelationships in dairy cattle. *J. Nutr.* 119:1128-1137.

Vlessis, A. A., and Mela-Riker, L. (1987). Selenite-induced NAD(P)H oxidation and calcium release in isolated mitochondria: Relationship to *in vivo* toxicity. *Molec. Pharmacol.* 31:643-646.

Wallace, E., Calvin, H. I., Ploetz, K., and Cooper, G. W. (1987). Functional and developmental studies on the role of selenium in spermatogenesis. Pages 181-196 *in* G.F. Combs, Jr., J. E. Spallholz, O. A. Levander and J. E. Oldfield, eds., *Selenium in Biology and Medicine*, Part A. Avi, New York.

Wallach, J. D., Lan, M., Yu, W. H., Gu, B., Yu, F. T., and Goddard, R. F. (1990). Common denominators in the etiology and pathology of visceral lesions of cystic fibrosis and Keshan disease. *Biol. Trace Elem. Res.* 24:189- 205.

Watanabe, C., and Suzuki, T. (1986). Sodium selenite-induced hypothermia in mice: Indirect evidence for a neural effect. *Toxicol. Appl. Pharmacol.* 86:372-379.

Watanabe, T., and Endo, A. (1991). Effects of selenium deficiency on sperm morphology and spermatocyte chromosomes in mice. *Mutat. Res.* 262:93-99.

Whiting, R. F., Wei, L., and Stich, H. F. (1980). Unscheduled

DNA synthesis and chromosome aberrations induced by inorganic and organic selenium compounds in the presence of glutathione. *Mutat. Res.* 78:159-169.

Wickens, D., Wilkins, M. H., Lunec, J., Ball, G., and Dormandy, T. L. (1981). Free-radical oxidation (peroxidation) products in plasma in normal and abnormal pregnancy. *Ann. Clin. Biochem.* 18:158-162.

Wilbur, C. G. (1980). Toxicology of selenium: A review. *Clin. Toxicol.* 17:171-230.

Willett, W. C., and Stampfer, M. J. (1986). Selenium and human cancer: Epidemiological aspects and implications for clinical trials. *J. Amer. Coll. Toxicol.* 5:29-36.

Willhite, C. C., Ferm, V. H., and Zeise, L. (1990). Route-dependent pharmacokinetics, distribution, and placental permeability of organic and inorganic selenium in hamsters. *Teratology* 42:359-371.

Yonemoto, J., Satoh, H., Himeno, S., and Suzuki, T. (1983). Toxic effects of sodium selenite on pregnant mice and modification of the effects by vitamin E or reduced glutathione. *Teratology* 28:333-340.

Zimmerman, A. W., and Lozzio, C. B. (1989). Interaction between selenium and zinc in the pathogenesis of anencephaly and spina bifida. *Zentbl. Kinderchir.* 44 (Suppl. 1): 48-50.

Zumkley, H. (1988). Clinical aspects of selenium metabolism. *Biol. Trace Elem. Res.* 15:139-146.

Chapter 8

Teratogenic Potential of Mycotoxins

R. V. Reddy and C. S. Reddy

Mycotoxins are secondary fungal metabolites produced in animal feed and human food ingredients. They have toxic effects on living organisms, including animals and humans and cells in culture. These secondary metabolites are products of reactions that branch off at limited number of steps, such as those involving acetate, pyruvate, malonate, mevalonate, schikimate, and amino acids (Steyn, 1977) and perform minor or no obvious function in the metabolic scheme of the mold. Of the more than 400 identified secondary fungal metabolites, just under 100 are toxic to mammals (Watson, 1985), among which only a few have been studied extensively.

The spores of mycotoxin-producing fungi are carried to the seed in the field where they vegetate and produce toxin. Unfavorable conditions such as drought and damage of seeds by insects or during mechanical harvesting can enhance mycotoxin production during both growth and storage. Toxin production can take place over wide range of moisture (10% to 33%), relative humidity (>70%), and temperature (4° to 35° C), depending on the fungal organism involved (Ciegler, *et al.*, 1981). Most of the mycotoxins are relatively heat resistant, so they persist in an active form in pelleted feeds or canned foods processed from contaminated ingredients (Pier, 1981). A wide variety of fungi may produce one or more of these secondary metabolites. From the standpoint of human and animal health, fungal genera *Aspergillus, Penicillium,* and *Fusarium* have received the most attention because of their frequency of occurrence in food and feed commodities. The chemical identity of some important mycotoxins is presented in Figure 1.

Because of widespread occurrence of mycotoxin-producing fungi, it is likely that numerous animal and human expo-

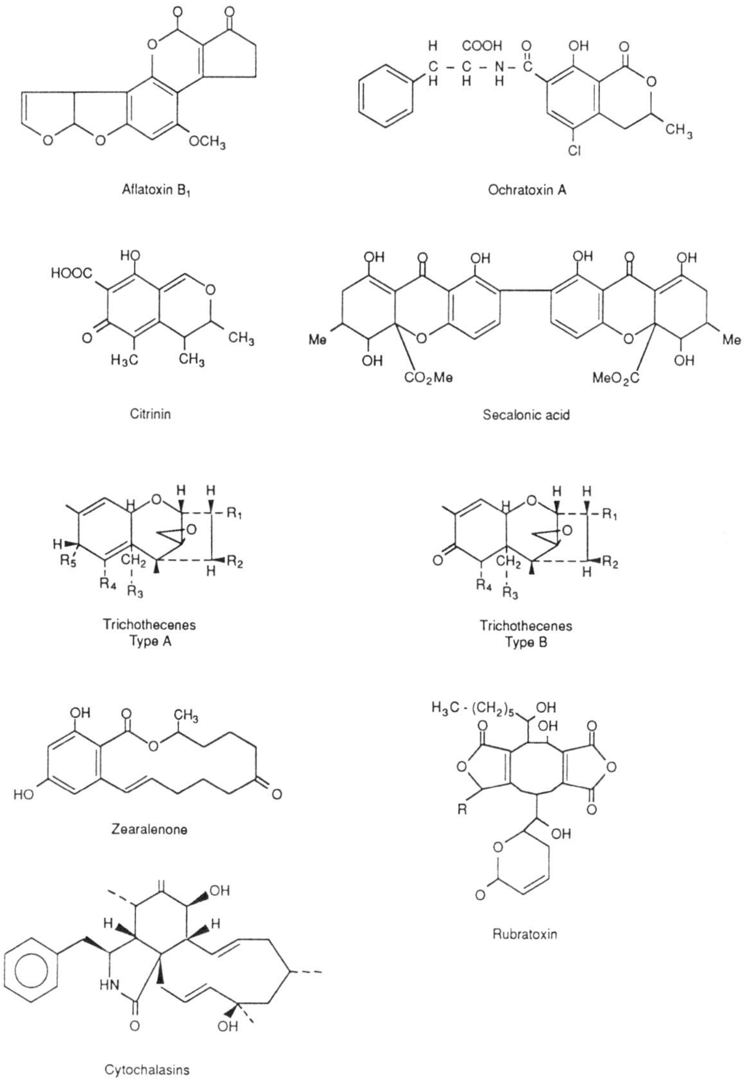

FIGURE 1. Structures of some commonly occurring mycotoxins.

sures occur in underdeveloped and developing countries where a lack of knowledge of proper cultivation, harvesting, and storage techniques can increase the likelihood of food contamination. In addition to contamination of foods derived from plants, mycotoxins and their metabolites can also occur in tissues of food animals exposed to mycotoxins in feeds. For example, mycotoxin aflatoxin B_1 (AFB$_1$) can be consumed by humans either directly from contaminated grain products or transferred indirectly through milk or meat products from AFB$_1$-exposed animals. Hsieh (1985) considers the carcinogenicity of aflatoxin M_1 (AFM$_1$) to be two orders of magnitude lower than that of AFB$_1$, which has a significant lifetime risk of liver cancer for adult humans.

Most mycotoxins are toxic after acute, subchronic, and chronic exposure, with the effects varying with species of the animal, dosage, and route. Many organ systems, including liver (AFB$_1$ and rubratoxin B), kidney (ochratoxin A and citrinin), hematopoietic system (T-2 toxin), reproductive system (ochratoxin A and secalonic acid D), endocrine system (zearalenone), and immune system (AFB$_1$ and T-2 toxin), are targets of adverse mycotoxic effects. Some commonly occurring mycotoxins, producing fungi, and their principal toxic effects are given in Table 1.

Teratogenesis

Living things are more sensitive to the adverse influence of environment during early developmental stages. As gestation progresses from conception through delivery, many changes occur in the mother, placenta, embryo, or fetus. Ingestion of mycotoxin-contaminated foods during pregnancy, especially during organogenesis, is a direct and early threat to the embryo and fetus. The period of organogenesis is from implantation until 8 to 12 weeks of gestation in the human, from implantation until 14 to 15 days in the rat and mouse. During this time, the conceptus undergoes rapid and complex changes characterized by the division, migration, and formation of organ rudiments. Within the period of organogenesis, individual organ systems possess highly specific periods of vulnerability to teratogenic insult. For example, administration of a teratogen on day 10 of rat gestation would result in brain and eye defects, with a small incidence

TABLE 1. Some Commonly Occurring Mycotoxins, Producing
Fungi, Their Source and Principal Toxic Effects

Mycotoxin	Major producing organisms	Source of fungi	Principal toxic effects
AFB₁	*Aspergillus flavus* *Aspergillus parasiticus*	Ground nuts	Hepatotoxic, carcinogenic, immunosuppressive
Citreoviridin	*Penicillium citreoviride*	Rice	Neurotoxic
Citrinin	*Penicillium viridicatum* *Penicillium citrinum*	Corn	Nephrotoxic
Cyclopiazonic acid	*Penicillium cyclopium*	Ground nuts	Nephrotoxic, enterotoxic
Cytochalasins	*Aspergillus clavatus* *Phoma* sp., *Phomosis* sp. *Hoeniscium* sp.	Rice, potatoes, pecans, tomatoes	Cytotoxic, teratogenic
Ochratoxin A	*Aspergillus ochraceous* *Penicillium viridicatum*	Legumes, cereals	Nephrotoxic, teratogenic, immunosuppressive
Patulin	*Penicillium urticae*	Apple juice	Mutagenic, carcinogenic, pulmonary toxicant
Penicillic acid	*Penicillium* spp.	Corn	Mutagenic, carcinogenic
Rubratoxin	*Penicillium rubrum*	Corn	Hepatotoxic, teratogenic, immunosuppressive
Secalonic acids	*Aspergillus aculeatus* *Penicillium oxalicum*	Rice, corn	Cardiotoxic, teratogenic, lung irritant
Sporidesmins	*Pithomyces chartarum*	Pasture grasses	Hepatotoxic, causes photo-sensitization
Sterigmatocystin	*Aspergillus flavus*	Mammals	Mutagenic, carcinogenic, and hepatotoxic
Trichothecenes	*Fusarium* spp.	Corn	
T-2 toxin			Necrosis of liver, intestine and kidney, hematopoietic system, immunosuppressive
Vomitoxin			Food refusal, vomiting, hemorrhaging throughout body
Fumitremorgens A and B	*Aspergillus fumigatus*	Rice	Neurotoxic
Penitrems A, B, and C	*Penicillium cyclopium*	Peanuts, cheese	Neurotoxic
Ergotoxins	*Claviceps purpurea* *Claviceps paspali*	Grains and grasses	Gangrene, tremors, ataxia

of heart and skeletal malformations. Administration of the
same agent on day 11, however, leads predominantly to brain
and palate malformations. Exposure to teratogens during
lactation may also adversely affect the overall development
of organ systems including the immune, endocrine, reproductive, and central nervous systems which continue to develop
well into the fetal and postnatal period.

Mycotoxins have been examined for their teratogenicity mostly in laboratory animals and to a minor extent in domestic animals and birds. Results of these studies and a limited number of epidemiological studies have led to the identification of some fungal toxic metabolites from contaminated food material as teratogens. This review is an attempt by the authors to summarize available information on the teratogenicity of some commonly occurring mycotoxins.

Aflatoxin B_1

Aflatoxin B_1 (AFB_1), a secondary fungal metabolite produced by the fungi *Aspergillus flavus* and *Aspergillus parasiticus*, is one of the most potent hepato-carcinogens so far recognized. AFB_1-producing fungi are found worldwide (including in the United States) infecting corn, peanuts, and other crops (Hesseltine, 1974). Human beings are likely to be exposed to aflatoxins directly as a result of ingesting aflatoxin-contaminated food or indirectly through meat, milk, and milk products. It has been established that livestock consuming feed contaminated with aflatoxin excrete toxic metabolites such as AFM_1 in milk.

Exposure during mating, gestation, and lactation to a diet containing AFB_1 and B_2 (50 μg/day) has no effect on the estrus cycle of the adult female rat, litter size, or birth weight of pups. However, a significant increase in intrauterine fetal resorption in pregnant rats and a significant increase in the weaning weight of the pups were observed (Panda, *et al.*, 1970).

Aflatoxin has been reported to be embryotoxic and teratogenic in domestic as well as laboratory animals. Among laboratory animals, the Golden hamster appears to be the most susceptible and mice relatively resistant to the teratogenicity of aflatoxins (Hayes, 1981). Intraperitoneal injection of 4 mg/kg of aflatoxin into pregnant hamsters on day 8 of gestation resulted in fetal death, resorption of some fetuses, and malformations such as anencephaly, disorganization of the cranial end of the neural tube, and ectopia cordis. If the treatment was given on day 13, when organogenesis was almost complete, no malformed fetuses and only a few dead or resorbed fetuses were present (Elis & DiPaolo, 1967). These authors also reported that an aflatoxin and DNA mixture was nine times less teratogenic to the fetuses than the same dose (4 mg/kg) of AFB_1 alone. Histologic examination showed severe toxic effect on the livers of both mothers and offspring after exposure to AFB_1 alone compared to those receiving AFB_1-DNA mixture, suggesting that the AFB_1-DNA adduct might not cross the placenta, and/or the release of aflatoxin from the complex might be limited.

Butler & Wrigglesworth (1966) reported that aflatoxins retarded rat fetal growth when mycotoxin exposure occurred late in the pregnancy. This effect was observed when the toxin was given early in pregnancy. Single intraperitoneal administration of AFB_1 (300 μg) caused fetal death with hemorrhage at the uteroplacental junction, whereas repeated small doses resulted in fetal growth retardation (Le Breton, *et al.*, 1964). Recently, Sharma & Sahai (1987) observed dose-dependent reductions in fetal body weight following the administration of aflatoxin (75% AFB_1 and 25% B_2; 0.7 to 7 mg/kg) on day 8 of pregnancy and fetal injury such as enlarged head and wrinkled skin following exposure later in the pregnancy (day 16). Administration of aflatoxin to rats on days 17 and 19 of pregnancy caused increased synthesis of total lipids and fatty acids, and decreased synthesis of phosphatidyl choline in 21-day-old fetal lungs (Das, *et al.*, 1978).

Aflatoxin B_1 exposure did not induce any malformations in C3H mice, but fetal death and resorption did occur (DiPaolo, *et al.*, 1967). However, in pregnant CBA mice, a single oral dose of AFB_1 (4 mg/kg) caused grossly observable fetal malformations. The malformations, including exencephaly, open eyelids, and protrusion of intestines, occurred in about 11% of the fetuses exposed on day 8, but not following exposure on day 9 (Arora, *et al.*, 1981).

Aflatoxin is embryotoxic and teratogenic in chick embryos treated at early stages of development both *in vivo* and *in vitro* (Legator, 1969; Verrett, *et al.*, 1964; Joshi & Joshi, 1981).

Early stages of development, especially the primitive streak stage, were found to be the most susceptible (Basir & Adekunle, 1970). When AFB_1 was added to *in vitro* embryo cultures, the embryos showed various malformations together with toxin-arrested mitosis. The abnormal embryos showed overall retardation of growth as well as structural anomalies in the somites, heart, and the brain. The authors Joshi & Joshi (1981) concluded that aflatoxin-induced teratogenesis was due to a reduction in cell proliferation during early morphogenesis.

It has been reported that aflatoxin can induce growth retardation in chick embryos, independently of time or mode of toxin administration (Verrett, *et al.*, 1964; Smith, *et al.*, 1975), whereas malformations were induced only when the compound was injected into the yolk sac (Verrett, *et al.*, 1964), but not if the compound was injected via the air chamber (Buddingh, 1952). Recently, Khan, *et al.* (1989) reported the toxicity of AFB_1 (26, 81, and 216 ng/egg) to chicken embryos via the air cell route. Exposure to aflatoxin resulted in decreased hatchability and death of most of the embryos before the 12th day of development.

Applegren and Arora (1983) reported that, by administration of ^{14}C-labeled AFB_1 to pregnant mice, the fetuses in late pregnancy showed a distinct uptake of radioactivity in the pigment layer of the eyes and to some extent in the nasal mucosa. In the fetal liver, very small amounts of radioactivity were found, although the maternal liver had very high concentrations.

Previously published work on humans from Nigeria indicated very infrequent transplacental transfer of AFB_1, and only aflatoxin M_1, M_2, and B_3 were found (Lamplugh, *et al.*, 1988). Recently, Denning, *et al.* (1990) quantified the presence of aflatoxin in human cord sera obtained immediately after birth and in maternal serum obtained immediately after parturition. Seventeen of the cord sera (48%) and two of the mothers' sera (6%) contained detectable aflatoxin. The highest concentration among the cord sera was 13.6 nmol/ml (mean value for group was 3.1 nmol/ml). The highest value among the mothers' sera was 1.22 nmol/ml. These authors concluded that a possible important factor contributing to the high concentration of AFB_1 in cord sera is the fetal excretion of the toxin in the urine.

Ochratoxin A

Ochratoxin A (OA), a dihydroisocoumarin derivative linked over a 7-carboxy group to l-phenylalanine by an amide bond, is a nephrotoxic secondary metabolite produced by various species of fungal genera *Aspergillus* and *Penicillium* (Scott, *et al.*, 1972). In several regions of Yugoslavia, Romania, and Bulgaria, a chronic and fatal human disease, Balkan endemic nephropathy, has been described (Hult, *et al.*, 1982). High prevalence of OA in foodstuffs from some of the villages where the disease has occurred (Krogh, *et al.*, 1977), as well as in the serum of some patients with the disease (Hult, *et al.*, 1979), strongly suggest that this mycotoxin may be a public health problem.

Ochratoxin A has been implicated in natural outbreaks of swine and cattle abortion (Still, *et al.*, 1971). However, when swine were fed a mixture of OA and OB from days 21 to 28 of pregnancy, no obvious gross abnormalities were seen in either the reproductive tract of adult sows or in their fetuses (Shreeve, *et al.*, 1977). This may be because of the relatively small window of exposure (days 21 to 28) during the 115-day gestation period. Still, *et al.* (1971) also reported experimentally induced reproductive toxic effects of OA that included a marked increase in the number of dead or resorbed fetuses in pregnant rats at oral doses of 6.25, 12.5, or 25 mg/kg body weight given on day 10 of pregnancy.

More & Galtier (1974) corroborated the reproductive toxicity (embryotoxicity and teratogenicity) of OA, reporting that this mycotoxin caused an increase in the number of resorptions and a decrease in fetal body weights when given intraperitoneally and orally to pregnant rats at 4 or 5 mg/kg body weight, respectively, for 2 to 8 consecutive days. They observed fetal hemorrhage, edema, and coelocomy, but no skeletal or visceral anomalies. The malformation, coelocomy, was attributed to the effects of OA on carbohydrate metabolism (Pitout, 1968). Reduced litter size, stunted growth, and higher incidence of hydrocephalus were observed in F_1 generation female rats exposed to 5 mg/kg of OA orally for 2 or 4 days beginning at day 8 of pregnancy. No effects were observed in F_2 animals (More & Galtier, 1975).

Brown, *et al.* (1976) treated pregnant rats with daily doses of 0.25, 0.5, 0.75, 1, 2, 4, or 8 mg/kg body weight of OA on days 6 to 15 of gestation. The high dose levels (4 and 8 mg/kg) were toxic (maternal mortality) to the dams. There were no signs of toxicity in dams given 1 or 2 mg/kg. Multiple doses of 1 mg/kg or more were embryocidal, 0.75-mg/kg/day doses were embryotoxic and teratogenic, and doses of 0.25 to 0.5 mg/kg were mainly teratogenic. Many gross and skeletal malformations, including open eyes, deformed snouts, and skeletal defects (wavy ribs and agenesis of the vertebrae) were observed.

Mayura, *et al.* (1982b) confirmed the embryotoxicity and teratogenicity of OA in rats. In this study, OA was injected as a single dose subcutaneously in rats on one of several gestation days (4 to 10). A single dose of 5 mg/kg resulted in complete resorption of fetuses, and 2.5 mg/kg given on any gestation day from 4 through 8 produced 80% to 100% incidence of fetal resorption. Treatment (1.75 mg/kg) on gestational days 4, 5, 6, or 7 resulted in increased fetal resorptions and decreased fetal weights. Fetal weights were depressed after treatment on day 8. No effects were observed in rats when exposed on day 9 or 10 of gestation. The highest number of resorptions, greatest depression of fetal weights, and largest number of malformations occurred when OA was injected on days 5, 6, or 7. External hydrocephaly, omphalocoel, and anophthalmia were the major gross malformations. Internal hydrocephaly and a shift in position of the esophagus were the main internal soft tissue defects. Major skeletal defects involved sternebrae, vertebrae, and ribs. Lower doses (0.5 or 1.0 mg/kg) failed to produce any embryotoxicity and malformations. These authors observed certain defects that were not reported by others, such as ectopia cordis, hydrocephaly, and a shift in position of the esophagus. The list of birth defects observed is given in Table 2. The dietary protein deficiency may increase the suscepti- bility of the animal to the teratogenic effects of OA, with major increased susceptibility related to skeletal develop- ment. Complete rehabilitation took place after the replace- ment of the very low protein diet (5% normal protein) with a normal protein diet (Mayura, *et al.*, 1983).

TABLE 2. Fetal Malformations In Rats Associated With Ochratoxin A[1]

External

External hydrocephaly
Omphalocele
Ectopia cordis
Anophthalmia
Hematoma
Micrognathia
Short snout
Curled tail
Protruded tongue

Internal soft tissue

Internal hydrocephaly
Microphthalmia
Hydronephrosis
Anophthalmia
Shift in position of esophagus
Ectopic kidney
Renal agenesis
Cryptorchid testes
Situs inversus
Right sided arch of aorta

Skeletal

Bipartite sternebrae
Sternebrae agenesis
Bipartite vertebral centra
Rudimentary rib
Fused ribs
Missing ribs
Extra ribs
Incomplete ossification of skull bones
Broken ribs
Branched ribs
Asymmetrical arrangement of ribs
Wavy ribs

[1] Source: Mayura, *et al.*, 1982b.

Ochratoxin A and citrinin have been found to occur together in mold-contaminated foods. When injected as a single subthreshold teratogenic dose, OA (1 mg/kg) or citrinin (30 mg/kg) produced minimal effects on embryos and fetuses. However, when OA and citrinin were administered concurrently, enhanced prenatal toxicity, gross, soft tissue, and skeletal malformations were observed (Mayura, *et al.*, 1984a). These authors also reported that the teratogenicity of OA was enhanced in impaired renal function rats as compared to sham-operated rats. This enhanced toxicity may be related to higher circulating levels of OA available for fetal delivery because of a significantly reduced renal reserve, which results in less OA excreted via urine than in non-renal-impaired animals (Mayura, *et al.*, 1984c).

Studies were also performed (Mayura, *et al.*, 1989) to determine the *in vitro* effects of OA on post-implantation rat embryos. A concentration (0 to 300 μg/ml)-dependent reduction in yolk sac diameter, crown rump length, somite number count, and protein and DNA content was observed. OA treatment also resulted in an increase in the incidence of defective embryos. Malformations included growth retardation, hypoplasia of the telencephalon, poor flexion, stunted limb bud development, underdeveloped sensory primordia, and decreased mandibular and maxillary size. In addition, OA-induced necrosis of embryonal mesodermal structures was reported.

Prenatal mortality and a variety of gross and skeletal defects occurred in mice following treatment with OA (5 mg/kg) on one of days 7 to 12 of gestation (Hayes, *et al.*, 1974). The most striking malformations affected the cranio-facial region and included median facial cleft, exencephaly, and polydactyly.

Hood, *et al.* (1976b) reported various gross malformations and no skeletal defects in fetuses from OA-treated hamsters. Gross malformations included short snouts, hydrocephalus, short tails, and limb defects.

Ochratoxin A also has significant effect on chicken embryo. Choudhury & Carlson (1973) reported that 0.05 μg of

OA per egg resulted in 50% embryonic mortality when administered via the air cell. Ochratoxin injection (0.005 to 0.007 µg/egg) after 48, 72, and 96 hr of incubation led to the following malformations on day 8: short and twisted limbs, short and twisted necks, microphthalmia, exencephaly, everted viscera, and reduced body size (Gilani, *et al.*, 1978). Microscopic examination of whole embryos treated at 48 hr showed ventricular spinal defects, aortic stenosis, and malformations of the valves.

Various explanations have been suggested by many workers to explain the teratogenic mechanism of OA. More and Galtier (1974) proposed that since OA inactivates phosphorylase β-kinase (Pitout, 1968) and impairs glycolysis in maternal liver, many of the effects may be due to decreased concentration of glucose available to developing fetuses. Suzuki, *et al.* (1975) reported that OA increased serum glucose in rats and caused marked depletion of hepatic glycogen stores. They attributed the glycogen depletion to inhibition of active transport of glucose into the liver, suppression of glycogenesis, and acceleration of glycogenolysis. Hood, *et al.* (1976b), on the other hand, suggested that OA might have a direct effect on the fetus, rather than having its action mediated through an effect on the dam. OA also inhibited mitochondrial respiration (Moore & Truelove, 1970; Meisner & Chan, 1974), providing another potential mechanism for its teratogenic effects. OA inhibits protein synthesis by competition with amino acid phenylalanine in the phenylalanyl-tRNA synthetase-catalyzed reaction (Bunge *et al.*, 1978; Creppy, *et al.*, 1979). Studies were conducted to determine the efficacy of phenylalanine in preventing or diminishing the teratogenic effects of OA in rats (Mayura, *et al.*, 1984b). In this study, pregnant rats were injected on gestation day 7 with a single dose of OA (1.75 mg/kg) alone or in combination with phenylalanine (20 mg/kg). The incidence of OA-induced fetal malformations (gross and skeletal) was significantly diminished in the presence of phenylalanine, suggesting impaired amino acid balance as a possible mechanism of teratogenic action. The molecular basis for teratogenic effects of OA appears to be very complex and may involve multiple pathways of metabolism.

Citrinin

Citrinin, a 3R-trans-4,-6-dihydro-8-hydroxy-3,4,5-trimethyl-6-oxo,3H-2-benzopyran-7-carboxylic acid, is a secondary fungal metabolite which has been found to contaminate human food and animal feed. It is obtained from cultures of several species of *Penicillium*. The mycotoxin has been detected in samples of wheat, oats, barley, and rye. Indian groundnuts infected with *Aspergillus flavus*, *Penicillium citrinum*, and *Aspergillus terreus* also contained citrinin in addition to aflatoxins (Subramanyam & Rao, 1974). The most important pathologic change caused by citrinin in experimental and farm animals is kidney damage.

Citrinin is embryocidal, fetotoxic, and a mildly teratogenic compound. Mice exposed to citrinin (30 or 40 mg/kg) on gestation day 6, 7, 8, or 9 exhibited reduced fetal weight gain and increased fetal and maternal mortality. No increase in fetal abnormalities was observed (Hood, *et al.*, 1976a).

The teratogenicity of single doses of citrinin was determined in rats after administration of 35 mg/kg subcutaneously on gestation days 3 to 15 (Reddy, *et al.*, 1982b). Relatively high maternal mortality was associated with this treatment regimen, mortality on certain days of gestation exceeding 50%. Weight gain for the surviving animals was reduced for the initial 48 hr, but was similar to that of controls subsequently.

No significant effects of citrinin were observed on the number of implants. Fetuses from dams given citrinin were significantly smaller than those from controls. No major gross or skeletal malformations were found in fetuses born to mothers receiving citrinin at a dose of 35 mg/kg. The major internal soft tissue malformations seen were enlarged kidneys (day 11), internal hydrocephalus (days 7, 11, and 15), and cleft palate (day 12). The combination of citrinin with OA,

another nephrotoxin, increased the occurrence of malformations (Mayura, *et al.*, 1984a).

After subcutaneous treatment of pregnant dams with [14]C-
labeled citrinin on day 12 of gestation, disappearance of
radioactivity from serum was rapid, and by 12 hr most had
disappeared (Reddy, *et al.*, 1982a). Citrinin is excreted mostly
as the parent compound along with two metabolites. Absence
of metabolites and the presence of the parent compound in
the fetus suggested that the embryocidal and fetotoxic effects
of citrinin may be due to the direct effects of this mycotoxin.

Secalonic Acids

Secalonic acids (SA) are a group of diastereomeric fungal
metabolites belonging to the ergochrome group which were
initially isolated and identified by Aberhart, *et al.* (1965) and
Franck, *et al.* (1966) from cultures of *Claviceps purpurea*.
Secalonic acids A(SAA), B(SAB), C(SAC), D(SAD, Figure
1), E(SAE), F(SAF), and G(SAG) have been isolated and
identified from a variety of substrates (including corn) contaminated by *Aspergillus ochraceus*, *Phoma terrestris*, *Penicillium oxalicum*, *A. aculeatus*, and *Pyrenochaeta terrestris*
(see review by Reddy & Reddy, 1991). Due to high yields of
the toxin (1.9 to 3.5 g/kg of corn) in laboratory grown cultures
(Steyn, 1970; Ciegler, *et al.*, 1980) and its occurrence in grain
(corn) dust in storage elevators in the southern and midwest-
ern United States at levels as high as 24.8 mg/kg (Ehrlich, *et
al.*, 1982; Bullerman, 1983), SAD has drawn particular attention in terms of its toxic effects, including teratogenicity.

Intraperitoneal administration of SAD in pregnant mice on
days 7 to 15 of gestation resulted in a dose-dependant reduction in maternal weight gain, an increase in resorptions, a
decrease in the number of live fetuses and in their weights,
and an increase in malformations including cleft palate, cleft
lip, open eyelids, missing phalangeal ossification centers, and
shortened mandibles as reported by Reddy, *et al.* (1981)
(Table 3). The minimum teratogenic dose for SAD given in
NaHCO$_3$ (5% w/v) was 6 mg/kg, and 100% resorptions

TABLE 3. Incidence of Cleft Palate and Other Reproductive Effects in Mice Following Intraperitoneal Doses of Secalonic Acid D in DMSO or Sodium bicarbonate[2,5]

| | Dose of SAD (mg/kg in | | | | | | | | |
| | DMSO | | | | NaHCO₃ | | | | |
Parameter	0	5	10	15	0	5	6	8	10
Implants	13.6	12.4	13.8	12.9	13.0	13.5	13.4	12.9	13.0
Resorption (% of implants)	8.8	5.7	23.2[3]	99.5[3]	11.9	20.7	22.0	76.2[3]	98.7[3]
Live fetuses (% of implants)	91.2	94.3	76.8[3]	0.5[4]	88.1	79.3	78.0	23.8[3]	1.3[4]
Fetal body weight (average, g)	1.34	1.21[3]	1.08[3]	0.73[4]	1.30	1.13[3]	1.14[3]	0.87[3]	1.02[4]
Cleft palate (% of live fetuses)	0	8	53[3]	100[4]	0	7	46[3]	73[3]	100[3]

[2] SAD was administered either DMSO (10% v/v in NaHCO₃) or in 5% (w/v) NaHCO₃ on days 7 through 15 of gestation
[3] Significantly different from respective control for the same parameter (p <0.05)
[4] Statistics not done because data represent pups from one dam
[5] Data from Reddy, et al. (1981)

occurred at 10 mg/kg. Interestingly, when dimethylsulfoxide (DMSO, 10% v/v in NaHCO$_3$) was used as the solvent, the teratogenicity of SAD was substantially reduced. When given in NaHCO$_3$, 10 mg/kg of SAD produced 100% cleft palate in live fetuses, whereas when given in DMSO this dose only produced 53% incidence of cleft palate (Table 2). Although Mayura, *et al.* (1982a) were able to produce teratogenic effects in rats following a single subcutaneous dose of SAD on various gestation days, the spectrum of malformations bore no resemblance to those seen in mice. In addition to fetal resorptions, lower body weight of pups, malformations such as anophthalmia, exencephaly, limb and tail defects, hydronephrosis, tracheo-esophageal fistula, and renal agenesis were seen. Whether these differences reflect difference in species or the route of administration is unclear. In chick embryos, SAD ranked 14 among the 22 mycotoxins tested for toxic effects (Vesely, *et al.*, 1985). Secalonic acid-D was among the eight teratogenic mycotoxins tested in the chick embryo system. The same group (Vesely, *et al.*, 1985) isolated *P. oxalicum* from corn, which produced SAD both on wheat as well as in liquid culture. Strong teratogenic effects, including high frequency of microphthalmia and bilateral beak fissure, were produced by SAD in chick embryos. The ED$_{50}$ values for 2-, 3-, and 4-day-old chicken embryos were 0.9, 2.8, and 3.8 µg of SAD, respectively.

Teratogenic influences of SAD are not limited to structural visceral and skeletal malformations. St. Omer & Reddy (1985) reported that a single 25 mg/kg dose of SAD, intraperitoneally on day 11 of gestation to pregnant mice, produced delays in postnatal growth, teeth eruption, and ontogeny of various parameters including righting reflex, swimming behavior, negative geotaxis, and hindlimb grip strength. Associated with these effects, a reduction in dopamine levels in the forebrain also was seen. A previously non-teratogenic dose of 15 mg/kg, intraperitoneally on day 11, resulted in postnatal growth depression and altered negative geotaxis.

Mechanism of Secalonic Acid D-Induced Cleft Palate

During normal development, mesenchymal cells from the neural crest migrate to the oral cavity and, in association with craniopharyngeal ectoderm, form palatal shelves that grow vertically downward from the medial aspect of the maxillary process. Then at a critical time during development, these shelves elevate above the tongue and make contact in the midline before fusion to form the secondary palate. The complex and precisely timed sequence of events needed for normal palatogenesis makes this structure vulnerable to abnormal development under the influence of a wide variety of chemicals that are capable of including a diverse array of biochemical and morphological changes in the palate tissue. Structural abnormality within the shelves, small size shelves failing to meet at the midline following elevation, reduction in the internal shelf force (osmotic or of neuromuscular origin) that could lead to a delay or failure of elevation of the shelves, interference with epithelial fusion, post-fusion rupture, and failure of mesenchymal consolidation and differentiation can all lead to abnormal palatogenesis (Ferguson, 1988). Understanding the mechanisms of cleft-palate induction by chemical agents in experimental animals can go a long way to suggest preventive and therapeutic approaches to minimize the incidence and human impact of this common malformation. The mechanisms of teratogenicity presented here were also reviewed earlier (Reddy & Reddy, 1991).

Shelf development in mice begins at embryonic day 12 and ends at around day 14.5 of gestation with elevation and fusion. In order to evaluate the effect of SAD on shelf size and morphology, Reddy, *et al.* (1986) first established that an optimally teratogenic dose of SAD when given on day 11 (day 12 when the day of vaginal plug is considered as day 1) of gestation failed to alter palatal morphology, cell density, mitotic index and cell proliferation (using uptake of ^{3}H-thymidine as an index) at various stages during palate development. Subsequently, however, morphological studies (Eldeib

& Reddy, 1988a) demonstrated that the SAD-exposed shelves fail to elevate above the tongue at a time when 100% of the control shelves have undergone elevation and fusion. This suggests failure of elevation as the sole factor in SAD-induced cleft palate.

A transient rise occurs in 3',5'-cyclic adenosine monophosphate (cAMP) levels in the normal developing palate, lasting for up to 2 days, around the time of palate elevation and fusion (Greene & Pratt, 1979). Alteration of the normal pattern of cAMP levels in palate cells by a variety of agents including caffeine (Schreiner, et al., 1986), an agent not known to affect fusion, and the fact that the rise lasts for up to 2 days, whereas the elevation and fusion process may only last a few hours at the most, suggest that the biochemical processes contributing to basal cAMP patterns in the palate may be crucial for normal palatogenesis and that these processes are associated not only with palate epithelial fusion, as generally accepted, but with many other pre- and possibly post-fusion events. It is also clear that a disruption of basal pattern of cAMP levels in palate would lead to abnormal palatogenesis. Events regulating palatal basal cAMP levels, which when modified by teratogens may lead to cleft palate, include prostaglandin (PG) synthesis. The cleft-palate teratogen hydrocortisone (glucocorticoids) has been shown to inhibit both the transient rise in cAMP (Pratt, et al., 1980) and phospholipase-mediated arachidonic acid (AA) release and thus PG synthesis (Gupta, et al., 1985).

Our recent studies (Eldeib & Reddy, 1988a) indicate that SAD similarly inhibits the embryonic palatal cAMP levels on days 13.5 and 14 of gestation, followed by a rebound increase on day 15.5 (corresponds to 12 to 25 hr post-fusion in controls). In addition, cyclic GMP levels, which showed a diurnal pattern in control palates, also showed early reduction followed by later increase in treated palates, similar to cAMP (Figure 2). Whether glucocorticoids affect cGMP in the developing palate is a question that needs to be answered.

Serotonin is a neurotransmitter shown to stimulate palate mesenchymal cells (Zimmerman, et al., 1983), which sug-

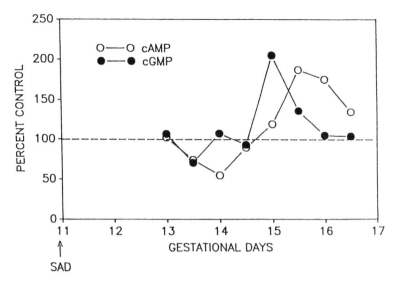

FIGURE 2. Secalonic Acid D-induced changes (% of control) in palatal cyclic nucleotide patterns in mice (from Eldeib & Reddy, 1988a).

gests a relevance to the effects of SAD on cGMP. Parallelism of SAD-induced biochemical changes with those of glucocorticoids seems appropriate in view of the recent demonstration that a single SAD-treatment at the optimal dose on gestation day 11 elevated maternal plasma corticosterone levels (Figure 3) by more than 400% and 300% on days 12 and 13 of gestation, respectively, over the controls (Eldeib & Reddy, 1990). The relevance of such an effect to SAD-induced cleft palate was suggested by a complete prevention of the plasma corticosterone elevation by the protective agent, DMSO (20% w/v in 5% $NaHCO_3$). The specific role of this response in teratogenesis was suggested by a lack of corticosterone elevation following a similar single dose in males.

Our earlier studies (Eldeib & Reddy, 1988b) have demonstrated that DMSO is optimally protective when included in the solvent at 20% (w/v). Simultaneous administration of DMSO (20%) not only reduced the incidence SAD-induced cleft palate from 45% to 7% (Eldeib & Reddy, 1988a), but also significantly reduced the entry of ^{14}C-SAD-derived radioactivity into fetal tissues and all maternal tissues other than

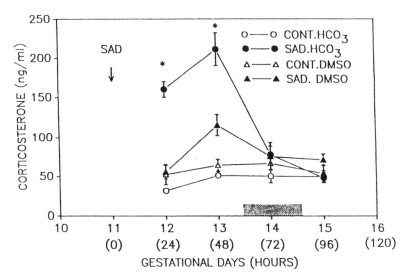

FIGURE 3. Maternal plasma corticosterone elevation following secalonic acid D exposure (arrow) in pregnant mice and its prevention by dimethyl sulfoxide. Asterisk means significantly different (p<0.01) from all other groups on the same day. Shaded area on the abscissa represents time of palate elevation and fusion (from Eldeib & Reddy, 1990).

the liver. A 220% increase in SAD-derived radioactivity was seen in maternal liver, concomitant with reduced fecal and urinary elimination of SAD. The role of reduced SAD uptake by the fetus in DMSO-treated animals and the reduction of SAD-induced cleft palate by DMSO needs to be determined.

The foregoing discussion suggests that SAD-induced teratogenicity may be mediated by elevated maternal corticosterone, and the data by Tzartzatou, *et al.* (1981) provide evidence to support the mechanistic involvement of inhibited AA release and PG synthesis in glucocorticoid-induced cleft palate. However, our unpublished studies showed that repeated subcutaneous doses of AA, ranging from 100 to 250 mg/kg, administered simultaneously with subcutaneous doses of hydrocortisone or intraperitoneal doses of SAD, failed to reduce both hydrocortisone as well as SAD-induced cleft palate, which suggests the irrelevance of the AA pathway in SAD-induced cleft palate. In most normal tissues, the roles of cAMP and cGMP are antagonistic to each other

(Goldberg, et al., 1974), and hence their levels are affected in opposite direction by various stimuli. The fact that SAD affects both nucleotides downward in pre-fusion palates may suggest an actual depletion of ATP and GTP levels during the critical development period. Kawai, et al. (1983) demonstrated increased O_2 consumption and decreased respiratory control index and P/O ratio, both of which are indicative of uncoupling of oxidative phosphorylation, in rat liver mitochondrial preparations by SAD, with total uncoupling at 70 μM. In addition, SAD also suppressed 2,4-dinitrophenol-stimulated ATPase activity, but did not affect latent ATPase activity.

Our unpublished data suggest that glucose-6-phosphate dehydrogenase in adult mouse liver and accessory sex organs may also be inhibited by SAD. The uncoupling effect seems to be closely associated with the lipophilicity and the acid dissociation properties of SAD with a pK value of 6.0 (Nakamura, et al., 1983). Ionization of the phenolic group in the xanthone ring releases protons from the 1- or 8-hydroxy group or both at the physiological pH and causes the uncoupling effect which results in deficient synthesis of ATP and GTP, the two substrates for the respective cyclases. The progression of these reactions in embryonic mouse palate and the uncoupling effect of SAD in this tissue need to be studied. The fact that other secalonic acids possess the same structure suggests that they all may be uncouplers and possibly teratogens.

These studies strongly suggest that SAD-induced cleft palate may, at least partly, be mediated through SAD-induced elevations in maternal plasma corticosterone. Recent evidence suggests that unlike its anti-inflammatory activity, the teratogenicity of glucocorticoids, and thus SAD, may be mediated through mechanisms other than the inhibition of phospholipase A_2, which, in turn, leads to a sequence of events leading to reduced synthesis of PG. Although the subsequent events are unclear at this time, the reduced magnitude of the cAMP message caused by SAD could, for example, translate to a subthreshold stimulus (biochemical nature unknown) for elevation of palate shelves and thus failure of elevation and fusion.

Trichothecenes

Trichothecene mycotoxins are produced by several families of pathogenic fungi, such as *Fusarium, Trichothecium, Myrothecium, Cephalosporium, Stachybotrys, Trichoderma, Cylindrocarpon, and Verticimonosporium* species (Ueno, 1983). Some examples of trichothecene mycotoxins include T-2 toxin, neosolaniol, HT-2 toxin, nivalenol, fusarenon-X, deoxynivalenol, and crotocin. These compounds are acutely toxic, inhibit protein synthesis (Lafarge-Frayssinet, *et al.*, 1979; Ueno, *et al.*, 1973; McLaughlin, *et al.*, 1977), and are immunosuppressants (Rosenstein, *et al.*, 1979 and 1981; and Taylor, *et al.*, 1985).

The reproductive toxicity of trichothecenes has been recently reviewed (Magnus, 1989). The available data show that maternally toxic doses of trichothecenes are also embryotoxic. Fetal death is the most common result in both birds and mammals (Magnus, 1989). Although embryotoxicity of these mycotoxins is high, only deoxynivalenol is implicated as being teratogenic. In this review, discussion will be limited to T-2 toxin, diacetoxyscirpenol (DAS) and deoxynivalenol (DON).

T-2 Toxin.

Both maternal and fetal mortality were observed (Stanford, *et al.*, 1975) when mice were exposed intraperitoneally to T-2 toxin (0.5, 1.0, and 1.5 mg/kg) on one of days 7 to 11 of gestation. Effects on fetus included decreased survival and growth. Among the surviving pups from dams treated at 1.0 or 1.5 mg/kg on day 10, 37% were grossly malformed and 42% had skeletal malformations. Gross malformations included exencephaly, open eyelids, and retarded jaws.

Administration of T-2 toxin to mice, subcutaneously or in the feed, resulted in abortions on day 10 of gestation and an increase in the frequency of resorptions (Ito, *et al.*, 1980). Teratogenic effects were not apparent from these studies.

After oral administration of a single dose (3.0 mg/kg) of T-2 toxin to CD-1 mice on gestation days 7, 8, 10, 11, and 12 of pregnancy, 17% maternal mortality following vaginal hemorrhage was observed (Rousseaux, *et al.*, 1985). The exact cause of hemorrhage with subsequent death seen in some dams is not known. Blakley, *et al.* (1987) also reported that oral administration of the toxin (1.5 mg/kg) to pregnant CD-1 mice on gestation day 11 resulted in embryotoxicity. At the dose levels tested (0 to 4 mg/kg), T-2 toxin was embryotoxic, but not a teratogen in CD-1 mice. The lack of any specific type of defect in the presence of embryolethality and considerable maternal mortality indicate that the action of T-2 toxin on fetal development is possibly mediated through maternal toxicity. Recently, Bean, *et al.* (1990) confirmed the maternotoxic and embryolethal effects as well as the lack of teratogenicity of T-2 toxin in the rat following repeated exposure to up to 3 mg/kg daily of T-2 toxin throughout organogenesis (gestation days 6 to 15).

In hens, egg production is reduced by acute exposure to T-2-contaminated feed (Shlosberg, *et al.*, 1984). Subchronic exposure of birds to different levels (0.5 to 8.0 ppm) of T-2 toxin resulted in a decrease in egg production, fertility of eggs, and hatchability. There was no increase in malformations among T-2-exposed chicks (Chi, *et al.*, 1977; Wyatt, *et al.*, 1975). In swine, T-2 has been shown to cause abortions, runting, and stillbirths (Weaver, *et al.*, 1978a,b).

Deoxynivalenol (Vomitoxin)

Khera, *et al.* (1982), reported the teratogenic effect of vomitoxin in mice. In this study, 0.5 to 15 mg/kg vomitoxin was administered once daily by gastric intubation for four consecutive days (days 8 through 11) of pregnancy. Vomitoxin caused vaginal bleeding and diarrhea in mice from high dose groups. The incidence of resorptions was 100% at the 10 and 15 mg/kg doses and 80% at the 5 mg/kg dose. The number of live fetuses and average fetal weight were significantly decreased. Vomitoxin also caused visceral and skeletal malformations, including cleft palate, exencephaly, syndactylia, hypoplastic cerebellum, lumbar vertebrae with fused arches, absent or fused ribs, and missing or fused sternebrae.

In laboratory rats, low levels of DON (5 ppm in feed) fed throughout pregnancy did not adversely affect pregnancy or cause birth defects (Morrisey, 1984). Khera, *et al.* (1984) fed rats at 0.25, 0.5, or 1.0 mg/kg body weight for 6 weeks and then mated them. The mated females, maintained on their respective diets for the entire period of pregnancy, were killed the last day of pregnancy. The dam's weight gain was reduced; no other adverse effect was observed. Similar effects were observed by other workers (Morrisey & Vesonder, 1985).

Feeding a diet contaminated with DON did not affect hens adversely (Hamilton, *et al.*, 1985). All parameters of fertility were normal, including the number of eggs laid, the incidence of dead and abnormal embryos, and the weight and survival of chicks at hatching.

Diacetoxyscirpenol

Diacetoxyscirpenol was not maternotoxic to Sprague-Dawley rats at 2, 3, and 6 mg/kg. However, the highest dose caused 100% resorptions. At low dose, surviving pups showed a variety of malformations including hydrocephaly and exencephaly (Mayura, *et al.*, 1985). Diacetoxyscirpenol is also toxic to avian reproduction (Allen, *et al.*, 1982).

In summary, trichothecene mycotoxins are embryotoxic and cause some teratogenic effects. However, these effects were seen at maternally toxic doses. The role of maternal toxicity in the induction of malformations needs to be clarified.

Zearalenone

Zearalenone (ZEN) is a toxic metabolite produced by

members of the *Fusarium* group. It has been detected in a variety of agricultural commodities, such as hay, corn, pig feed, sorghum, diary rations, and barley. In different years, 1% to 17% of corn samples contained detectable levels of ZEN (Bennett & Shotwell, 1979). Zearalenone and its derivatives produce estrogenic effects in farm animals and laboratory animals. In a recent outbreak of precocious pubertal changes in young children in Italy (Fara, *et al.*, 1979) and Puerto Rico (Saenz de Rodriguez, 1984), ZEN or zeralanol was considered as a possible causative agent (Saenz de Rodriguez, 1984; Saenz de Rodriguez, *et al.*, 1985). The effects seen included premature thelarche (development of breasts before age 8), premature pubarche, prepubertal gynecomastia, and precocious pseudopuberty.

Zearalenone caused reproductive disturbances in laboratory animals. Mirocha, *et al.* (1968, 1971) reported signs of estrogenic effects such as enlarged uteri and mammary glands, vulvo-vaginitis, and testicular atrophy in the rat, mouse, and guinea pig. Among domestic animals, swine appear to be the most sensitive, exhibiting signs of hyperestrogenic syndrome — swollen and edematous vulva, hypertrophic myometrium, vaginal cornification, and prolapse in extreme cases (Osweiller, *et al.*, 1985), infertility, pseudopregnancy, nymphomania, and constant estrus. In the offspring, there was decreased body weight and juvenile hyperestrogenism (Chang, *et al.*, 1979).

No teratogenic effects were seen when mice were given ZEN orally once on day 8 or 9 of pregnancy at levels of up to 20 mg/kg body weight (Arora, *et al.*, 1981, 1983). Ruddick, *et al.* (1976) reported significant decrease in maternal weight gain, decreased fetal weights, and increased incidence of some minor skeletal anomalies (delayed ossification, missing or malappositioned sternal plates, short ribs, extra ribs, and wavy ribs) in the fetuses of rats given ZEN daily during the period of major organogenesis (days 6 to 15). No visceral malformations were observed.

The toxicity of ZEN (0.1, 1, and 10 mg/kg body weight) was studied in two generations of Wister rats over approximately 10 months (Becci, *et al.*, 1982). Zearalenone in the diet at the highest dose level caused maternal toxicity, decreased fertility, and a decrease in the number of live born pups per litter in both first and second generations. The reproductive effects seen with ZEN were attributable to its estrogenic activity. Based on the published data, ZEN is not a teratogenic mycotoxin.

Rubratoxins

Rubratoxin A and B, anhydrides of gluconic acid, are two closely related toxic metabolites of *Penicillium rubrum and Penicillium purpurogenum*, both common soil fungi. Rubratoxin B is primarily a hepatotoxic mycotoxin, which is reported to be teratogenic in mice (Hood, *et al.*, 1973) and chickens (Gilani, *et al.*, 1979).

In mice, single i.p. administration of rubratoxin B in propylene glycol and water (1:1, v/v), on one of gestation days 6 to 12 at dosages of 0.4 to 1.2 mg/kg resulted in growth retardation, embryonic death, and fetal anomalies. Fetal malformations included exencephaly, malformed pinnae, malformed jaws, umbilical hernias, and open eyelids. No skeletal malformations were observed (Hood, *et al.*, 1973). Similar results were also reported by Koshakji, *et al.* (1973), but they also observed a high incidence of internal hydrocephalus, hydronephrosis, and cleft palate.

Recently, Hood (1986) reported the effects of concurrent prenatal exposure to rubratoxin B and T-2 toxin in CD-1 mice. These mycotoxins were given individually or together by intraperitoneal injection to pregnant CD-1 mice at doses of 0.5 (T-2 toxin), and 0.4 (rubratoxin B) mg/kg on day 10 of gestation. The combination resulted in an increased adverse effect at the doses used on both fetal weight and mortality of the conceptus in comparison with either treatment given alone. T-2 toxin given alone resulted in gross malformations characterized by tail and limb defects, and the incidence of these malformations were not increased by the addition of rubratoxin B.

Cytochalasins

Cytochalasins are highly substituted perhydroisoindol-1-one compounds fused with a macrocyclic ring (usually carbocyclic, but occasionally a lactone or a cyclic carbamate; Natori, 1977). Fifty-four compounds belonging to the group have so far been isolated (Natori & Yahara, 1991). Two cytochalasin mycotoxins, cytochalasin D and chaetoglobosin A, are known to be teratogenic. In pregnant mice, intraperitoneal administration of cytochalasin D at dosages of 0.4 to 0.9 mg/kg on gestation days 7 through 11 resulted in ex- or anencephaly, hypognathia, and axial skeletal defects. These malformations were strain dependent (C57Bl/6 and Balb/C had birth defects, and no malformations were observed in the Swiss-Webster strain). However, in all strains, a significantly increased resorption rate was found (Shepard & Greenaway, 1977). The embryolethality and teratogenicity of cytochalasins D and E vary from strain to strain, with cytochalasin D being relatively more teratogenic than cytochalasin E (Austin, *et al.*, 1982).

Conclusions

Although mycotoxins, by definition, are not nutritionally important to human and animal health, their importance stems from the fact that their presence in food and feed commodities and thus their teratogenic effects cannot be totally prevented for many reasons. *First*, that fungal-resistant varieties of crops are unavailable for cultivation in most cases. *Second*, man's inability to control weather patterns and prevent drought will promote fungal infestation of crops, probably for generations to come. *Third*, the constant increase in demand for world food production due to uncontrollable growth in world population will necessitate continued use of mechanical harvesting procedures that damage crops and promote fungal infestations and toxic production during storage. *Fourth*, development of a data base on the teratogenicity of heretofore uninvestigated mycotoxins and development of processing methodologies to inactivate dietary mycotoxins are likely to lag severely behind other priority areas of research. *And finally,* the exposure to these mycotoxins in the general population (especially those responsible for the population explosion in the developing countries) will continue unchecked due to the unavailability of mycotoxin-free food commodities as well as due to the failure of helpful current research findings to reach these very same populations in need of such information.

The information presented in this review attests to the lack of emphasis received by this group of teratogens despite the unavoidable nature of almost a lifetime of exposure in populations at risk. In addition to their potential adverse effects on human and animal conceptus, several mycotoxins produce malformations common to many nutritional, hormonal, and other toxic chemicals (secalonic acid D-induced cleft palate, for example), thus providing animal models to study mechanisms of pathogenesis of common human malformations. Mycotoxins as a group deserve enhanced emphasis in identifying their role in human maldevelopment, up to 70% or more of which appears to be contributed by environmental factors.

References

Aberhart, D. J., Chem, Y. S., de Mayo, P., and Stothers, J. B. (1965). NMR studies. VII. Mold metabolites. 4. Isolation & constitution of some ergot pigments. *Tetrahedron* (London) 21:1417-1420.

Allen, N. K., Jevne, R. L., Mirocha, C. J., and Lee, Y. W. (1982). The effect of a *Fusareum roseum* culture and diacetoxyscirpenol on reproduction of white leghorn females. *Poult. Sci.* 61:2172-2175.

Appelgren, L. E., and Arora, R. G. (1983). Distribution Studies of ^{14}C-labeled AFB_1 and ochratoxin A in pregnant mice. *Vet. Res. Commun.* 7:141-144.

Arora, R. G., Frolen, H., and Nilsson, A. (1981). Interference of mycotoxins with prenatal development of the mouse. I. Influence of AFB_1, ochratoxin A, and zearalenone. *Acta Vet. Scand.* 22:524-534.

Arora, R. G., Frolen, H., and Fellner-Feldegg, H. (1983). Inhibition of ochratoxin A teratogenesis by zearalenone and diethylstilbestrol. *Food Chem. Toxicol.* 21:779-783.

Austin, W. L., Wind, M., and Brown, K. S. (1982). Differences in the toxicity and teratogenicity of cytochalasins D and E in various mouse strains. *Teratology* 25:11-18.

Basir, O., and Adekunle, A. (1970). Teratogenic action of AFB_1, palmotoxin B_o and plamotoxin G_o in the chick embryo. *J. Pathol.* 102:49-51.

Bean, M. S., Mayura, K., Clement, B. A., Edwards, J. F., Harvey, R. B., and Phillips, T. D. (1990). Studies of prenatal development in the rat following oral exposure to T-2 toxin. *Toxicologist* 10:124.

Becci, P. J., Johnson, W. D., Hess, F. G., Gallo, M. A., Parent, R. A., and Taylor, J. M. (1982). Combined two-generation reproduction teratogenesis study of zearalenone in the rat. *J. Appl. Toxicol.* 2:201-206.

Bennett, G. A., and Shotwell, O. L. (1979). Zearalenone in cereal grains. *J. Amer. Oil Chem.* 56:812-819.

Blakley, B. R., Douglas, S. H., and Rousseaux, C. G. (1987). Embryotoxic effects of prenatal T-2 toxin exposure in mice. *Can. J. Vet. Res.* 51:399-403.

Brown, M. H., Szczech, G. M., and Purmalis, B. P. (1976). Teratogenic and toxic effects of ochratoxin A in rats. *Toxicol. Appl. Pharmacol.* 37:331-338.

Buddingh G. J. (1952). Bacterial and mycotic infections of the chick embryos. *Ann. NY Acad. Sci.* 55:282-287.

Bullerman, L. (1983). Health hazards of dust and pesticides reported at annual meeting. *Grain Qual. Newslett.* 5:3.

Bunge, I., Dirheimer, G., and Roschenthaer, R. (1978). *In vivo* and *in vitro* inhibition of protein synthesis in *Bacillus stearothermophillus* by ochratoxin A. *Biochem. Biophys. Res. Commun.* 83:398-405.

Butler, W. H., and Wrigglesworth, J. S. (1966). Effects of AFB_1 on the pregnant rats. *Brit. J. Exp. Pathol.* 47:242-247.

Chang, K., Kurtz, J. H., and Mirocha, C. J. (1979). Effects of the mycotoxin zearalenone on swine reproduction. *Amer. J. Vet. Res.* 40:1260-1267.

Chi, M. S., Mirocha, C. J., Kurt, H. J., Weaver, G., Bates, F., and Shimoda, W. (1977). Effects of T-2 toxin on reproductive performance and health of laying hens. *Poult. Sci.* 56:628-637.

Choudhury, H., and Carlson C. W. (1973). The lethal dose of ochratoxin to chick embryos. *Poult. Sci.* 52:1202-1203.

Ciegler, A., Hayes, A. W., and Vesonder, R. F. (1980). Production and biological activity of secalonic acid D. *Appl. Environ. Microbiol.* 39:285-287.

Ciegler, A., Burmeister, H. R., Vesondes, R. F., and Hesseltine C. W. (1981). Mycotoxins. Occurrence in the environment. Pages 1-50 *in* R. C. Shank, ed., *Mycotoxins and Nitroso Compounds: Environmental Risks,* Vol. I. CRC Press, Boca Raton, FL.

Creppy, E. E., Lugnier, A. A. J., Fasiolo, F., Heller, K., Roschenthaler, R., and Dirheimer, G. (1979). *In vitro* inhibition of yeast phenylalanyl-t-RNA synthetase by ochratoxin A. *Chem. Biol. Interact.* 24:257-261.

Das, S. K., Nair, R. C., Patthey, H. L., and Mabodile, M. U. K. (1978). The effects of AFB_1 on rat fetal lung lipids. *Biol. Neonat.* 33:283-288.

Denning, D. W., Allen, R., Wilkinson, A. P., and Morgan M. R. A. (1990). Transplacental transfer of aflatoxin in human. *Carcinogenesis* 11:1033-1035.

DiPaolo, J. W., Elis, J., and Erwin, H. C. (1967). Teratogenic response by hamsters, rats, and mice to AFB_1. *Nature* (London) 215:638-639.

Ehrlich, K. C., Lee, L. S., Ciegler, A., and Palmgren, M. S. (1982). Secalonic acid D: Natural contaminant of corn dust. *Appl. Environ. Microbiol.* 44:1007-1008.

Eldeib, M. M. R., and Reddy, C. S. (1988a). Secalonic acid D-induced changes in palatal cyclic AMP and cyclic GMP in developing mice. *Teratology* 37:343-352.

Eldeib, M. M. R., and Reddy, C. S. (1988b). A mechanism of dimethylsulfoxide protection against the teratogenicity of secalonic acid D in mice. *Teratology* 38:419-425.

Eldeib, M. M. R., and Reddy, C. S. (1990). Role of maternal plasma corticosterone levels in the teratogenicity of secalonic acid D in mice. *Teratology* 41:137-146.

Elis, J., and DiPaolo, J. A. (1967). AFB_1 induction of malformations. *Arch. Pathol.* 83:53-57.

Fara, G. M., Del Corvo, G., Bernuzzi, S., Bigatello, A., DiPietro, C., Scaglioni, S., and Chimello, G. (1979). Epidemic of breast enlargement in an Italian school. *Lancet* 2:295-297.

Ferguson, M. W. (1988). Palate development. *Development* 103(suppl.):41-60.

Franck, B., Gottschalk, E. M., Ohmsorge, U., and Huper F. (1966). Trennung, structor undabsolute konfiguration der diastereomeren secalonsauren A, B, und C. *Chem. Berl.* 99:3842-3862.

Gilani, S. H., Bancroft, T., and Reily, M. (1978). Teratogenecity of ochratoxin A in chick embryos. *Toxicol. Appl. Pharmacol.* 46:543-546.

Gilani, S. H., Bancroft, J., and Reilly, M. (1979). Rubratoxin B and chicken embryogenesis: An experimental study. *Environ. Res.* 20:199-204.

Goldberg, N. D., Haddox, M. K., Estensen, R., White, J. G., Lopez, C., and Hadden , J. W. (1974). Evidence for dualism between cGMP and cAMP in regulation of cell proliferation and other cellular processes. Pages 247-262 *in* L. Lichenstein and C. Parker, eds., *Cyclic AMP in Cell Growth and Immune Response.* Springer-Verlag, New York.

Greene, R. M., and Pratt, R. M. (1979). Correlation between cyclic-AMP levels and cytochemical localization of adenyl cyclase during development of secondary palate. *J. Histochem. Cytochem.* 27:924-931.

Gupta, C., Katsumata, M., and Goldman, A. S. (1985). H_2 histocompatibility region influences the inhibition of arachidonic acid cascade by dexamethasone and phenytoin in mouse embryonic palates. *J. Craniofac. Genet. Dev. Biol.* 5:277-285.

Hamilton, R. M., Thompson, B. K., Trenholm, H. L., Fiser,

P. S., and Greenhalgh, R. (1985). Effects of feeding white Leghorn hens diets that contain deoxynivalenol (vomitoxin)-contaminated wheat. *Poult. Sci.* 64:1840-1852.

Hayes, A. W. (1981). Mycotoxins and abnormal fetal development. Pages 41-66 *in* A. W. Hayes, ed., *Mycotoxin, Teratogenicity, and Mutagenicity.* CRC Press, Boca Raton, FL.

Hayes, A. W., Hood, R. D., and Lee, H. L. (1974). Teratogenic effects of ochratoxin A in mice. *Teratology* 9:93-97.

Hesseltine, C. W. (1974). Natural occurrence of mycotoxins in cereals. *Mycopathol. Mycol. Appl.* 53:141-153.

Hood, R. D. (1986). Effects of concurrent prenatal exposure to rubratoxin B and T-2 toxin in the mouse. *Drug Chem. Toxicol.* 9:185-190.

Hood, R. D., Innes, J. E., and Hayes, A. W. (1973). Effect of rubratoxin on prenatal development in mice. *Bull. Environ. Contam. Toxicol.* 10:200-207.

Hood, R. D., Hayes, A. W., and Scammell, J. G. (1976a). Effects of prenatal administration of citrinin and viriditoxin to mice. *Food Cosmet. Toxicol.* 14:175-178.

Hood, R. D., Naughton, M. J., and Hayes, A. W. (1976b). Prenatal effects of ochratoxin A in hamsters. *Teratology* 13:11-14.

Hsieh, D. P. H. (1985). An assessment of liver cancer risk posed by aflatoxin M_1 in the western world. Pages 521-528 *in* J. Lacey, ed., *Trichothecenes and Other Mycotoxins.* John Wiley, New York. p.521-528.

Hult, K., Hoekby, E., Gatenbeck, S., Plestina, R., and Ceovic, S. (1979). Ochratoxin A and Balkan endemic nephropathy. IV. Occurrence of ochratoxin A in humans. *Separatchuck aus Chem. Rundscou* 35:32.

Hult, K., Plestina, R., Habazin-Novak, V., Radic, B., and Ceovic, S. (1982). Ochratoxin A in human blood and Balkan endemic nephropathy. *Arch. Toxicol.* 51:313-321.

Ito, Y., Ohtsubo, K., and Saito, M. (1980). Effects of fusarenon-X, a trichothecene produced by *Fusarium nivale*, on pregnant mice and their fetuses. *Japan J. Exp. Med.* 50:167-172.

Joshi, M. S., and Joshi, M. V. (1981). Effect of AFB₁ on early embryonic stages of the chick *Gallus domesticus* cultured *in vitro*. *Indian J. Exp. Biol.* 19:528-531.

Kawai, K., Nakamuru, T., Maebayashi, Y., Nozawa, Y., and Yamazaki, M. (1983). Inhibition by secalonic acid D of oxidative phosphorylation and CA^{2+}-induced swelling of mitochondria isolated from rat livers. *Appl. Environ. Microbiol.* 46:794-796.

Khan, B. A., Hussain, S. S., and Ahamad, M. A. (1989). Toxicity of AFB₁ to chick embryo. *Pakistan J. Sci. Indust. Res.* 32:353-354.

Khera, K. S., Whalen, C., Angers, G., Vasonder R. F., and Kuiper-Goodman, T. (1982). The embryotoxicity of 4-deoxyniralenol (vomitoxin) in mice. *Bull. Environ. Contem. Toxicol.* 29:487-491.

Khera, K. S., Arnold, D. L., Whalen, C., Angers, G., and Scott, P. M. (1984). Vomitoxin (4-deoxynivalenol): Effects on reproduction of mice and rats. *Toxicol. Appl. Pharmacol.* 74:345-356.

Koshakji, R. P., Wilson, B. J., and Harbison, R. D. (1973). Effects of rubratoxin B on prenatal growth and development in mice. *Res. Commun. Chem. Pathol. Pharmacol.* 5:584-592.

Krogh, P., Hold, B., Plestina, R., and Coevic, S. (1977). Balkan (endemic) nephropathy and foodborne ochratoxin A: Preliminary results of a survey of foodstuffs. *Acta Pathol. Microbiol. Scand.* B85:238-240.

Lafarge-Frayssinet, C., Lespinats, G., Lafont, P., Loisillier, F., Mousset, S., Rosenstein, Y., and Frayssinet, C. (1979). Immunosuppressive effects of fusarium extracts and trichothecenes: Blastogenic response of murine splenic and thymic cells to mitogens. *Proc. Soc. Exp. Biol. Med.* 160:302-311.

Lamplugh, S. M., Hendrickse, R. G., Apeagyei, F., and Mwanmut, D. D. (1988). Aflatoxins in breast milk, neonatal, blood, and serum of pregnant women. *Brit. Med. J.* 296:968.

Le Breton, E., Frayssinet, C., Lafarge, C., and DeRecondo, A. M. (1964). Aflatoxin — mecarisme de l'action. *Food Cosmet. Toxicol.* 2:675-677.

Legator, M. S. (1969). Biological assay for aflatoxins. Pages 107-149 *in* L. A. Goldblatt, ed., *Aflatoxins.* Academic Press, New York.

Magnus, F. B. (1989). Reproductive toxicology of trichothecenes. Pages 143-159 *in* V. R. Beasley, ed., *Trichothecene Mycotoxicosis: Pathologic Effects,* Vol. 1. CRC Press, Boca Raton, FL.

Mayura, K., Hayes, A. W., and Berndt. W.O. (1982a). Teratogenicity of secalonic acid D in rats. *Toxicology* 25:311-322.

Mayura, K., Reddy, R. V., Hayes, A. W., and Berndt W. O. (1982b). Embryocidal, fetotoxic, and teratogenic effects of ochratoxin A in rats. *Toxicology* 25:175-185.

Mayura, K., Hayes, A. W., and Berndt, W. O. (1983). Effects of dietary protein on teratogenicity of ochratoxin A in rats. *Toxicology* 27:147-157.

Mayura, K., Parker, R., Berndt, W. O., and Phillips, T. D. (1984a). Effect of simultaneous prenatal exposure to ochratoxin A and citrinin in the rat. *J. Toxicol. Environ. Health* 13:553-561.

Mayura, K., Parker, R., Berndt, W. O., and Phillips, T. D. (1984b). Ochratoxin A-induced teratogenesis in rats: Partial protection by phenylalanine. *Appl. Environ. Microbiol.* 46:1186-1188.

Mayura, K., Stein, A. F., Berndt, W. O., and Phillips, T. D. (1984c). Teratogenic effects of ochratoxin A in rats with impaired renal function. *Toxicology* 32:277-285.

Mayura, K., Smith, E., Heidelbaugh, N., and Phillips, T. D. (1985). Diacetoxyscirpenol induced prenatal dysmorphogenesis in the rats. *Toxicologist* 5:187.

Mayura, K., Edwards, J. F., Maull, E. A., and Phillips, T. D. (1989). The effect of ochratoxin A on postimplantation rat embryos in culture. *Arch. Environ. Contam. Toxicol.* 18:411-415.

McLaughlin, C. S., Vaughn, M. H., Cambell, I. M., Wei, C. M., Stafford, M. E., and Hansen, B. S. (1977). Inhibition of protein synthesis by trichothecenes. Pages 263-273 *in* J. V. Rodricks, C. W. Hesseltine, and M. A. Mehlman, eds., *Mycotoxins in Human and Animal Healh.* Pathotox Publishers, Park Forest, IL.

Meisner, H., and Chan, S. (1974). Ochratoxin A, an inhibitor of mitochondrial transport systems. *Biochemistry* 13: 2795-2800.

Mirocha, C. J., Christensen, C. M., and Nielson, G. H. (1968). Physiologic activity of some fungal estrogens produced by fusarium. *Cancer Res.* 28:2319-2322.

Mirocha, C. J., Christensen, C. M., and Nielson, G. H. (1971). F-2 (Zeralenone) oestrogenic mycotoxin from *Fusarium.* Pages 107-138 *in* S. Kadis, A. Ciegler, and A. J. Ajl, eds., *Microbial Toxins*, Vol. VII. Academic Press, New York.

Moore, J. H., and Truelove, B. (1970). Ochratoxin A: Inhibition of mitochondrial respiration. *Science* 168:1102-1103.

More, J., and Galtier, P. (1974). Toxicit'e de l'ochratoxine A. I. Effect embryotoxique et teratogene chez le rat. *Ann Rech. Vet.* 5:167-178.

More, J., and Galtier, P. (1975). Toxicite de l'ochratoxine A. II. Effects du taitement sur la descendance (F_1 et F_2) de rattes intoxiquees. *Ann. Rech. Vet.* 6:379-389.

Morrissey, R. E. (1984). Teratological study of Fischer rats fed diet containing added vomitoxin. *Food Chem. Toxicol.* 22:453-457.

Morrissey, R. E., and Vesonder, R. F. (1985). Effect of deoxynivalenol (vomitoxin) on fertility, pregnancy, and postnatal development of Sprague-Dawley rats. *Appl. Environ. Microbiol.* 49:1062-1066.

Nakamura, T., Kawai, K., Nozawa, Y., Maebayashi, Y., and Yamazaki, M. (1983). The biological activity of secalonic acid D from *Aspergillus ochraceus.* Effects on mitochondrial reactions. *Proc. Japan. Assoc. Mycotoxicol.* 16:4-7.

Natori, S. (1977). Toxic cytochalasins. Pages 559-581 *in* J.

V. Rodricks, C. W. Hesseltine, and M. A. Mehlman, eds., *Mycotoxins in Human and Animal Health.* Pathotox Publishers, Park Forest South, IL

Natori, S., and Yahara, I. (1991). Cytochalasins. Pages 291-336 *in* R. P. Sharma and D. K. Salunhke, eds., *Mycotoxins and Phytoalexins.* CRC Press, Boca Raton, FL.

Osweiller, G. D., Carson, T. L., Buck, W. B., and Van Gelder, V. A. (1985). *Clinical and Diagnostic Veterinary Toxicology*, 3rd ed. Kendall-Hunt, Dubuque, IA. 512 pp.

Panda, P. C., Sreenivasamurthy, V., and Parpia, H. A. B. (1970). Effect of aflatoxin on reproduction in rats. *J. Food Sci. Technol.* 7:20-22.

Pier, A. C. (1981). Mycotoxins and animal health. *Adv. Vet. Sci. Comp. Med.* 25:185-243.

Pitout, M. J. (1968). The effect of ochratoxin A on glycogen storage in the rat liver. *Toxcol. Appl. Pharmacol.*, 13:299-306.

Pratt, R. M., Salomon, D. S., Diewert, V. M., Erickson, R. P., Burns, R., and Brown, S. (1980). Cortisone-induced cleft palate in the brachymorphic mouse. *Teratogen. Carcinogen. Mutagen.* 1:15-23.

Reddy, C. S., Reddy, R. V., Hayes, A. W., and Ciegler, A. (1981). Teratogenicity of secalonic acid D in mice. *J. Toxicol. Environ. Health* 7:445-455.

Reddy, C. S., Hanumaiah, B., Hayes, T. G., and Ehrlich, K. C. (1986). Developmental stage specificity and dose response of SAD-induced cleft palate and the absence of cytotoxicity in the developing mouse palate. *Toxicol. Appl. Pharmacol.* 84:346-354.

Reddy, C. S., Reddy, R. V., Hayes, A. W., and Ciegler, A. (1981). Teratogenicity of secalonic acid D in mice. *J. Toxicol. Environ. Health* 7:445-455.

Reddy, C. S., and Reddy, R. V. (1991). Secalonic acids. Pages 167-190 *in* R. P. Sharma & D. K. Salunkhe, eds., *Mycotoxins and Phytoalexins.* CRC Press, Boca Raton, FL.

Reddy, R. V., Hays, A. W., and Berndt, W. O. (1982a).

Disposition and metabolism of ^{14}C-citrinin in pregnant rats. *Toxicology* 25:161-174.

Reddy, R. V., Mayura, K., Hays, A. W., and Berndt, W. O. (1982b). Emryocidal teratogenic and fetotoxic effects of citrinin in rats. *Toxicology* 25:151-160.

Rossenstein, Y., Lafarge-Frayssinet, C., Lespinats, G., Loisillier, F., Lafont, P., and Frayssinet, C. (1979). Immunosuppressive activity of *Fusarium* toxins. Effects of antibody synthesis and skin grafts of crude extracts, T-2 toxin and diactoxyscirpinol. *Immunology* 36:111-117.

Rossenstein, Y., Kretschmer, R. R., and Lafarge-Frassinet, C. (1981). Effect of *Fusarium* toxins, T-2 toxin, and diactoxyscirpinol on murine T-dependent immune responses. *Immunology* 44:555-560.

Rousseaux, C. G., Nicholson, S., and Schieffer, H. B. (1985). Fatal placental hemorrhage in pregnant CD-1 mice following one oral dose of T-2 toxin. *Can. J. Exp. Med.* 49:95-98.

Ruddick, J. A., Scott, P. M., and Harwig, J. (1976). Teratological evaluation of zearalenone administrated orally to the rat. *Bull. Environ. Contam. Toxicol.* 15:678-681.

Saenz de Rodriguez, C. A. (letter) (1984). Environmental hormone contamination in Puerto Rico. *New Engl. J. Med.* 310:1741.

Saenz de Rodriguez, C. A., Bongiovanni, A. M., and Conde de Borrego, L. (1985). An epidemic of precocious development in Puerto Rican children. *J. Pediatr.* 107:393-396.

Schreiner, C. S., Zimmerman, E. F., Wee, E. L., and Scott, Jr., W. (1986). Caffeine effects on cyclic AMP levels in the mouse embryonic limb and palate in vitro. *Teratology* 34:21-27.

Scott, P. M., Van Walbeek, W., Kennedy, B., and Anyeti, D. (1972). Mycotoxins (ochratoxin A, citrinin and sterigmatocystin) and toxigenic grains and agricultural products. *J. Agric. Food Chem.* 20:1103-1109.

Sharma, A., and Sahai, R. (1987). Teratological effects of aflatoxin on rats. *Indian J. Anim. Res.* 21:35-40.

Shepard, T. H., and Greenaway, J. C. (1977). Teratogenicity of cytochalasin D in the mouse. *Teratology* 16:131-136.

Shlosberg, A., Weisman, Y., Handji, V., and Yagen, B. (1984). A severe reduction in egg laying in a flock of hens associated with trichothecene mycotoxins in the feed. *Vet. Hum. Toxicol.* 26:384-386.

Shreeve, B. J., Patterson, D. S. P., Pepin, G. A., Roberts, B. A., and Wrathhall, A. E. (1977). Effect of feeding ochratoxin to pigs during early pregnancy. *Brit. Vet. J.* 133:412-417.

Smith, J. A., Adekunle, A. A., and Bassir, O. (1975). Comparative histopathological effects of AFB_1 and Palmotoxins B_o abd G_o on some organs of the newly hatched chick (*Gallus domesticus*). *Toxicology* 3:177-185.

St. Omer, V. E. V., and Reddy, C. S. (1985). Developmental toxicity of secalonic acid D in mice. (abstr.) *Toxicologist* 5:106.

Stanford, G. K., Hood, R. H., and Hayes, A. W. (1975). Effects of prenatal administration of T-2 toxin to mice. *Res. Commun. Chem. Pathol. Phamacol.* 10:743-746.

Steyn, P. S. (1970). The isolation, structure, and absolute configuration of secalonic acid D, the toxic metabolic of *Penicillium oxalicum. Tetrahedron* 26:51-57.

Steyn, P. S. (1977). Mycotoxins excluding aflatoxin, zearalenone, and the trichothecenes. Pages 419-467 *in* J. V. Rodricks, C. W. Hesseltine and M. A. Mehlman, eds., *Mycotoxins in Human and Animal Health.* Pathotox, Park Forest South, IL.

Still, P. E., MacKlin, A. W., Ribelin, W. E., and Smalley, E. B. (1971). Relationship of ochratoxin A to fetal death in laboratory and domestic animals. *Nature* (London), 234:563-564.

Subramanyam, P., and Rao, A. S. (1974). Occurrence of aflatoxins and citrinin in groundnuts at harvest in relation to pod condition and kernel moisture. *Curr. Sci.* 43:707-710.

Suzuki, S., Satoh, T., and Yamazaki, M. (1975). Effect of

ochratoxin A on carbohydrate metabolism in rat liver. *Toxicol. Appl. Pharmacal.* 32:116-122.

Taylor, M. J., Reddy, R. V., and Sharma, R. P. (1985). Immunotoxicity of repeated low level exposure to T-2 toxin, a trichothecene mycotoxin, in CD1 mice. *Myco. Res.* 1:57-64.

Tzartzatou, G. G., Goldman, A. S., and Bontwell, W. S. (1981). Evidence of a role of arachidonic acid in glucocorticoid-induced cleft palate in rats. *Proc. Soc. Exp. Biol. Med.* 166:321-324.

Ueno, Y. (1983). Trichothecenes: Chemical, biological, and toxicological aspects. *In: Developments in Food Science.* Elsevier, New York. 313 pp.

Ueno, Y., Jakajima, M., Sakai, K., Ishii, K., Sato, N., and Shimada, N. (1973). Comparative toxicology of trichothecenes: Inhibition of protein synthesis in animal cells. *J. Biochem.* 74:285-296.

Verrett, J. M., Marhac, J. P., and McLaughlin Jr., J. (1964). The use of chicken embryo in the assay of aflatoxin toxicity. *J. Assoc. Off. Anal. Chem.* 47:1003-1006.

Vesely, D., Vesela, D., and Jelinek, R. (1985). Toxic and teratogenic effects of mycotoxins on chick embryos. *Cesk Hyg.* 30:493-498.

Watson, D. H. (1985). Toxic fungal metabolites in food. *CRC Crit. Rev. Food Sci.Nutri.* 22:177-198.

Weaver, G. A., Kurtz, H. J., Mirocha, C. J., Bates, F. Y., Behrens, J. C., and Robinson T. S. (1978a). Effect of T-2 toxin on porcine reproduction. *Can. Vet. J.* 19:310-314.

Weaver, G. A., Kurtz, H. J., Mirocha, C. J., Bates, F. Y., Behrens, J. C., Robinson, T. S., and Gripp, W. F. (1978b). Mycotoxin-induced abortions in swine. *Can. Vet. J.* 19: 72-74.

Wyatt, R. D., Doerr, J. A., Hamilton, P. B., and Burmeister, H. R. (1975). Egg production, shell thickness, and other physiological parameters of laying hens affected by T-2 toxin. *Appl. Microbiol.* 29:641-645.

Zimmerman, E. F., Clark, R. L., Ganguli, S., and Verkatasubramaniyam, K. (1983). Serotonin regulation of cell motility and metabolism. *J. Craniofac. Genert. Dev. Biol.* 3:371-385.

Chapter 9

Natural Products and Congenital Malformations: Structure-Activity Relationships

Richard F. Keeler, William Gaffield and Kip E. Panter

This paper discusses teratogens from poisonous plants that induce malformations in domestic livestock. We consider here why and how frequently livestock encounter poisonous plants; how and why the plants are a hazard; how we know that some are teratogenic; what logistic problems we have found in testing plants or derivatives in livestock for teratogenicity; and what protocols we have therefore adopted. We consider structural relationships of compounds that have been positively incriminated or are highly suspect as responsible for congenital malformations induced in livestock or laboratory animals by members of the *Veratrum, Lupinus, Conium,* and *Nicotiana* plant genera along with related synthetic and naturally-occurring analogs. From these data, we speculate on the structural features present in responsible compounds that are essential to teratogenicity and speculate as to probable teratogenicity of structurally related compounds that are known to be ingested by man and animals.

Preliminary Perspectives

In most countries, domestic livestock are allowed to graze freely on forage from uncultivated rangelands for a large share of their feed intake. The forage on these ranges is comprised of native plants, many of which may be classified as poisonous to animals. Episodes of plant-induced toxicoses in grazing livestock are commonplace. Many poisonous plants are quite palatable to grazing livestock, and, as a general rule, these animals do not avoid poisonous plants.

The incidence of plant-induced toxicosis is highly variable

in grazing animals for numerous reasons. Major factors that account for the differences include: (a) marked variations in plant abundance from one location to another, (b) variations in concentrations of toxic compounds, (c) variations in experience with the plants among animals, and (d) variations in the amount of plant ingested. In any given year, some ranches may suffer from an inordinately high incidence (ca. 10-20%) of poisonous plant-induced toxicoses, while other ranches are spared serious losses. However, very few ranches escape problems over an extended number of years. With the aid of information from contacts over several decades with ranchers, land management agencies, extension and research personnel, the USDA's Poisonous Plant Research Laboratory has estimated that approximately 5% of all grazing livestock have serious encounters with poisonous plants each year, and 1-2% die or are otherwise lost to production (Keeler, 1979a).

Expressions of toxicoses in livestock from poisonous plant ingestion cover the spectrum of signs (Kingsbury, 1964) because of the great variability of toxic compounds ingested. Thousands of different poisonous species worldwide are grazed by animals, and some of the poisonous genera contain dozens of different toxic compounds (Kingsbury, 1964; Everist, 1974; Keeler & Laycock, 1988). The notoriously toxic *Lupinus* genus serves as an appropriate example (Kingsbury, 1964). About 70 known quinolizidine alkaloids and a few piperidine alkaloids comprise the presumed toxic repertoire of the genus. There are several dozen species within that genus each of which may contain a dozen or more quinolizidine alkaloids. Piperidine alkaloids are found in a few of the species (Keeler, 1989).

In recent years, it has become apparent that congenital malformations are prominent among the expressions of toxicoses from poisonous plant ingestion by pregnant livestock (Keeler, 1975). In particular, malformations of the spinal column, the limbs, and the cephalic regions have been common.

In a strict sense, some of the malformations might be classified as deformations and therefore be called deformities rather than malformations. However, for this review, all deformities shall be called malformations, and reasons for the distinction will be noted in appropriate sections.

Several different plant genera have been definitively incriminated as responsible agents for mammalian malformations, and several other genera have been suspected because of epidemiologic or other evidence (Keeler, 1975, 1983, 1984c). The incidence of livestock congenital malformations has been estimated as 1-3% of all births (Leipold, *et al.*, 1972; Priester, *et al.*, 1970; Dennis & Leipold, 1979), closely approximating human statistics (Keeler, 1988). We speculate that perhaps one-third of all congenital malformations in livestock are poisonous plant-induced.

Many teratogens in poisonous plants have been identified by administration of either the plant or derived compounds to experimental animals (Keeler, 1975, 1983, 1984c). Most of the relevant terata data has been obtained from studies on domestic livestock. Some of the logistic problems faced in terata testing in livestock include size, lengthy gestation period, housing requirements and inordinately large dosage requirements by such animals (Keeler, 1983). These logistic constraints often dictate the experimental design that must be employed. Recommended terata testing protocols using large groups of these big animals at several dosage levels simply cannot be followed. Consequently, our standard protocol tests for teratogenicity in livestock at dosage levels of the suspected poisonous plant or compound that induce the same degree of toxicosis displayed by intoxicated animals from herds on the range in which malformed offspring are later found. Thus, dosage levels are employed that duplicate the relevant natural dosage which induce the malformations. It is often uncertain whether the ensuing congenital malformations result from a direct effect upon the embryo or fetus or whether they are due to secondary effects arising from maternal toxicity. Furthermore, when testing in laboratory animals as a substitute for domestic livestock, we sometimes adhere to the same protocol even though the studies are not curtailed by logistic constraints.

Examples of Current State of Knowledge on Malformations and Responsible Compounds

Cephalic Malformations Induced By Veratrum

Cyclopia and related facial malformations in newborn lambs were common many years ago in parts of Idaho (Binns, et al., 1959, 1960, 1962). The malformed offspring were usually single or double globe cyclopics with or without a proboscis above the centrally located eye. Other common defects were anophthalmia, cebocephalia or mandibular hyperplasia accompanied by maxillary or premaxillary hypoplasia. Incidence of malformed offspring in some ranching operations exceeded 20%. Feeding trials with plants common to the areas grazed by the pregnant ewes demonstrated that the plant *Veratrum californicum* was responsible for the condition (Binns, et al., 1963) when ingested by pregnant ewes on the 14th day of gestation (Binns, et al., 1965). Oral administration of extracts and compounds isolated from the plant demonstrated that three jerveratrum alkaloids jervine, cyclopamine (11-deoxojervine), and cycloposine (3-glucosyl-11-deoxojervine) (Figure 1) induced malformations in sheep and laboratory animals that were similar to natural cases (Keeler, 1975, 1978, 1979a; Keeler & Binns, 1968).

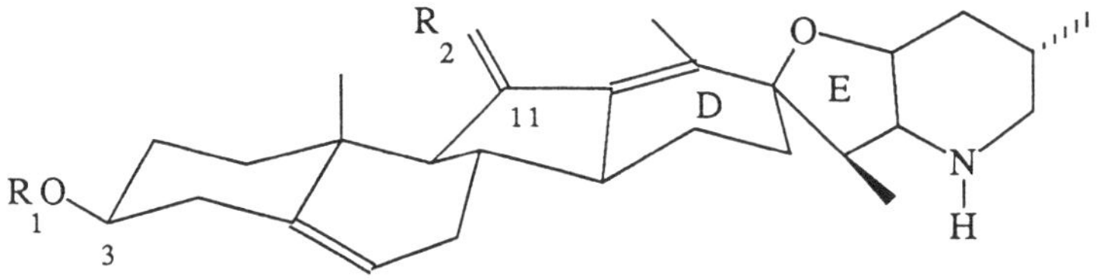

R_1=H, R_2=O   JERVINE

R_1=H, R_2=H_2 CYCLOPAMINE

R_1=GLC, R_2=H_2 CYCLOPOSINE

FIGURE 1. Structure of the *Veratrum* alkaloid teratogens jervine, cyclopamine and cycloposine.

The three teratogenic alkaloids are closely related C-nor-D-homo steroids bearing a fused furanopiperidine moiety attached *spiro* at carbon 17 of the steroid framework. Other *Veratrum* alkaloids tested, including veratramine and muldamine, did not induce either cyclopia or related cephalic malformations in sheep (Keeler, 1975, 1978, 1979a; Keeler & Binns, 1968).

In hamsters, cyclopamine and jervine induced a high incidence of exencephaly, encephalocele, harelip, cleft palate and cebocephaly (Keeler & Binns, 1968). At high dosages, muldamine induced some malformations (Brown & Keeler, 1978a).

Spirosolane alkaloids found widely in the *Solanum* genus are structurally related to the teratogenic *Veratrum* alkaloids (Figure 2) and for that reason were tested in the hamster assay for teratogenicity. Although solasodine was teratogenic, neither tomatidine nor the nitrogen-free solasodine analog diosgenin induced terata (Keeler, *et al.*, 1976). The significance of the nitrogen atom to hamster teratogenicity was demonstrated by lack of activity of diosgenin which contains an oxygen atom instead of an amino group. Assay of various jervine analogs by Brown (Brown & Keeler, 1978b) established that a basic nitrogen atom with a free electron pair was most critical in conferring teratogenicity to *Veratrum* alkaloids. On removal of the free electron pair of N-methyljervine by methylation, the resultant N-methylmethiodide of jervine did not induce terata. The piperidine nitrogen atom of the teratogenic *Veratrum* and spirosolane alkaloids is constrained to project α with respect to the steroidal plane because of the spiro connection between rings D & E in the jerveratrum teratogens or rings E & F in the spirosolane teratogen (Keeler, *et al.*, 1976), possibly in an appropriate position to interact with the active site in embryonic tissue.

The solanidane alkaloids of potatoes and other plants are less closely related to the teratogenic *Veratrum* and spirosolane alkaloids. They are based on the C_{27}-carbon steroid skeleton of cholestane with a tertiary nitrogen atom shared by rings E & F. Important examples include solanidine,

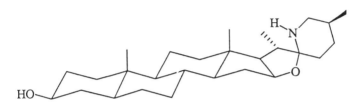

SOLASODINE

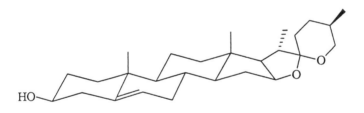

TOMATIDINE

DIOSGENIN

FIGURE 2. Structures of solasodine, tomatidine, and diosgenin.

demissidine and their glycosides (Figure 3). Several synthetic isomers of solanidine and demissidine epimeric at C-22 and C-25 (Sato & Ikekawa, 1961) provide a series of conformational epimers projecting the lone electron pair on the nitrogen either in the α or β direction with respect to the steroidal plane. Brown & Keeler (1978c) believed that the teratogenicity of the tertiary nitrogen-containing N-methyljervine sug-

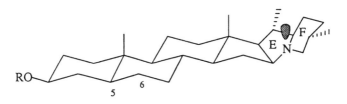

R =H, 5α H   DEMISSIDINE
R=H, $\Delta^{5,6}$ SOLANIDINE

SOLANIDANE GLYCOSIDES;
R=VARIOUS SUGARS; EITHER 5 αH OR $\Delta^{5,6}$

FIGURE 3. Structures of solanidine, demissidine, and their glycosides.

gested that solanidanes with nitrogen bonding capabilities α to the steroidal plane should be active. Epimers of 22S, 25R configuration were noted to have the nitrogen electron pair projecting α whereas those of 22R, 25S configuration project the lone pair toward the ß face (Figure 4). Two 22S, 25R epimers whose amino nitrogen project α were very teratogenic while the naturally occurring 22R, 25S epimer (demissidine) tested was not significantly teratogenic (Brown & Keeler, 1978c). The primary 22R, 25S epimer (solanidine) was not tested. Renwick, who had hypothesized in 1972 that potatoes (possibly their alkaloids) were teratogenic, reported in 1984 that isolated solanidine glycosides α-solanine and α-chaconine (presumably of 22R, 25S configuration) induced terata in hamsters (Renwick, et al., 1984). This was surprising to us in view of our earlier findings on the non-teratogenicity of demissidine (Brown & Keeler, 1978c). However, recent studies (Gaffield, et al., 1992) have established with certainty that not only are the alkaloid glycosides α-solanine and α-chaconine teratogenic in hamsters, but also that both 22R, 25S aglycone epimers (solanidine & demissidine) are teratogenic in hamsters albeit at markedly different incidences. Higher doses are required for the 22R, 25S alkaloids than were found to be necessary for terata induction by Brown's synthetic 22S, 25R epimers.

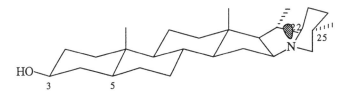

(22*R*, 25*S*)-5α H-SOLANIDAN-3β-OL (DEMISSIDINE)

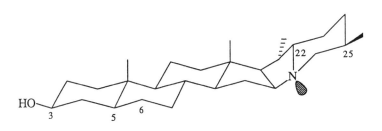

(22*S*,25*R*)-5αH-SOLANIDAN-3β-OL

(22*S*,25*R*)-SOLANID-5,6-ENE-3β-OL

FIGURE 4. Configuration of 22*S*, 25*R* and 22*R*, 25*S* solanidane epimers.

Skeletal and Palate Malformations from Quinolizidine Alkaloid-Containing *Lupinus Spp.*

Crooked calf disease, a congenital malformation in calves that usually affects limbs and spinal column, and sometimes palates, is induced by maternal ingestion principally during the 40th-70th days of gestation of quinolizidine alkaloid-containing members of the *Lupinus* genus, such as *L. sericeus* and *L. caudatus* (Shupe, *et al.*, 1967a, 1968). In natural outbreaks, incidence may exceed 30% of newborn calves (Shupe, *et al.*, 1967a, 1967b). Based on epidemiologic evidence and feeding trial evidence with semipurified alkaloid preparations, the teratogen is believed to be the quinolizidine alkaloid (-)-anagyrine (Figure 5) (Keeler, 1973a, 1973b,

1976). The condition could not be induced in sheep or hamsters (Keeler, 1984b). Three epimeric forms of the suspected teratogen are known to exist in nature: (-)-anagyrine, (+)-thermopsine and (-)-thermopsine (Figure 5) (Keeler, 1989). Whether there are inhibitive or additive effects among these three epimers remains to be established; however, they would be difficult to determine because of the aforementioned logistic problems inherent in terata studies of large livestock species.

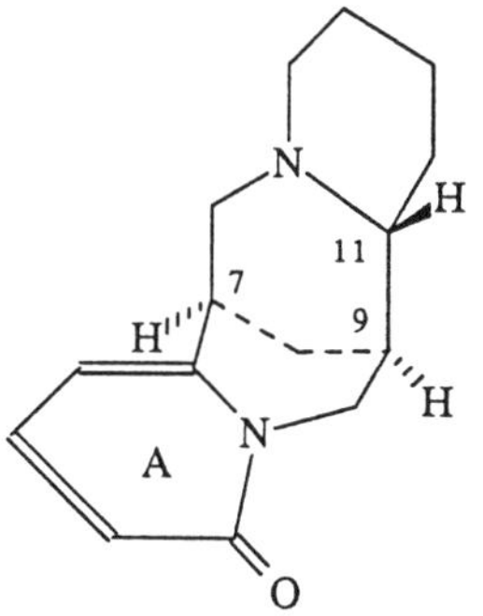

(-)-ANAGYRINE

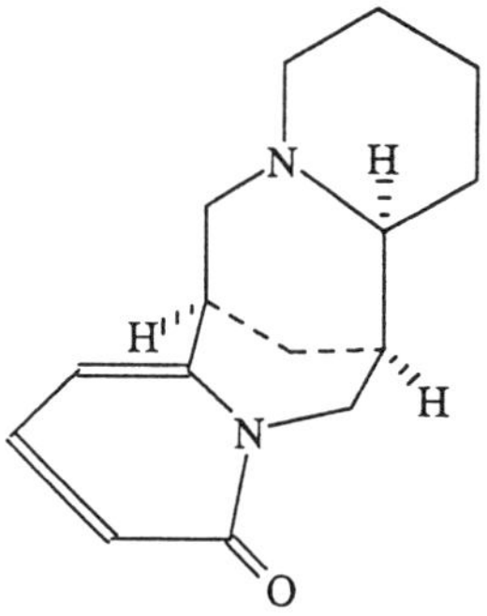

(-)-THERMOPSINE 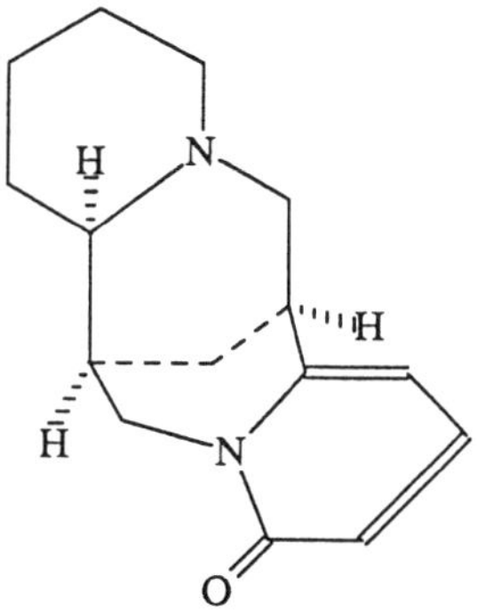   (+)-THERMOPSINE

FIGURE 5. Naturally occurring epimers of the quinolizidine alkaloids anagyrine and thermopsine.

Skeletal and Palate Malformations from Piperidine Alkaloid-Containing Conium maculatum

A congenital malformation in calves indistinguishable from *Lupinus*-induced crooked calf disease is induced by maternal ingestion of *Conium maculatum*. The principal insult period for either plant species is during the 40th-70th days of gestation (Keeler & Balls, 1978). Two piperidine alkaloids (Figure 6) are believed to be responsible — coniine (based on administration of the pure compound) and γ-coniceine (based on epidemiologic evidence) (Keeler, 1974; Keeler & Balls, 1978). Several livestock classes are susceptible to the teratogenic action of the plant and its teratogens: cattle (Keeler, 1974; Keeler & Balls, 1978), pigs (Panter, *et al.*, 1983), goats (Panter, *et al.*, 1990a,b), and to a reduced extent, sheep (Panter, *et al.*, 1988a,b). Limbs, spinal column and palate are the anatomical sites of the teratogenic effects.

CONIINE   γ-CONICEINE

FIGURE 6. The teratogenic piperidine alkaloids coniine and γ-coniceine.

Skeletal and Palate Malformations from Pyridine and Piperidine Alkaloid-Containing Nicotiana Spp.

A congenital malformation in piglets, primarily affecting the limbs, was reported in sows (Crowe, 1969; Menges, *et al.*, 1970) ingesting waste tobacco stalks. Crowe & Swerczek (1974) induced the effect experimentally by feeding stalks or leaf filtrates; however, the pyridine alkaloid nicotine (Figure 7), which is the principal plant alkaloidal constituent, did not induce the effect (Crowe, 1978). Because anabasine [2-(3-pyridyl) piperidine] (Figure 7) meets the structural requirements for teratogenicity that we had found earlier to be essential among piperidine analogs of coniine, we speculated

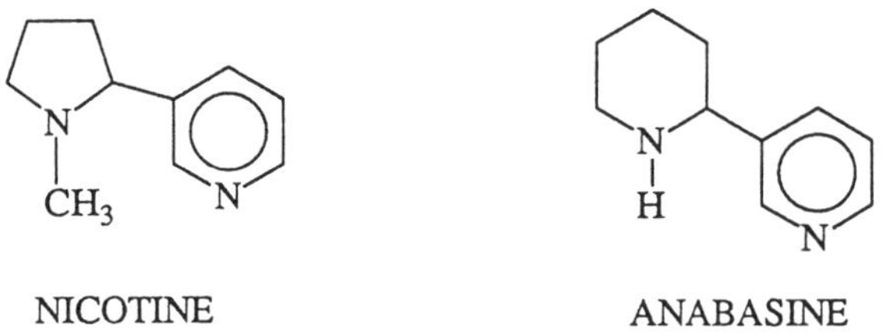

NICOTINE   ANABASINE

FIGURE 7. The tobacco alkaloids nicotine and anabasine.

that this minor tobacco alkaloid was more likely to be the teratogen than nicotine. Earlier experiments with coniine analogs (Keeler & Balls, 1978) had shown that both chain length and degree of ring unsaturation affected teratogenicity in calves. Whereas neither 2-ethylpiperidine nor 2-methylpiperidine was teratogenic, 2-propylpiperidine (coniine) induced malformations. Coniine with a fully saturated ring and γ-coniceine (Figure 6) with a single double bond in the heterocyclic ring were teratogenic; however, the fully unsaturated pyridine ring compound conyrine was not. These results suggested that saturated or nearly saturated α-substituted piperidines, whose α-substituent was at least propyl in length or bulk, might be teratogenic. The results implicated anabasine as more likely to prove teratogenic than nicotine. Anabasine was isolated from *Nicotiana glauca* as a racemic mixture and the alkaloid induced limb malformations in piglets that were clinically indistinguishable from those induced by *N. tabacum* or *N. glauca* plant material (Keeler, 1979b; Keeler, *et al.*, 1984). Pure anabasine also induced a high incidence of cleft palate (Keeler & Crowe, 1985).

Piperidines that appeared to satisfy the apparent structural requirements for teratogenicity had been found by the mid-1980s in a variety of plants important to man and animals including the *Punica, Duboisia, Sedum, Withania, Carica, Hydrangea, Dichroa, Cassia, Prosopis, Genista, Ammodendron, Lupinus, Liparia*, and *Collidium* genera (Keeler & Crowe, 1985). Among the above, plants of the genus *Lupinus* were particularly interesting. Few species of the *Lupinus* genus have been reported to contain piperidine alkaloids (Keeler, 1989). The alkaloids are absent from *L. caudatus* and

L. sericeus, the usual crooked calf disease inducers (Keeler, 1973a, 1973b; Keeler & Panter, 1989). Nonetheless, at least two of the lupins that do contain piperidine alkaloids are frequently found on certain cattle grazing areas. One of them is *Lupinus formosus*.

Skeletal and Palate Malformation from Piperidine-containing *Lupinus spp.*

The alkaloid composition of *L. formosus* (Keeler & Panter, 1989) had been reported by Fitch, *et al.* (1974) to be low in quinolizidines but rich in piperidine alkaloids. Piperidine alkaloids found by them (and which we suspect as potentially teratogenic) included hystrine, ammodendrine, N-methylammodendrine, N-acetylhystrine, anabasine, N-methylanabasine and N-methylpelletierine. Our analysis of *L. formosus* collections from a different location (Keeler & Panter, 1989) showed seven major and nine minor components in the total alkaloid fraction. All seven major and five of the nine minor components, representing all but 3% of the fraction, were identified by mass spectrometric fragmentation patterns and GC retention times. The mixture of alkaloids included several potentially teratogenic piperidine alkaloids (particularly a very large amount of ammodendrine) (Figure 8), and several non-teratogenic quinolizidine alkaloids, in addition to a trace (at non-teratogenic levels) of the known quinolizidine teratogen anagyrine. The alkaloids reported by Fitch and coworkers (Fitch, *et al.*, 1974) and by us in *L. formosus* (Keeler & Panter, 1989) are compared in Table 1.

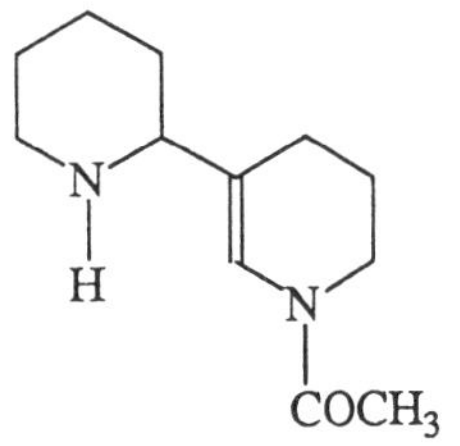

AMMODENDRINE

FIGURE 8. The piperidine alkaloid ammodendrine from *Lupinus formosus*.

TABLE 1. Comparison of Alkaloids Identified in *Lupinus formosus* as Reported by Fitch, *et al.* (1974) (F.D.D.) and by Keeler & Panter (1989) (K.P.)

Alkaloid	F.D.D. (g/kg)	K.P. (g/kg)
Hystrine	2.3	0.043
Ammodendrine	3.9	0.946
N-methylammodendrine	0.8	0.049
N-acetylhystrine	0.1	0.022
Anabasine	Trace	No
N-methylanabasine	Trace	No
N-methylpelletierine	Trace	No
Lupinine	Trace	No
Smipine	0.03	0.074
α-Isolupanine	No	0.011
5,6-Dehydrolupanine	No	0.016
Lupanine	No	0.595
N-methylalbine	No	0.101
Wink's No. 9	No	0.213
Multiflorine	No	0.234
Anagyrine	No	0.024

Administration of the plant to experimental calves induced severe crooked calf disease with limb, spinal and palate involvement. The malformations are presumed to have been induced by ammodendrine both because of its very high plant concentration and because it satisfies the presumed structural requirements for teratogenicity among piperidines.

Structure-Activity Relationships

All of the aforementioned teratogenic compounds from plants have one common structural feature, *i.e.*, they are piperidine ring-containing compounds. Is the piperidine ring the common structural aspect that confers teratogenicity, and do all of the compounds undergo metabolic conversion to a common proximal teratogen? If this question were answered affirmatively, a rather similar pattern of terata expression would be expected from all of the alkaloids if administration protocols were used that assured identical site of action, insult times and levels. Plants whose teratogens are apparently the simple α-substituted piperidine alkaloids as well as those whose teratogen is apparently the quinolizidine alkaloid anagyrine do exhibit a similar pattern of terata expression; however, the steroidal alkaloid teratogens exhibit a much different pattern of terata expression.

We speculate that, in cattle, anagyrine undergoes intra-ruminal metabolic conversion to a compound with ring A opened providing an α-substituted piperidine that serves as proximal teratogen. The lack of teratogenicity of quinolizid-ine-containing lupin plants or their extracts in sheep possess-ing different rumen flora or in monogastric hamsters (Keeler, 1984a) adds credence to this possibility. Various mechanism studies with piperidine, quinolizidine and steroidal alkaloid-containing plants or compounds therefrom do not suggest a common mechanism of terata induction.

Review of Studies on Mechanisms of Terata Induction

Panter, *et al.* (1983, 1990a) hypothesized that multiple congenital contractures involving limbs, spinal column, and neck (similar to those described herein) may arise from restricted fetal movement induced by certain plant constitu-ents when consumed by or administered to the dam during susceptible gestational periods. Furthermore, cleft palate may result from mechanical interference imposed by the tongue between the palatine shelves if there is lack of mouth, jaw, and tongue movement during critical developmental periods (Panter, *et al.*, 1985). Ultrasound measurements showed that fetal movement in livestock was reduced when animals were fed either *Conium maculatum* containing the teratogens co-niine and γ-coniceine or *Nicotiana glauca* containing anabas-ine (Panter, *et al.*, 1988b, 1990a, 1990b). Reduced fetal movement was believed to have resulted from placental trans-fer of the piperidine alkaloids resulting in induction of a sedative or anesthetic effect in the fetus that over a prolonged period of gestation could induce malformations (Panter, *et al.*, 1988b, 1990b).

A somewhat related suggestion was made by Finnell and coworkers (Finnell, *et al.*, 1991) that crooked calf disease induced by anagyrine might arise through lack of fetal movement imposed by a severely contracted uterine space induced by a toxic effect of anagyrine on the dam rather than on the fetus. These workers also correctly stated that crooked calf disease should more properly be referred to as a deformity rather than a malformation because the effects occur after limb bud initiation during the period when there is normally a great deal of fetal movement. Clearly, if movement were curtailed deformities, could result.

The nature of the malformations in calves from cows gavaged *Lupinus formosus*, whose teratogen is believed to be ammodendrine, from day 40 to day 70 of gestation, offers particularly strong evidence in favor of a lack of fetal movement hypothesis. A deformed rib cage depression accommodated the calf's head in near perfect fit, and the "at rest" position due to spinal curvature was with the head in that depression as though movement had been restricted over a protracted period. However, the action of the teratogen appears to be directly on the fetus rather than a result of maternal toxicity because fetal movement reduction continues between doses for a very much greater duration than do signs of overt toxicity in the dam.

To date, mechanism studies of jerveratrum steroidal alkaloids have suggested two alternate mechanisms of action quite unlike the proposed mechanism of action for piperidines that involves reduced fetal movement. Experiments by Campbell, *et al.* (1984) showed that, prior to differentiation, exposure of limb bud mesenchyme cells to the *Veratrum* teratogen *in vitro* suppressed subsequent accumulation of cartilage proteoglycan; however, treatment after differentiation had no such effect. Campbell, *et al.* (1987), using culture systems representing sequential stages of chondrocyte development, further showed that jervine compromises rapidly developing chondrogenic precursors.

A possible alternative mechanism was suggested by Sim and coworkers (Sim, *et al.*, 1984, 1985). The Australian researchers proposed that catecholamine-secreting cells in embryonic neuroepithelium are a specific target for the expression of steroidal alkaloid teratogenicity. Experiments showed that cyclopamine significantly decreased the acetylcholine- or nicotine-mediated ATP release (Sim, *et al.*, 1984, 1985), suggesting that jerveratrum alkaloids may act upon the nicotine receptor, perhaps by competitive binding. These observations were consistent with the earlier reported effect of *Veratrum* teratogens on the embryonic cranial neuroepithelium (Sim, *et al.*, 1983).

Thus, while there may be a degree of mechanism of action similarity in the proximal teratogen(s) among α-substituted piperidine and quinolizidine aikaloids, that similarity does not extend from those classes to the steroidal alkaloid teratogen class. Mechanism of action differences may even prevail among members of the steroidal alkaloid class itself, judging from their reported differences in expression of teratogenic effects (Keeler, 1984a). Finally, there appears to be no reason to presume proximal teratogen structural similarities between α-substituted piperidine teratogens and steroidal alkaloid teratogens that are related merely by the presence of piperidine rings in their molecular structure.

Conclusion

Several alkaloids from poisonous plants have been positively incriminated or are highly suspect as teratogens responsible for malformations in livestock. The compounds are piperidine, quinolizidine and steroidal alkaloids. Based on expressions of malformations and proposed mechanisms of action, some of them may actually be metabolized to common or similar proximal teratogens. It is doubtful, however, that all fit that category as isolated and ingested, even though they do share a common feature — presence of simple or complex piperidine rings.

References

Binns, W., Anderson, W. A., and Sullivan, D. J. (1960). Futher observations on a cyclopian-type malformation. *J. Amer. Vet. Med. Assoc.* 137:515-521.

Binns, W., James, L. F., Shupe, J. L., and Everett, G. (1963).

A congenital cyclopian-type malformation in lambs induced by maternal ingestion of a range plant, *Veratrum californicum. Amer. J. Vet. Res.* 24:1164-1175.

Binns, W., James, L. F., Shupe, J. L., and Thacker, E. J. (1962). Cyclopian-type malformation in lambs. *Arch. Environ. Health* 5:106-108.

Binns, W., Shupe, J. L., Keeler, R. F., and James, L. F. (1965). Chronologic evaluation of teratogenicity in sheep fed *Veratrum californicum. J. Amer. Vet. Med. Assoc.* 147:839-842.

Binns, W., Thacker, E. J., James, L. F., and Huffman, W. T. (1959). A congenital cyclopian-type malformation in lambs. *J. Amer. Vet. Med. Assoc.* 134:180-183.

Brown, D., and Keeler, R. F. (1978a). Structure-activity relation of steroid teratogens. 1. Jervine ring system. *J. Agric. Food Chem.* 26:561-563.

Brown, D., and Keeler, R. F. (1978b). Structure-activity relation of steroid teratogens. 2. N-Substituted jervines. *J. Agric. Food Chem.* 26:564-566.

Brown, D., and Keeler, R. F. (1978c). Structure-activity relation of steroid teratogens. 3. Solanidan epimers. *J. Agric. Food Chem.* 26:566-569.

Campbell, M., Brown, K. S., Saunders, B., Hassell, J., Horigan, E., and Keeler R. F. (1984). Early mesenchymal differentiation as the target of teratogenic *Veratrum* alkaloids. *Teratology* 29:22A.

Campbell, M., Horton, W., and Keeler, R. F. (1987). Comparative effects of retinoic acid and jervine on chondrocyte differentiation. *Teratology* 36:235-243.

Crowe, M. W. (1969). Skeletal anomalies in pigs associated with tobacco. *Mod. Vet. Pract.* 69:54-55.

Crowe, M. W. (1978). Tobacco-a cause of congenital arthrogryposis. Pages 419-427 *in* R. F. Keeler, K. R. Van Kampen and L. F. James, eds., *Effects of Poisonous Plants on Livestock.* Academic Press, New York.

Crowe, M. W., and Swerczek, T. M. (1974). Congenital arthrogryposis in offspring of sows fed tobacco (*Nicotiana tabacum*). *Amer. J. Vet. Res.* 35:1071-1073.

Dennis, S. M., Leipold, H. W. (1979). Ovine congenital defects. *Vet. Bull.* 49:233-239.

Everist, S. L. (1974). *Poisonous Plants of Australia.* Angus & Robertson, Melbourne. 966 pp.

Finnell, R. H., Gay, C. G., and Abbott, L. C. (1991). Teratogenicity of rangeland *Lupinus*: The crooked calf disease. Pages 27-39 *in* R. F. Keeler and A. T. Tu, eds., *Handbook of Natural Toxins: Toxicology of Plant and Fungal Compounds*, Vol. 6. Dekker, New York.

Fitch, W. L., Dolinger, P. M., and Djerassi, C. (1974). Alkaloid studies. LXVIII. Novel piperidyl alkaloids from *Lupinus formosus. J. Org. Chem.* 39:2974-2979.

Gaffield, W. and Keeler, R. F. (1992). Unpublished observations.

Gaffield, W., Keeler, R. F., Baker, D. C., and Stafford, A. E. (1992). Studies on the *Solanum tuberosum* sprout teratogen. Pages 418-422 *in* L. F. James, R. F. Keeler, P. R. Cheeke, E. M. Bailey and M. P. Hegarty, eds., *Proceedings: Third International Symposium on Poisonous Plants.* Iowa State Univ. Press, Ames, IA.

Keeler, R. F. (1973a). Lupin alkaloids from teratogenic and nonteratogenic lupins. I. Correlation of crooked calf disease incidence with alkaloid distribution determined by gas chromatography. *Teratology* 7:23-30.

Keeler, R. F. (1973b). Lupin alkaloids from teratogenic and nonteratogenic lupins. II. Identification of the major alkaloids by tandem gas chromatography-mass spectrometry in plants producing crooked calf disease. *Teratology* 7:31-35.

Keeler, R. F. (1974). Coniine, a teratogenic principle from *Conium maculatum* producing congenital malformations in calves. *Clin. Toxicol.* 7:195-206.

Keeler, R. F. (1975). Toxins and teratogens of higher plants. *J. Nat. Prod.* (Lloydia) 38:56-86.

Keeler, R. F. (1976). Lupin alkaloids from teratogenic and nonteratogenic lupins. III. Identification of anagyrine as the probable teratogen by feeding trials. *J. Toxicol. Environ. Health* 1:887-898.

Keeler, R. F. (1978). Cyclopamine and related steroidal alkaloid teratogens: Their occurrence, structural relationship, and biologic effects. *Lipids* 13:708-715.

Keeler, R. F. (1979a). Congenital defects in calves from maternal ingestion of *Nicotiana glauca* of high anabasine content. *Clin. Toxicol.* 15:417-426.

Keeler, R. F. (1979b). Toxins and teratogens of the Solanaceae and Liliaceae. Pages 59-82 *in* A. D. Kinghorn, ed., *Toxic Plants*. Columbia University Press, Irvington-on-Hudson, NY.

Keeler, R. F. (1983). Naturally occurring teratogens from plants. Pages 161-199 *in* R. F. Keeler and A. T. Tu, eds., *Handbook of Natural Toxins: Plant and Fungal Toxins*, Vol. 1. Dekker, New York.

Keeler, R. F. (1984a). Mammalian teratogenicity of steroidal alkaloids. Pages 531-562 *in* W. D. Nes, G. Fuller and L.-S. Tsai, eds., *Isopentenoids in Plants: Biochemistry and Function*. Dekker, New York.

Keeler, R. F. (1984b). Teratogenicity studies on non-food lupins in livestock and laboratory animals. Pages 301-304 *in* L. Lopez Belido, ed., *Proceedings of the Second International Lupine Conference*. Publicaciones Agrarias, Madrid.

Keeler, R. F. (1984c). Teratogens in plants. *J. Anim. Sci.* 58:1029-1039.

Keeler, R. F. (1988). Livestock models of human birth defects, reviewed in relation to poisonous plants. *J. Anim. Sci.* 66:2414-2427.

Keeler, R. F. (1989). Quinolizidine alkaloids in range and grain lupins. Pages 133-167 *in* P. R. Cheeke, ed., *Toxicants of Plant Origin*, Vol. 1, "Alkaloids." CRC Press, Boca Raton, FL.

Keeler, R. F., and Balls, L. D. (1978). Teratogenic effects in cattle of *Conium maculatum* and Conium alkaloids, and analogs. *Clin. Toxicol.* 12:49-64.

Keeler, R. F., and Binns, W. (1968). Teratogenic compounds of *Veratrum californicum* (Durand). V. Comparison of cyclopian effects of steroidal alkaloids from the plant and structurally related compounds from other sources. *Teratology* 1:5-10.

Keeler, R. F., and Crowe, M. W. (1985). Anabasine, a teratogen from the *Nicotiana* genus. Pages 324-333 *in* A. A. Seawright, M. P. Hegarty, L. F. James and R. F. Keeler, eds., *Plant Toxicology.* Queensland Poisonous Plants Comm., Yeerongpilly, Australia.

Keeler, R. F., Crowe, M. W., and Lambert, E. A. (1984). Teratogenicity in swine of the tobacco alkaloid anabasine isolated from *Nicotiana glauca. Teratology* 30:61-69.

Keeler, R. F., and Laycock, W. A. (1988). Use of Plant Toxin Information in Management Decisions. Pages 347-362 *in* L. F. James, M. H. Ralphs and D. B. Nielsen, eds., *The Ecology and Economic Impact of Poisonous Plants on Livestock Production.* Westview Press, Boulder, CO.

Keeler, R. F., and Panter, K. E. (1989). The piperidine alkaloid composition and relation to crooked calf disease-inducing potential of *Lupinus formosus. Teratology* 40: 423-432.

Keeler, R. F., Young, S., and Brown, D. (1976). Spina bifida, exencephaly, and cranial bleb produced in hamsters by the *Solanum* alkaloid solasodine. *Res. Commun. Chem. Pathol. Pharmacol.* 13:723-730.

Kingsbury, J. M. (1964). *Poisonous Plants of the United States and Canada.* Prentice-Hall, Englewood Cliffs, NJ. 626 pp.

Leipold, H. W., Dennis, S. M., and Huston, K. (1972). Congenital defects in cattle. Nature, cause, and effect. *Adv. Vet. Sci. Comp. Med.* 16:103-150.

Menges, R. W., Selby, L. A., Marienfeld, C. J., Aue, W. A., and Greer, D. L. (1970). A tobacco related epidemic of congenital limb deformities in swine. *Environ. Res.* 3: 285-302.

Panter, K. E., Bunch, T. D., and Keeler, R. F. (1988a). Maternal and fetal toxicity of poison-hemlock (*Conium maculatum*) in sheep. *Amer. J. Vet. Res.* 49:281-283.

Panter, K. E., Bunch, T. D., Keeler, R. F., and Sisson, D. V. (1988b). Radio ultrasound observations of the fetotoxic effects in sheep from ingestion of *Conium maculatum* (poison-hemlock). *J. Toxicol., Clin. Toxicol.* 26:175-187.

Panter, K. E., Keeler, R. F., Buck, W. B., and Shupe, J. L. (1983). Toxicity and teratogenicity of *Conium maculatum* in swine. *Toxicon* (*Suppl.*) 3:333-336.

Panter, K. E., Keeler, R. F., and Buck, W. B. (1985). Induction of cleft palate in newborn pigs by maternal ingestion of poison hemlock (*Conium maculatum*). *Amer. J. Vet. Res.* 46:1368-1371.

Panter, K. E., Keeler, R. F., Bunch, T. D., and Callan, R. J. (1990a). Congenital skeletal malformations and cleft palate induced in goats by ingestion of *Lupinus, Conium* and *Nicotiana* species. *Toxicon* 28:1377-1385.

Panter, K. E., Bunch, T. D., Keeler, R. F., Sisson, D. V., and Callan, R. J. (1990b). Multiple congenital contractures (MCC) and cleft palate induced in goats by ingestion of piperidine alkaloid-containing plants: Reduction in fetal movement as the probable cause. *J. Toxicol., Clin. Toxicol.* 28:69-83.

Priester, W. A., Glass, A. G., and Waggoner, N. S. (1970). Congenital defects in domestic animals: General considerations. *Amer. J. Vet. Res.* 31:1871-1879.

Renwick, J. H. (1972). Hypothesis: Anencephaly and spina bifida are usually preventable by avoidance of a specific but unidentified substance present in certain potato tubers. *Brit. J. Prev. Soc. Med.* 26:67-88.

Renwick, J. H., Claringbold, W. D. B., Earthy, M. E., Few, J. D., and McLean, C. S. (1984). Neural-tube defects produced in Syrian hamsters by potato glycoalkaloids. *Teratology* 30:371-381.

Sato, Y., and Ikekawa, N. (1961). Chemistry of the spiroaminoketal side chain of solasodine and tomatidine: V. The synthesis of the isomeric solanidanones. *J. Org. Chem.* 26:1945-1947.

Shupe, J. L., Binns, W. James, L. F., and Keeler, R. F. (1967a). Lupine, a cause of crooked calf disease. *J. Amer. Vet. Med. Assoc.* 151:198-203.

Shupe, J. L., James, L. F., and Binns, W. (1967b). Observations on crooked calf disease. *J. Amer. Vet. Med. Assoc.* 151:191-197.

Shupe, J. L., Binns, W., James, L. F., and Keeler, R. F. (1968). A congenital deformity in calves induced by the maternal consumption of lupin. *Aust. J. Agric. Res.* 19:335-340.

Sim. F. R. P., Livett, B. G., Browne, C. A., and Keeler, R. F. (1985). Studies on the mechanism of *Veratrum* teratogenicity. Pages 344-348 *in* A. A. Seawright, M. P. Hegarty, L. F. James and R. F. Keeler, eds., *Plant Toxicology.* Queensland Poisonous Plants Comm., Yeerongpilly, Australia.

Sim, F. R. P., Livett, B. G., Browne, C. A., Moore, S. E., Keeler, R. F., and Thorburn, G. D. (1984). Effect of 11-deoxojervine on catecholamine secretion by adrenal chromaffin cells. *Teratology* 30:50A.

Sim, F. R. P., Matsumoto, N., Goulding, E. H., Denny, K. H., Lamb, J., Keeler, R. F., and Pratt, R. M. (1983). Specific craniofacial defects induced by jervine in the cultured rat embryo. *Teratog. Carcinog. Mutagen.* 3:111-121.

Chapter 10

Cyanide Containing Foods and Potential For Fetal Malformations

R. P. Sharma

A considerable number of plant species that are used as food for man or animal contain traces of cyanide containing compounds. There are perhaps 2000 species of higher plants that produce cyanide (Conn, 1981). Some of the cyanide containing crops serve as a major source of food to a large human population, particularly in the tropics. The acute toxic effects of cyanide are well known, although the chronic effects of long-term ingestion are still unclear. A variety of diseases, including atoxic neuropathy, have been linked to continued intake of foods high in cyanide contents (Osuntokun, 1973). In addition, there is evidence that a high prevalence of goiter in African countries is related to cyanide containing diets. A brief description of foods that have a potential for toxic effects related to their cyanide contents and the possibility of birth defects that have been shown in animal models and are suspected in populations exposed to cyanide-containing foods is presented in this chapter. The need for considering cyanide in foods, particularly with factors such as less than desirable caloric intake, is discussed in relation to possible effects on pregnancy outcome.

Cyanide Containing Foods

Cassava. Cassava is the fourth most important source of calories in the tropics (Cock, 1982). The plant (*Manihot esculenta* Crantz) occurs as a shrub, propagates vegetatively, and has fleshy roots rich in starch. Commonly referred to "*manioc*," it is consumed as a principal source of carbohydrates in parts of Africa lying south of Sahara and Ethiopia and north of Zimbabwe. In several South Asian tropical countries, it is commonly referred to as *tapioca*. It has been a basic staple of native Indians and perhaps cultivated for 4000 years in the Americas. It is also known by several other names, *e.g., mandioca* or *aipim* in Brazil, or as *yuca* in Spanish-speaking American countries. Most of these terms often refer to a particular type of preparation made out of the starchy flour rather than its source. It has been used by native Americans and Africans either as an uncooked vegetable or after baking or boiling (Jones, 1959). It is also used as a paste or meal manufactured out of fine whitish flour.

Cassava is a good source of food energy, better than potatoes, sweet potatoes or yams, on a calories-per-unit weight basis. Compared to other starchy roots, it is also rich in calcium and vitamin C. It could well provide nearly all the dietary requirement of iron and a major portion of water soluble vitamins. However, it is a relatively poor source of sulfur-containing amino acids, and certain varieties (or other parts of the plant) may contain undesirable levels of prussic acid (hydrogen cyanide). In fact, the reason that it does not provide sufficient amounts of sulfur-containing amino acids is that these form thiocyanates with the free cyanide during various methods of food preparation (*e.g.*, cooking). The source of natural cyanide is the cyanogenic glycoside linamarin, found in considerable amounts in bitter cassava. The structure of linamarin is shown in Figure 1.

Cassava may contain varying amounts of bound (in glycoside form) or free cyanide depending on the variety, conditions of activation, or processing method used. The "bitter varieties" (high cyanide containing) may have over 600 parts per million (ppm) cyanide (dry matter basic), whereas the "sweet" cassava contains much less (Gomez, *et al.*, 1980). The cyanide content of cassava from selected reports are listed in Table 1. Traditional methods of preparation, *i.e.*, sun-drying, boiling, fermentation, etc, eliminate most of the free cyanide. Although much of the free hydrocyanic acid can be eliminated by processing of food, the thiocyanate or cyano-glycoside contents are relatively stable.

TABLE 1. Cyanide Contents of Various Varieties of Cassava

Clone or Variety	Hydrocyanic Acid Content mg/kg Dry Matter	References
Tabouca	103[1]	DeBruijn, 1973
461	686[1]	DeBruijn, 1973
CMC 40	436 ± 111[2]	Gomez, et al., 1984
CMC 84	772 ± 167	Gomez, et al., 1984
M Col 22	540 ± 97	Gomez & Valdivieso, 1985
M Col 1684	1034 ± 160	Gomez & Valdivieso, 1985

[1] Calculated from μg/g fresh weight reported, assuming 35% dry matter relative to fresh weight.

[2] Mean ± S.E.M.

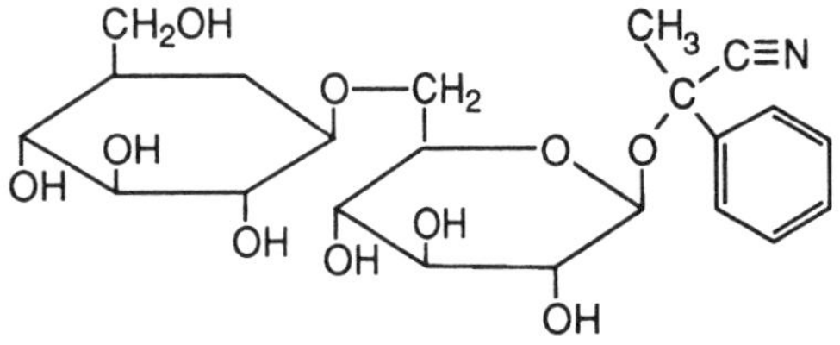

Amygdalin

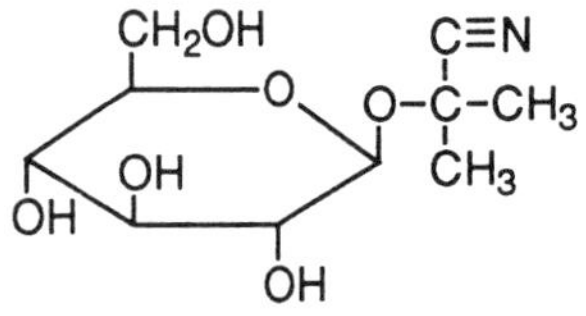

Linamarin

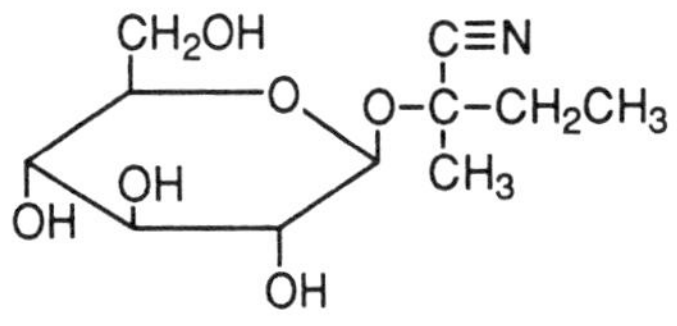

Lotaustralin

FIGURE 1. Structures of selected cyanogenic glycosides present in foods. Amygdalin is the major constituents of laetrile (obtained from peach pits or bitter almonds), whereas the other two, linamarin and lotaustralin are found in bitter cassava.

Other Food Sources of Cyanide

Cyanogenic glycosides have been found in a variety of other natural products, most of which are considered inedible due to their inherent toxicity. However, many cases of cyanide poisoning are reported by consumption of such substances. Among the most notable are wild lima beans (which contain linamarin), that have as much as 4,000 ppm of cyanide in fresh mature seeds (Conn, 1979). Only the wild small black lima beans grown in Central America contain these high levels of cyanide; the large white variety commonly used in Europe and North America has much less (1-2% of that found in the wild type) of cyanide.

Almond (*Prunus amygdalus*) is another example of an edible commodity that may have toxic levels of the cyanogenic glycoside amygdalin. Most edible almonds have either none or little cyanide, although the "bitter" varieties may contain considerable amounts. Other members of the same Rosaceace family, *e.g.*, apricot, cherry, plum, peach also contain cyanogenic compounds. Fortunately, the pulp of the ripe fruit, in most cases, has no cyanide and is perfectly good to eat. However, the pits, such as those of peach or apricot, contain the same cyanogenic glycoside as in almonds. In the 1970s, the extract from the pits of peaches (referred to as laetrile) achieved notoriety as a cure for certain types of cancer and was consequently subjected to several scientific studies (Willhite, 1982). Cases of cyanide poisoning after eating bamboo plant have also been reported (Baggchi & Ganguli, 1943).

Sorghum vulgare is cultivated for both human and animal consumption. The grain, used by people in many tropical countries, is harmless. The plant, particularly young shoots and leaves, have lethal levels of cyanide and when grazed by animals have caused severe economic losses. The same is true for certain varieties of white clover.

Cyanogenic Glycosides

Most of the cyanide contained in natural foods occur in the form of cyanogenic glycosides. These compounds, either by treatment with acid or by the action of appropriate hydrolytic enzymes, release free cyanide in the form of hydrocyanic acid. The acid environment in the human stomach thus favors release of free cyanide after consumption of food containing cyanogenic glycosides. Certain foods, *e.g.*, lima beans, contain the enzyme linamarase (a β-glucosidase) which can liberate cyanide during soaking. It is, therefore, considered unsafe to soak these beans without taking appropriate measures to remove free cyanide.

Amygdalin is perhaps the best known of cyanogenic glycosides and is present in bitter almonds. Similar substances, *i.e.*, linamarin and lotaustralin, are the glycosides found in cassava. Chemical structures of these compounds are shown in Figure 1. Amygdalin is a diglucoside and releases prunasin (a monoglucoside) after the action of β-glucosidase. The same enzyme can liberate mandelonitrile (cyanide containing benzaldehyde), which by the action of hydroxynitrile lyase will liberate hydrocyanic acid and benzaldehyde. The cyanoglucosides present in cassava are principally monoglucosides that can liberate free cyanide and acetone by the action of linamerase and lyase. The rate of cyanide liberation depends on the pH and presence of enzymes, and, therefore, may depend on the species of animal ingesting the cyanogenic compound-containing foods.

Studies in rats indicated that amygdalin is not absorbed as such after oral administration; much of it is hydrolyzed by the gut flora (Strugala, *et al.*, 1986). The walls of proximal jejunum converted amygdalin to prunasin, which is partially absorbed. Cyanide liberation from amygdalin occurs primarily by the gut micraflora. A similar observation was reported for dogs where no unchanged amygdalin was absorbed after oral treatment, but nearly half of the prunasin was systemically absorbed (Rauws, *et al.*, 1982).

Toxic Effects of Cyanide-Containing Foods

The lethal action of cyanide is due to the inhibition of cytochrome oxidase in mitochondrial respiration. A variety of metalloenzymes are susceptible to the inhibitory action of cyanide, and cytochrome oxidase in the brain is believed to be most susceptible. However, consumption of cyanide containing foods rarely causes acute symptoms in people. Most toxicities are associated with accidental ingestion of peach pits or chokecherry or in animals after the ingestion of young sorghum plants or other cyanide containing vegetation.

For a long time, cyanide was not considered to be a chronic poison because the animal body is capable, within limits, of metabolizing cyanide. The toxicity of foods containing cyanogenic glycosides, other than acute effects of cyanide, has become apparent only in the last few decades. One of the effects of cyanide in food is to bind sulfur-containing amino acids, thus producing thiocyanate. An excess of thiocyanate in food results in a depressed uptake of iodine by the thyroid gland that subsequently may cause symptoms of iodine deficiency, including goiter. Cretinism in children of Idjwi Island of the Congo, associated with a deficiency of dietary iodine, is worsened by eating cassava (Miller, 1974). Other human diseases associated with the abnormal detoxication of cyanide and long term ingestion of cyanogenic foods include retrobulbar neuritis, inherited optic atrophy and deficiency of vitamin B_{12} (Wilson, 1973).

The ataxic neuropathy prevalent in West African countries has been associated with high cassava diets (Osuntokin, 1973). In Nigeria, it was characterized by lesions of the skin, mucous membranes, optic and auditory nerves, spinal cord and peripheral nerves. It was suggested that the thiocyanate content of the Nigerian diet is low; however, the cyanide in cassava is generally high. The prevalence of disease is associated with the intensity of cassava cultivation and not with either iodine or vitamin B_{12} status. The higher presence of goiter in the population was related to plasma thiocyanate levels. Increasing the intake of hydroxocobalamin, riboflavin or cystine had no beneficial effect, and there was no evidence of genetic predisposition for the disease.

In an epidemiologic study, Cliff, *et al.* (1986a) compared cassava consumption, cyanide exposure and ankle clonus (convulsive spasms involving the ankle joint) rate in children of Mozambique. All of these parameters were higher in children from an area with a high prevalence of spastic peresis related to cyanide exposure from cassava, compared to children from neighboring areas where no peresis was reported. The urinary thiocyanate excretion was higher in children with clonus than those without clonus. The authors suggested that exposure to cyanide from cassava was the cause of lesions in cortico-spinal tracts. In a subsequent report (Cliff, *et al.*, 1986b), the same group of investigators reported on the circulating hormones and urinary excretion of iodine in individuals affected by spastic paraperesis. A normal excretion of iodine suggested an adequate intake of this element. The ratio for T3/T4 was raised indicating an adaptation to the antithyroid effect of cyanide from cassava. The thiocyanate excretion in urine increased, suggesting a high intake of cyanide containing compounds. It was, therefore, proposed that the thyroid gland adapts to the toxic effects of cyanide if the iodine intake is adequate.

Konzo, a distinct form of myelopathy characterized by spastic paraperesis, is frequent in rural Zaire. According to Tylleskar, *et al.*, (1992), the affected population consumes high amounts of cyanide due to insufficient soaking of cassava roots. In children affected with paraperesis, urinary excretion of thiocyanate was markedly elevated; urinary thiocyanate in affected children was 757 µmole/l compared to 50 µmole/l in unaffected children, suggesting a higher intake of cyanide. A casual relationship of blood cyanide concentration and deficient sulfur intake was reported with the disease. The authors suggested that the underlying causes of konzo are poverty and food shortage; however, the disease can be prevented with a minor improvement in food processing methods, *i.e.*, long soaking (three days) of cassava roots prior to consumption to reduce its cyanide contents. The report indicated a casual relationship between cyanide ingestion and birth defects and is highly indicative of a potential problem in newborns exposed to cyanide.

The incidence of endemic goiter in Eastern Nigeria is also related to high cassava consumption (Ekpechi, 1973). The antithyroid action of cassava was established in man and animals, both in epidemiologic studies and experimentation with rats (Delange, et. al., 1973).

Potential of Birth Defects After Cyanide Consumption

Interest in cyanide inducing congenital malformations actually arose while testing the safety of cyanide containing compounds used in manufacturing commercial products. Aliphatic nitrites are used in the manufacturing of certain types of plastics, synthetic fibers, resins, dyes, and pharmaceuticals. Some are used as agricultural insecticides. Many of these were found to be teratogenic when tested in laboratory animals (Willhite, et al., 1981). The effects of various aliphatic nitriles were associated with an increase in urinary thiocyanate and were alleviated by a simultaneous treatment with sodium thiosulfate, suggesting that these were mediated by liberation of cyanide from the toxic compounds.

Doherty, et al. (1982) evaluated the teratogenicity of sodium nitrile after slow infusion in Syrian golden hamsters. The treatment was carried out by subcutaneous implantation of osmotic minipumps and resulted in a high rate of embryonic resorption and dose-related induction of congenital malformations. The common anomalies seen were neural tube defects, including exencephaly and encephalocele. Simultaneous treatment with thiosulfate alleviated these effects. The type of malformations induced by cyanide were similar to those produced by acrylonitrile or propionitrile in the study reported above (Willhite, et al., 1981).

Exposure of pregnant hamsters to acetonitrile via inhalation, intraperitoneal injection or oral gavage produced severe axial skeletal disorders in the offspring (Willhite, 1983). The induction of skeletal and neural disorders was attributed to the *in vivo* liberation of free cyanide. The congenital defects produced by several other natural and synthetic compounds capable of producing cyanide have been reported.

Because of the popularity of laetrile as a possible cure for cancer, Willhite (1982) studied the congenital malformations produced by amygdalin, the principal constituent of laetrile. Oral treatment with amygdalin induced malformations typical of those produced by the cyanide; the intravenous injections of similar doses were ineffective. This suggested that amygdalin liberates cyanide in the gastrointestinal tract because of the presence of bacterial glycosidases. Mammalian tissues are unable to hydrolyze amygdalin to toxic levels of free cyanide. The incidence of abnormalities was dose-related in a relatively narrow dose range (200-300 mg/kg orally). Prunasin, a metabolite of amygdalin and also a constituent in laetrile, has same effect. The effects were nearly abolished by an intraperitoneal injection of 300 mg/kg of sodium thiosulfate. Blood and tissue cyanide or thiocyanate levels were elevated in animals orally treated with amygdalin. The teratogenicity of laetrile was evident after a single large dose, which suggests that long-term use of this substance, if taken orally, may lead to a possible unfavorable pregnancy outcome.

Treatment of Sprague-Dawley rats with 10% ground apricot kernels containing various levels of cyanide had no effect on their reproductive performance (Miller, *et al.*, 1981). Blood thiocyanate levels did increase in female rats after five months of feeding kernels having high cyanide content; no such increase was found in males. Urinary thiocyanate excretion also increased in both sexes when placed on high cyanide diets. The offspring were apparently not evaluated for any subtle malformations.

The human data after chronic ingestion of cyanide containing food and its effects on pregnancy are not available. Congenital anomalies in farm animals have been associated with ingestion of cyanogenic plants by pregnant females. In a case report, four out of seven pregnant mares grazing on hybrid Sudan grass pasture gave birth to dead foals that exhibited ankylosis of the joints (Prichard & Voss, 1967). In Warren County, Missouri, an outbreak of congenital malformations in swine was related to the consumption of wild black cherries (*Prunus serotina*) by pregnant sows (Selby, *et al.*, 1971). A calf had abnormal mammary glands after the mother had ingested a liberal amount of bamboo leaves (*Bambusa arundinacea*) during the gestation period (Alikutty & Aleyas, 1978).

Tewe & Manner (1981) reported on the reproductive performance of pigs given different levels of cyanide. Pregnant Yorkshire gilts were given low cyanide cassava supplemented with various levels of potassium cyanide. In the high cyanide group (500 mg/kg of diet), the fetal thiocyanate content increased along with pathological changes in the thyroid gland. No effects of cyanide supplementation were observed on performance of mothers or lactation. Similarly, Gomez, *et al.* (1983) found no effects of cassava cultivars with high cyanide on the performance (growth rate) of pigs or broilers. Because the cassava used in this study had been sun-dried, the authors proposed that sun-dried cassava is a suitable animal feed.

Cassava has long been suspected as a cause of various congenital human malformations in areas of Nigeria where cassava is used as a staple diet (Singh, 1981). Scientific reports confirming such association are not available. Singh (1981) conducted a preliminary study on rats fed milled cassava powder during the first 15 days of gestation. An increased incidence of open eye, microcephaly, limb defects and growth retardation was reported. It was pointed out that the rat may not be the most suitable species because these animals are relatively resistant to the acute toxic effects of oral cyanide poisoning, perhaps due to a rapid renal clearance.

Because cyanide-induced teratology occurs in hamsters, Frakes, *et al.* (1985) evaluated the teratogenic potential of linamarin, the principal cyanoglucoside in cassava, and various cassava diets in this species. Linamarin was given to pregnant hamsters on day 8 of gestation as single oral doses of 70 to 140 mg/kg. The fetuses were examined after laparatomy on day 15 of gestation. The treatment with linamarin caused a dose-related incidence of cyanide intoxication in pregnant animals, characterized by dyspnea, ataxia, tremors and hypothermia; however, the symptoms were short lived and reversed in most animals within a few hours. A few animals at the high doses (120 and 140 mg linamarin per kg body weight) died because of the treatment. Skeletal defects were the primary observation in the offspring. Missing presacral vertebrae (at least one vertebra missing) and agenesis of one or both 13th ribs were common anomalies. Fusion of ribs, rib bifurcation, asymmetrical rib cage, and fusion of adjacent vertebrae were noticed. Supernumary ribs (rudimentary or full-length 14th rib) were noted in nearly half of the fetuses examined; however, this observation was common in control fetuses and was not considered treatment-related. It was concluded that linamarin present in cassava may not be a threat to the fetus unless the cassava was consumed in quantities large enough to overwhelm the cyanide detoxication capability of the mother. It is, of course, possible that there are other interacting factors related to the cassava diet that may pose a danger during pregnancy. The teratogenic potential of linamarin appears to be much less than that for amygdalin.

In a follow-up study, Frakes, *et al.* (1986a) evaluated the potential of cassava diets on hamster prenatal development. Groups of pregnant hamsters were provided either a low cyanide (sweet) cassava diet or a high cyanide (bitter) cassava diet. The cyanide contents of the two diets were 16 (*Llanera* variety) and 213 (CMC84 and MCol 1684) ppm of prussic acid on dry matter basis, respectively. The cassava diets were sun dried, a common method of processing cassava in South American countries, and were used as 80% cassava together with 20% standard laboratory chow. These mixed diets were used throughout the gestation period beginning day 3 of pregnancy. Since linamarin alone was not found to be highly teratogenic and the protein quality of food may be a contributing factor in the pregnancy outcome, an additional group was given a specially formulated diet. That diet was low in protein and simulated the cassava diets, except that it had no detectable amounts of cyanide. Subsequent analyses indicated the protein content of standard laboratory chow to be 24.5%, compared with 4.1% in the cassava diets and 4.2% in the formulated low protein diet.

The animals given low protein or cassava diets had reduced fetal weight compared to those on a regular diet. A low incidence of gross congenital malformations was associated with the cassava consumption, especially in those on a high cyanide content. Three fetuses had hydrocephalus in one dam fed the low cyanide diet, one fetus with encephalocele was observed in the high cyanide group. The low protein diet itself did not cause any fetal malformations. Retarded skeletal ossification was noticed in both low and high cyanide cassava groups but not in the low protein group. Sacrocaudal vertebrae, metatarsal bones, and sternebrae were the most sensitive indicators of impaired skeletal ossification. It was concluded that although the presence of linamarin (in cassava) or the dietary protein deficiency alone is not sufficient to induce fetal anomalies, a combination of protein starvation along with cyanide content of cassava diets may be the cause of developmental retardation in hamsters. Impoverished people in tropical developing countries subsist almost entirely on cassava diets. Because a cassava diet is generally low in its protein content and usually has a greater amount of cyanide than those used in the above described experiments, pregnant females subsisting primarily on cassava may have a potential risk of having low birth weight in babies and related developmental problems.

In the cassava feeding experiments mentioned above, there was a single case of cephalothoracophagus twins from a dam fed a high cyanide diet. Because of the lone incidence of this anomaly, it can not be ascertained that it was induced by either cyanide or other factors in the cassava diet. These twins were highly symmetrical, possessed a single head and thorax but divided abdomen and normally looking limb patterns (Willhite, *et al.*, 1985). Lordotic exencephaly was evident, a condition commonly associated in some other studies where cyanide containing compounds were administered. The internal abdominal organs, *i.e.*, kidneys, adrenals, ureters, bladders, and testes with external genitalia were present in normal positions in both abdomens. The twins in the upper part of the body possessed only one pharynx, a single larynx and trachea, a single thyroid, one esophagus and one stomach. Spleens and pancreas were also present in a single set. The twins exhibited an extensive diaphragmatic hernia, allowing protusion of abdominal organs into the thoracic cavity. The liver was separated into two regions, each with its own portal vein. Much of the upper gastrointestinal tract was shared, after the proximal ilium the intestines bifurcated into two lower digestive tracts. The incidence of such twinning is thought to be extremely rare and the contribution of cassava diet as a cause can not be totally eliminated.

Because the cyanogenic glycosides present in different plant sources, *e.g.*, amygdalin from almonds and peaches, and linamarin from cassava, produced different responses in hamsters in relation to congenital malformations, Frakes, *et al.* (1986b) investigated the rate of cyanide production from the two cyanogenic glycosides in this species. When the same amount (on a molar basis) of either linamarin or amygdalin was given orally to female hamsters, the blood cyanide levels after amygadalin achieved higher values than in individuals given linamarin. In the case of linamarin, cyanide in blood appeared earlier but stayed consistently lower than those after amygdalin. The total bioavailability of cyanide from the two cyanoglycosides appeared nearly similar. No differences in thiocyanate excretion were observed between the two groups. It was apparent that the peak blood level of cyanide, which was higher after amygdalin than after linamarin, may be responsible for retarded development of fetuses. The observation that the rate of cyanide formation by hamster intestinal tract glycosidase enzymes (derived from cecal tissues and contents) *in vitro* was higher in the case of amygdalin than that of linamarin, confirmed this hypothesis (Frakes, *et al.*, 1986b). Amygdalin exhibited a small lag period (less than 10 minutes) after which a high rate of metabolism was observed. The hamster's intestinal enzymes degraded prunasin (the monoglucoside derivative of amygdalin) at a much higher rate, suggesting that the initial lag in amygdalin breakdown was due to the formation of prunasin, which will cause a faster subsequent release of free cyanide. The apparent Km values of hamster cecal glycosidase enzymes were much lower for amygdalin than for linamarin; there was nearly four and one-half times more cyanide liberated when amygdalin was the substrate compared to linamarin. The differences in the teratogenic potential of amygdalin or linamarin in hamsters, therefore, can be explained on the basis of cyanide liberation in the gastrointestinal tract of this species. Whether higher mammals, like humans, have a different rate of cyanide liberation after cassava consumption (linamarin), is not known.

Conclusions

The information presented above indicates that the presence of cyanide in food may be a potential contributing factor in developmental anomalies. Cassava is a basic staple for more than 500 million people worldwide and has been suspected as a cause of human congenital defects. Appropriate epidemiologic studies are, thus, warranted to answer this question. Whether the higher incidence of cretinism, low birth weights and congenital goiter are associated with the cyanide content, or with any other dietary factors in cassava-eating countries, needs to be investigated. Consumption of other cyanide containing foods, particularly lima beans, and bamboo shoots, should be avoided during pregnancy. The risks of cyanide-containing feeds in animal management and feeding are perhaps better understood than they are in people.

References

Alikutty, K. M., and Aleyas, N. M. (1978). Amastia of rear quarters in a cow. *Mod. Vet. Pract.* 59:623.
Baggchi, K. N., and Ganguli, H. D. (1943). Toxicology of

young shoots of common bamboos (*Bambusa arundinacea* Willd). *Indian Med. Gaz.* 78:40-42.

Cliff, J., Essers, S., and Rosling, H. (1986a). Ankle clonus correlating with cyanide intake from cassava in rural children from Mozambique. *J. Trop. Pediatr.* 32:186-189.

Cliff, J., Lundquist, P., Rosling, H., Sorbo, B., and Wide, L. (1986b). Thyroid function in a cassava-eating population affected by epidemic spastic paraperesis. *Acta Endocrinol.* (Copenhagen) 113:523-528.

Cock, J. H. (1982) Cassava: A basic energy source in the tropics. *Science* 218:755-762.

Conn, E. E. (1979). Cyanogenic glycosides. *Intern. Rev. Biochem.* 27:21-43.

Conn, E. E. (1981). Unwanted biological substances in foods: Cyanogenetic glycosides. Pages 105-121 in J. C. Ayres and J. C. Kirschman, eds., *Impact of Toxicology of Food Processing.* AVI Publishing Co., Wesport, CT.

De Bruijn, G. H. (1973). The cyanogenic character of cassava (*Manihot esculenta).* Pages 43-48 *in* B. Nastel and R. MacIntyre, eds., *Chronic Cassava Toxicity.* International Development Research Center, Ottawa, Canada.

Delange, F., Van der Velden, M., and Ermans, A. M. (1973). Evidence of an antithyroid action of cassava in man and animals. Pages 147-151 *in* B. Nestel and R. MacIntyre, eds., *Chronic Cassava Toxicity.* International Development Research Center, Ottawa, Canada.

Doherty, P. A., Ferm, V. H., and Smith, R. P. (1982). Congenital malformations induced by infusion of sodium cyanide in the golden hamster. *Toxicol. Appl. Pharmacol.* 64:456-464.

Ekpechi, O. L. (1973). Endemic goitre and high cassava diets in Eastern Nigeria. Pages 139-145 *in* B. Nestel and R. MacIntyre, eds., *Chronic Cassava Toxicity.* International Development Research Center, Ottawa, Canada.

Frakes, R. A., Sharma, R. P., and Willhite, C. C. (1985). Developmental toxicity of the cyanogenic glycoside linamarin in the golden hamster. *Teratology* 31:241-246.

Frakes, R. A., Sharma, R. P., Willhite, C. C., and Gomez, G.

(1986a). Effect of cyanogenic glycosides and protein content in cassava diets on hamster prenatal development. *Fund. Appl. Toxicol.* 7:191-198.

Frakes, R. A., Sharma, R. P., and Willhite, C. C. (1986b), Comparative matabolism of linamarin and amygdalin in hamsters. *Food Chem. Toxicol.* 24:417-420.

Gomez, G., De La Cuesta, D., Valdivieso, M., and Kawano, K. (1980). Contenido de cianuro toal y libre en parenquima y cascara de raices de diez variedades promisorias de yuca. *Turrialba* 30:361-365.

Gomez, G., Valdivieso, M., Santos, J., and Hoyos, C. (1983). Evaluation of cassava (*Manihot esculenta*) root meal prepared from low cyanide or high cyanide containing cultavars in pigs and broilers. *Nutr. Res. Internat.* 28:693-704.

Gomez, G., Valdivieso, M., De LaCuesta, D., and Salcedo, T. S. (1984). Effect of variety and plant age on the cyanide content of whole root cassava chips and its reduction by sun drying. *Anim. Feed Sci., Technol.* 11:57-65.

Gomez, G., and Valdivieso, M. (1985). Effects of drying temperature and loading rates on cyanide elimination from cassava whole root chips. *J. Food Technol.* 20:375-382.

Jones, W. O. (1959). *Manioc in Africa.* Stanford University Press, Stanford, CA. 315 pp.

Miller, K. W., Andersen, J. L., and Stoewsand, G. S. (1981). Amygdalin metabolism and effect on reproduction of rats fed apricot (*Prunus armeniaca*) kernels. *J. Toxicol. Environ. Health* 7:457-468.

Miller, R. W. (1974). Susceptibility of the fetus and child to chemical pollutants. *Science* 184:812-814.

Osuntokun, B. O. (1973). Ataxic neuropathy associated with cassava diets in West Africa. Pages 127-138 *in* B. Nestel and R. MacIntyre, eds., *Chronic Cassava Toxicity.* International Development Research Center, Ottawa, Canada.

Pritchard, J. T., and Voss, J. L. (1967). Fetal ankylosis in horses associated with hybrid Sudan pasture. *J. Amer. Vet. Med. Assoc.* 150:871-873.

Rauws, A. G., Olling, M., and Timmerman, G. (1982). Pharmacokinetics of prunasin, metabolite of amygdalin. *J. Toxicol. Clin. Toxicol.* 19:851-856.

Selby, L. A., Menges, R. W., Houser, E. C., Flatt, R. E., and Case, A. A. (1971). Outbreak of swine malformations associated with the wild black cherry, *Prunus serotina. Arch. Environ. Health* 22:496-501.

Singh, J. D. (1981). The teratogenic effects of dietary cassava on the pregnant albino rat: A preliminary report. *Teratology* 24:289-291.

Strugala, G. J., Rauws, A. G., and Elbers, R. (1986). Intestinal first-pass metabolism of amygdalin in the rat in vitro. *Biochem. Pharmacol.* 35:2123-2128.

Tewe, O. O., and Manner, J. H. (1981). Performance and pathological changes in pregnant pigs fed cassava diets containing different levels of cyanide. *Res. Vet. Sci.,* 30:147-151.

Tylleskar, T., Banea, M., Bikangi, N., Cooke, R. D., Poulter, N. H., and Rosling, H. (1992). Cassava cyanogens and konzo, an upper motoneuron disease found in Africa. *Lancet* (339):208-211.

Willhite, C. C. (1982). Congenital malformations induced by laetrile. *Science* 215:1513-1515.

Willhite, C. C. (1983). Developmental toxicology of acetonitrile in the Syrian golden hamster. *Teratology* 27:313-325.

Willhite, C. C., Ferm, V. H., and Smith, R. P. (1981). Teratogenic effects of aliphatic nitriles. *Teratology* 23:317-323.

Willhite, C. C., Rossi, N. L., Frakes, R. A., and Sharma, R. P. (1985). Cranioschisis aperta with encephaloschisis in cephalothoracopagus hamster twins. *Can. J. Comp. Med.* 49:195-201.

Wilson, J. (1973). Cyanide and human disease. Pages 121-125 *in* B. Nestel and R. MacIntyre, eds., *Chronic Cassava Toxicity.* International Development Research Center, Ottawa, Canada.

Chapter 11

Substance Abuse and Pregnancy Outcome

R. P. Sharma and Y. W. Kim

The primary emphasis of this book is on dietary factors that are important in the outcome of pregnancy, including associated fetal malformations. However, other non-dietary factors such as drug use can contribute to complications during pregnancy. Extensive research has been published regarding the effects of addictive substances, and this chapter summarizes some of the major findings concerning the effects of chronic or habitual use of these chemicals during pregnancy.

Epidemiologic studies concerning the use of substances of abuse and possible effects on pregnancy of substances of abuse are often confounded. First, it is difficult to ascertain the amount of drug consumed; a user is seldom willing to admit to the actual extent of "abuse." Second, abuse is often associated with malnutrition and various psychological problems, which themselves can influence pregnancy. These confounding factors should be considered when evaluating these reports. Whenever possible, the experimental models used to evaluate the effects of such "abused" chemicals are briefly described. The term "abuse" here refers to chemicals which generally are "self-administered" and are not necessary for normal functioning. The social acceptability or the legal implications associated with the use of these substances are not considered here.

Substances of Abuse

The substances of abuse include alcohol, caffeine, nicotine, cannabis, cocaine, and opiates. The first three, alcohol, nicotine, and caffeine are legal to use. The illicit compounds are cannabis, cocaine and opiates. The term "abuse" connotes misuse, and condemnation or disapproval of users, particularly those using illicit substances. The substances tend to be addictive. The compulsive or self-destructive behavior often accompanies drug dependence, which can be defined as a psychic or physical state where the person is unable to function normally without the repeated use of the substance. A psychic or physical tolerance may or may not develop. Withdrawal symptoms associated with chemicals such as heroin can make the addictive persons continue to (ab)use the drug(s) and withdrawal can sometimes be life threatening.

The use of drugs by women during pregnancy can have profound effects on fetal development. Although the consumption of alcohol is generally acceptable in most societies, the use of alcohol by pregnant women places their fetuses at risk. Drugs such as cocaine, marijuana, and nicotine are known to decrease appetite and may result in malnutrition and ultimately low weight gain, both to the detriment of the fetus. Of the pregnant women who are drug addicts, the majority are from low socioeconomic levels and have a long history of drug abuse that is frequently associated with both psychiatric and medical illnesses. Unless these risks can be explained scientifically to these women, there will be little background to persuade avoidance of alcohol or drugs during pregnancy.

In pregnant women, drug dependency presents unique problems in terms of maternal-fetal conflicts. The drugs may act directly on the fetus by killing the embryo, inducing structural malformations, and/or reducing the growth rate, or indirectly by causing secondary effects such as premature abortion of the fetus by direct action on the mother. Because there are certain risks to the fetuses and the nature of the risks are preventable, the use of drugs during pregnancy has inherently provoked moral issues. It may seem quite reasonable to think that pregnant women should abstain from using drugs that may be harmful to the fetus. While there may be a reduction of alcohol, cigarette, and marijuana use during pregnancy, women may not alter their drug use patterns until the pregnancy is actually diagnosed (Adams, *et al.,* 1989).

Most women are unaware of their pregnancy until after two months and subsequent to the stage of fetal development that is most susceptible to chemical insult (Cohen, 1990). And, although women may be aware of the importance of drug abstinence for the sake of the fetus, the compulsive or addictive nature of some drugs compels them to continue to use them.

Many factors contribute to the complexity of risk assessment of drug use during pregnancy. Normally, all new pharmaceuticals and industrial chemicals such as pesticides, are investigated for developmental toxicity before their commercial use is approved. However, illicit drugs are neither tested, nor are these drugs consumed in a controlled manner in most addicted individuals. The simultaneous use of multiple drugs also hinders the evaluation of a particular drug. Much of the information on the risk of drug use is obtained from animal studies, and there are problems in extrapolating animal data to humans, particularly concerning the effects of drugs on behavior. In most cases, we learn about these effects outside of controlled studies (Hutchings, *et al.*, 1989). Reports of epidemiological excesses and horrific clinical outcomes may provide the rationale and scientific justification for basic research and may bias the descriptions of the effects of drugs on fetuses. The analyses and interpretations may reflect an investigator's approach and outlook. "Abuse" has pejorative connotations and is not used here; "use" is the term of choice.

The Developmental Processes and Teratology

Teratology is the study of abnormal development between conception and birth. Teratology was traditionally limited to gross structural malformations but now includes more subtle developmental anomalies such as intrauterine growth retardation, behavioral aberrations, demise, and other functional deficiencies (Dicke, 1989). The term "developmental toxicology" has emerged as the one that is more generic, encompassing all abnormal development that may result from exposure to chemical or physical agents prior to conception (*i.e.*, to either parent) until the time of puberty. Pregnancy outcomes in relation to drug uses being considered here lie in the realm of both of these fields. Also, the terms "teratology" and "developmental toxicology" are sometimes used interchangeably (Voorhees, 1989). More explicitly, teratology includes embryo/fetal toxic effects that are expressed as (1) death, malformation, growth disorder, or abnormal function, (2) a function of the organisms's genetic endowment and its environment, (3) a function of the dose of the agent reaching the target tissue, and (4) a function of the developmental stage of the organism at the time of insult. The developmental disorder results because of the molecular mechanisms of injury that exceed the compensatory influences of intracellular repair capacities and cell reserves. Any substance that may cause abnormal postnatal structure or function upon exposure during embryonic or fetal life is defined as a "teratogen" (Dicke, 1989). Susceptibility to teratogenesis varies during intrauterine development. Little teratogenesis occurs during the refractory period, the period from fertilization to differentiation of the three germ layers, but embryolethality may occur. The highest degree of sensitivity occurs during organogenesis, from days 18-60 of gestation, with the peak susceptibility to anatomic defects occurring approximately at 30 days (Cohen, 1990). As organogenesis advances, resistance to teratogenesis increases. The fetal period (2nd to 9th month) is characterized by histogenesis, and functional maturation and teratogenic interferences at this time consist mainly of growth retardation and functional disturbances (Dicke, 1989).

The etiology of congenital malformations is unknown in an estimated 65 to 70% of all cases. Of the remaining cases, heritable disorders account for 15 to 20%, while chromosomal disorders contribute an additional 5%. Environmental factors, such as drug exposure, congenital infections, and maternal systemic disorders, are presumed to be responsible for less than 10% of human malformations detected during the first year of life (Dicke, 1989). Most of the literature on drugs tends to exaggerate the occurrences of drug-induced teratogenesis.

Alcohol

The use, misuse, and abuse of alcohol is one of the major health problems in the United States. Alcoholism ranks as the third most prevalent public health problem in this society. The limited use of alcohol has been historically acceptable in many cultures and is sometimes encouraged. In the middle ages in Europe, it was considered a cure for a variety of illnesses and was called the *"elixir of life."* The limited therapeutic usefulness of alcohol has been recognized only recently.

Ethyl alcohol (ethanol) is a natural decomposition product of plant carbohydrates; the breakdown to alcohol is facilitated by the presence of yeast, which is either present naturally or deliberately added. Alcohol is a simple molecule (see Table 1) and mammalian cells can metabolize it to obtain caloric energy. The principal target organs of alcohol in the body are the cerebral and hepatic tissues. Pharmacologically, alcohol is a central nervous system depressant and produces effects similar to those of general anesthetics. The transient euphoric effects of alcohol are induced by depression of inhibitory mechanisms of the central nervous system. It is generally believed that ethyl alcohol's potency is due to its lipid solubility and hence ability rapidly to penetrate the blood-brain barrier. Since alcohol is 30 times more soluble in water than in fat, it is quickly distributed in water throughout the body after absorption. The average decrease in blood alcohol concentration is about 0.23 to 0.3 ounces per hour. The major pathway in the body for the initial biotransformation of alcohol involves the enzyme alcohol dehydrogenase, which is concentrated in the liver, where over 80% of absorbed alcohol is metabolized to chemically reactive acetaldehyde. Acetaldehyde is further oxidized to acetate, which then enters the energy-producing pathways and is ultimately excreted as carbon dioxide and water.

TABLE 1. Major Substances Of Abuse and
Related Effects on Pregnancy Outcome

Substance	Chemical Structure	Associated fetal malformations or effects on pregnancy
Ethanol	CH_3CH_2OH	Fetal alcohol syndrome (characterized by facial and cranial deformities, neuronal involvement) and alcohol related birth defects (including behavioral deficits)
Caffeine		Cleft palate, echodactyly, spontaneous abortions, reduced birth weight
Nicotine (tobacco)		Low birth weight, premature birth, perinatal mortality, congenital abnormalities (e.g., oral cleft, inguinal hernia, cleft palate)
Cannabinoids[1] (marijuana)		Intrauterine growth retardation
Cocaine		Growth retardation, microcephaly, other miscellaneous malformations
Heroin (Opiates)		Fetal withdrawal syndrome, reduced growth

[1] Structure shown is Δ^9-tetrahydrocannabinol.

Fetal Alcohol Syndrome (FAS) and Alcohol Related Birth Defects (ARBD)

Fetal alcohol syndrome (FAS) refers to a pattern of abnormalities occurring in afflicted children born to women who consume alcohol. FAS is characterized by dysfunctions in the central nervous system and a reduction in the intelligence (IQ). A diagnosis of FAS requires signs of abnormality in each of the following three categories (Sokol & Clarren, 1989):

(1) Prenatal and/or postnatal growth retardation
(2) Central nervous system dysfunction
(3) Characteristic facial and cranial deformities.

The facial and cranial deformities include short palpebral fissures (small eye openings), ptosis (drooping eyelids), microphthalmia (small eyes), midfacial hypoplasia (underdeveloped midface), epicanthal folds (skin folds across the inner corners of the eyes, an abnormality in Caucasians), underdeveloped philtrum (the depression just above the upper lip), abnormally shallow notch in the upper lip ("Cupid's bow"), an exaggerated space between the nose and the upper lip, and small head circumference (Jones & Smith, 1973). The diagnosis of FAS is subjective, and the relation between the phenotype and the behavior is highly variable. Patients with only some of these characteristics are sometimes diagnosed with alcohol-related birth defect (ARBD) (Day and Richardson, 1991). ARBD is associated with various anatomic or functional defects (Sokol & Clarren, 1989). Excessive drinking may also result in a higher incidence of spontaneous abortions and stillbirths. Alcohol use is also likely to disturb infant's sleep cycle after birth.

In the Western world, the estimated incidence of FAS is 0.33 cases per 1000 births in the general population. Whites have a slightly lower rate than blacks, 0.29 vs. 0.48 per 1000 (Abel & Sokol, 1991). These statistics suggest that FAS is a rare event in the offspring of alcoholic women and may be the result of additional factors such as genetic influences, smoking, life style, malnutrition, and prenatal care. Consumption of alcohol throughout pregnancy may also reduce birth weight, length, and head circumference of the offspring. Day & Richardson (1991) reviewed several papers related to alcohol intake and pregnancy and concluded that drinking before pregnancy and during pregnancy may or may not decrease birth weight, cause premature birth, or minor morphologic malformations. There is no consensus regarding the amount and time during gestation when alcohol adversely affects the fetus (Schenker, *et al.,* 1990). The etiology of FAS is, therefore, poorly understood.

FAS is generally associated with "heavy" drinking, which is defined as the consumption of two or more drinks per day or 14 or more drinks per week throughout pregnancy. A "drink" is further defined as the equivalent of one bottle of beer (360 ml; 2.5% v/v), one glass of wine (75 ml; 10% v/v), or one glass of distilled spirits (18 ml; 40% v/v)(Smith, *et al.*, 1991). There is no evidence that FAS occurs when women drink two or fewer drinks per day, are well nourished, and do not engage in other risk behaviors (Alpert & Zuckerman, 1991).

A fetus may be particularly sensitive to alcohol exposure during critical periods (Schenker, *et al.*, 1990, and references therein). In mice, *in utero* alcohol exposure during embryonic development corresponding to the organogenesis (first trimester equivalent) resulted in a variety of skeletal and visceral anomalies. Alcohol exposure at later stages (equivalent to second and third trimesters) caused behavioral deficits in the absence of overt physical defects. Episodic binge drinking that temporarily increases alcohol concentration might pose some risks to fetus, but there is no dose-response relationship for ethanol teratogenesis. Schenker, *et al.* (1990) reviewed the papers regarding critical exposure and suggested it was not possible to identify and demarcate a single critical exposure level for the wide range of alcohol's teratogenic actions. A moderate consumption of alcohol (such as one drink per day) has not been related to any adverse morphological or functional deficits in offspring.

The mode of action of alcohol in inducing FAS is not understood. Some of the proposed mechanisms for FAS are (1) fetal hypoxia, due to compromised blood flow to the placenta and fetus; a viable but unproven mechanism for FAS and lesser alcohol-induced abnormalities; (2) excessive production of certain prostaglandins; (3) a direct effect of ethanol on developing cells, especially of the central nervous system, altering net protein synthesis, neuronal membrane composition and/or neuronal process formation, and production of neurotropic factors needed for cell growth and interaction; (4) malnutrition (malnutrition *per se* is known to result in impaired fetal growth, a characteristic of infants with FAS); (5) effect of acetaldehyde, a metabolite of alcohol; (6) genetic predisposition (not all fetuses are affected, and the incidence of afflicted infants is astonishingly low); and (7) the role of other drugs. Women who drink heavily are also more likely to smoke, to use other drugs, especially marijuana and cocaine, and to be malnourished (Schenker, *et al.*, 1990; Alpert & Zuckerman 1991). Many other mechanisms have been proposed, including thiamine deficiency that occurs in adult alcoholics. Since the 1973 report of Jones & Smith (1973), about 3,000 papers have been published in relation to FAS (Anonymous, 1987).

FAS is viewed as an irreversible congenital malformation. Several authors have suggested that some symptoms of ARBD may be transient. Even moderate alcohol exposure (social drinking) may cause some handicaps in their offspring during infancy and childhood. The effects have been described as intellectual decrement, learning problems, attention and memory problems, fine and gross motor problems, and difficulty with organization and problem solving (Streissguth, *et al.*, 1989). A follow-up study of 61 adolescents and adults indicated that effects of FAS can be traced into adulthood (Streissguth, *et al.*, 1991). However, it is suggested that even the full-blown FAS patient can develop normally in a warm, caring environment where professional care is provided (Barbour, 1989).

Caffeine

Caffeine is a plant alkaloid found in coffee, tea, and cocoa. Cured coffee beans contain about 1% caffeine while dried tea leaves contain about 5% caffeine plus theophylline. Caffeine is listed in the Code of Federal Regulations as a multipurpose food substance that is *generally recognized as safe* (GRAS). The percentage of women who consume some caffeine during pregnancy ranges from 69-79% to 90-98% (Berger, 1988). In 1980, the U. S. Food and Drug Administration advised pregnant women to avoid or limit caffeine intake.

Caffeine (see Table 1 for chemical structure) is lipophilic, hence readily absorbed from the gut, and is distributed throughout the body including the placenta (Berger, 1988, and references therein). The half-life of caffeine increases from 2.5 hours in nonpregnant women to 10.5 hours during pregnancy. In humans, caffeine is metabolized by demethylation and oxidation to produce paraxanthine, 1-methylxanthine, and 1-methyluric acid.

Caffeine is a central nervous system stimulant, inhibits the enzyme phosphodiesterase, enhances the release of epinephrine and norepinephrine, and competes for binding to adenosine and benzodiazepine receptors (Al-Hachim, 1989, and references therein). Ingestion of 150 mg to 250 mg of caffeine, or the amount in about two cups of coffee, is sufficient to activate the central nervous system. At higher doses, about 500 mg, caffeine stimulates the autonomic centers of the brain, heart rate, and respiration. The high doses (1 to 10 g) can cause convulsions and respiratory failure.

Watkinson & Fried (1985) did not find significant relationships between caffeine use in birth weight and length, head circumference, ponderal index, Apgar scores, length of labor, or gestation. Miscarriages and premature births did not increase with caffeine use, even among those consuming more than 300 mg/day. Offspring of women who consumed more than 300 mg of caffeine daily had low birth weights and smaller head circumferences. In a 7-year study, Barr & Streissguth (1991) found that caffeine use during pregnancy did not affect height, weight, or head circumference or IQ at 7 years of age, and prenatal caffeine consumption had no adverse effects. However, other studies show that caffeine increased the incidence of spontaneous abortion, and reduced birth weights. There were a number of confounding factors, such as genetic difference, disease state, etc., which might have affected the findings. In most studies, however, caffeine intake is not associated with congenital malformations (see Berger, 1988, for review)

In mice and rats, fetal resorption occurred and fetal and placental weights decreased when 100 mg/kg/day or more of caffeine was administered (reviewed by Al-Hachim, 1989). Cleft palate and ectrodactyly occurred in rodents at doses between 50-300 mg/kg/day (equivalent to about 38 to 228 cups of coffee per day in man), a range that makes it extremely difficult to extrapolate to humans. Rats gavaged with 100 mg/kg/day of caffeine showed reduced ossification (Muther, 1988), although the method used to assess fetal ossification was questioned. To ingest an equivalent of 100 mg/kg/day of caffeine, a 60-kg human must consume approximately 50-70 cups of coffee per day, or at least 20 cups per day to correct for the metabolic body weight. A caffeine dose of 50 mg/kg/day did not cause malformations in rats.

Smoking

Cigarette smoke contains nearly 4,000 different compounds. The particulate matter, which constitute around 10% of smoke, is composed mainly of nicotine, water, and tar. Nicotine is suspended on tiny particles of tar. Tar contains various polycyclic aromatic hydrocarbon products, many of which are carcinogens. The aqueous constituents of smoke contain carbon monoxide, carbon dioxide, nitrogen oxides, cyanides and numerous other gases (Nash & Persaud, 1988).

Nicotine, an alkaloid from *Nicotiana tabacum,* is absorbed from the respiratory tract, buccal mucous membranes, skin and intestines. Absorption through the lungs is rapid so that nicotine moves into the arterial circulation quickly and reaches the brain within 10 seconds after it is inhaled. Nicotine is rapidly distributed throughout all body tissues and fluids. In the body, it has a half-life of 2-3 hours. In regular smokers, blood nicotine levels remain elevated for 8-12 hours and persist overnight. On average, about 70% of nicotine is converted to cotinine, which is then metabolized primarily to *trans*-3'-hydroxycotinine, and is excreted in the urine (Benowitz, 1991). Nicotine is a central nervous system stimulant and exerts its major action on all autonomic ganglion cells (Nash & Persaud, 1988).

Nicotine in the United States is the most abused substance, next to ethanol. According to a 1990 survey by the United States National Institute on Drug Abuse, 67 million individuals had used nicotine compared with 2.9 million who had used cocaine, and 12 million who had used marijuana within the month before the survey (London, 1991). Despite warnings that cigarette smoking is harmful to the fetus, cigarette smoking during pregnancy is still common. Even though the proportion of smokers may have decreased in the United States, the rate of smoking in the young white women, aged 18 to 24 years, has increased (Nash & Persaud, 1988). It is estimated that 20-30% of American women of child-bearing age smoke. Many female cigarette smokers quit smoking after they realize they are pregnant. However, about 25% of pregnant women in the United States smoke throughout pregnancy (Novello, 1990).

The influence of smoking on pregnancy outcome has been reviewed by Aaronson & Macnee, (1989) and Nash & Persaud (1988). Maternal smoking has been correlated with intrauterine growth retardation and may contribute 20-40% of the cases of low birth weight infants in the United States. It is speculated that smoking reduces birth weight directly by interfering with nutrition through depressing maternal weight gain or indirectly by decreasing maternal nutritional intake. Smoking reduces fertility, may cause spontaneous abortion, abruptio placenta, and premature rupture of the membranes. McIntosh (1984) reviewed the effects of smoking on 28 pregnancy-related outcomes (*i.e.*, bleeding, premature rupture of membranes, stillbirths) and concluded that 15-45% of unfavorable outcomes may be caused by smoking. Smoking may increase perinatal mortality, defined as reproductive loss after the 20th week of gestation and before the 7th day of life, but this effect was inconsistent. Smoking may increase congenital abnormalities, such as oral cleft and inguinal hernia. The results of one study indicated that smoking may increase cleft lip and cleft palate (Khoury, *et al.,* 1989), but like other epidemiologic studies, the results may have been affected by confounding factors.

Marijuana

Marijuana is prepared from the cannabis plant (*Cannabis*

saliva). The cannabis plant produces a group of chemicals called the cannabinoids, most potent of which are Δ^9-*trans*-tetrahydrocannabinol (Δ^9-THC), Δ^8-THC, Δ^9-*trans*-tetrahydrocannabinolic acid (THC acid), cannabinol (CBN), and cannabidiol (CBD). The primary psychoactive agent, Δ^9-THC, is concentrated in the resin of the plant; the flowering tops contain the highest concentration, the leaves contain less, and the fibrous stalks contain little.

Approximately 5 mg of Δ^9-THC is contained in one marijuana cigarette. The major psychoactive and physiologic effects usually appear within 2 to 3 minutes, peak within 10 to 20 minutes, and may last from 1.5-2 hours (Hollister, 1986). Forty-five minutes after oral administration, the plasma concentration of Δ^9-THC peaks and remains relatively constant for 4 to 6 hours (Levy & Koren, 1990). Almost all the Δ^9-THC is metabolized by the body. Δ^9-THC and its metabolites tend to bind to proteins and remain stored in body fat. Five days after a single injection of Δ^9-THC, 20% was stored, and 20% of its metabolites remained in the blood. It can take up to 30 days to eliminate completely a single dose. The biological half-life for Δ^9-THC in chronic users is 19 hours and the half-life of its metabolites is 50 hours. Δ^9-THC affects the electrical properties of nerve membranes, possibly by increasing membrane fluidity (Martin, 1986).

The placenta of some species of rodents is a partial barrier to the transmission of cannabinoids, and it may also be a barrier in humans. Maternal blood concentrations of Δ^9-THC are 2.5-6 times greater than those in fetal blood (Levy & Koren, 1990). Reports of teratogenic effects of cannabinoids in animals are inconsistent and are rarely controlled for drug-induced maternal undernutrition. Because these compounds depress food and water consumption, drug-related undernutrition may confound the results of these studies. Both marijuana extract and Δ^9-THC increase the rate of fetal resorption in pregnant mice, regardless of the route of administration. Except for two reports which also involved the use of other drugs, malformations have not been linked to marijuana use during pregnancy (Abel, 1985).

Several studies (Fried, 1989; 1991) show that marijuana use prior to or during pregnancy did not affect birth weight, birth length, or head circumference in children after correction for gestational length. In these studies, pregnant women were divided into irregular users (less than one marijuana cigarette per week), moderate users (more than five marijuana cigarettes per week), and heavy users (less than five marijuana cigarettes per week). In animals, intrauterine growth retardation is one of the most reliable effects associated with prenatal exposure to cannabinoids. Prenatal exposure to cannabinoids did not produce gross malformations in humans, and they occur in mice only following exposure to relatively high doses and following intraperitoneal route of administration. Cannabinoid exposure *in utero* increases fetal resorption rates in mice, but not in rats (Abel, 1985). Maternal food and water consumption and weight gain during pregnancy decrease following cannabinoid administration (Hutchings, *et al.*, 1989), which may account for many of the effects associated with prenatal exposure to cannabinoids, *e.g.*, increased resorption rate.

In an epidemiological study of 59 Jamaican children from birth to 5 years of age, there were no differences in physical and mental developmental of children born to marijuana using and matched control mothers (Hayes, *et al.*, 1991). Another study found no differences between the marijuana users and their matched (alcohol use, cigarette use, and family income) controls in incidence of miscarriage, type of presentation at birth, and the frequency of complications or major anomalies at birth (Fried, 1991).

Cocaine

Cocaine is an alkaloid derived from the leaves of the coca plant (*Erythroxylon coca*), which is indigenous to the Andes mountains of Peru and Bolivia. Cocaine was introduced into Europe around the 16th century. In the late 19th century, Sigmund Freud wrote an article named *"On Coca"* (Freud, 1884), in which he encouraged the use of cocaine. From 1866 to 1903, the widely consumed soft drink "Coca-Cola" contained cocaine. Passage of the Harrison Act of 1914 banned the use of drugs, such as cocaine. Around 1970, there was an explosive resurgence of cocaine use in the United States.

Coca paste, extracted from the leaves of the coca plant, contains approximately 80% cocaine. The paste is converted to hydrochloride salt and usually mixed with other compounds, such as sugar. The purity of this mixture is around 40%. This product is snorted or injected intravenously. The product can be further processed into a freebase by removing hydrochloric acid with sodium bicarbonate and then recrystallized with ether. The resulting product is a highly purified form of cocaine that has a lower melting point (98°C) than cocaine salt (195°C). The product is commonly called "*crack*" or "*rock*" and is smoked (*freebasing*). The vapors produced when a piece of this cocaine "*crack*" or "*rock*" is heated, are inhaled (Waldorf, *et al.*, 1991).

Cocaine is rapidly metabolized by serum and hepatic cholinesterases to inactive metabolites, benzoylecgonine and ecgonine methyl ester, which are excreted in the urine. Cocaine is lipophilic and rapidly traverses most biological membranes. It passes through the blood-brain barrier. Cocaine concentrations in the brain are 4 or 20 times higher than in plasma because biotransformation of cocaine is slower in the brain. The estimated half-life of cocaine varies from 9.6 hours after an intravenous injection, 0.9 hours after oral use, and 1.3 hours after intranasal use (Wiggins, *et al.*, 1989). Thirty to 90 minutes after cocaine is administered to pregnant rats, the concentration of cocaine in the fetal brain was 109-1512% of that in the blood.

Cocaine interferes with presynaptic catecholamine reuptake, resulting in its accumulation at the postsynaptic site, thereby increasing the sympathetic tone with clinical manifestations of hypertension, tachycardia, cardiac arrhythmias, and convulsions. The enhanced sympathetic tone may also cause hyperglycemia, hyperpyrexia and mydriasis (Farrar & Kearns, 1989). Cocaine quickly causes a feeling of euphoria and produces powerful positive reinforcing qualities, probably because of its effect on the mesocortical dopaminergic pathways. Chronic use of the drug can, however, result in abnormalities of the dopaminergic pathways, leading to psychiatric complications. Chronic use impairs serotonin biosynthesis because of decreased uptake of tryptophan, which may enhance the excitatory effects of dopamine and decrease the need for sleep.

The adverse effects of cocaine on pregnancy outcome can be summarized as growth retardation, malformations such as microcephaly, and neurobehavioral effects (Farrar & Kearns, 1989; Dow-Edwards, 1991). Cocaine use can cause abruptio placentae, stillbirth, or premature delivery. These complications may be related to the intense vasoconstriction produced by cocaine, which in turn increases maternal blood pressure and decreases placental blood flow. Chasnoff, *et al.* (1985) reported that there were two abruptio placentas, an infant with prune-belly syndrome (a major malformation of the genitourinary tract), bilateral hydronephrosis and bilateral cryptorchidism in 12 cocaine-exposed pregnancies. However, the birth weights, Apgar scores, and head circumferences of cocaine babies were not significantly different from controls. In another report, there were four malformed infants (prune-belly syndrome, transverse distal limb reduction, jejunal atresia and bowel infarction, and imperforate anus, horseshoe kidney, clubfoot, and amniotic band defect) in 70 cocaine-exposed pregnancies (MacGregor, *et al.*, 1987). In this study, 24 pregnant women used only cocaine while others also used marijuana, opiates, and other illicit substances. Chasnoff, *et al.* (1988) reported on multiple drug exposures with or without cocaine. Among cocaine users (50 infants), nine infants had malformations (two ileal atresias and seven malformations of the genitourinary tract). Among the non-cocaine group exposed to other multiple drugs (30 infants), only one infant exhibited fetal alcohol syndrome.

In another study of 75 cocaine pregnancies (Chasnoff, *et al.*, 1989), a group of 23 involved exposures during the first trimester and there were two ileal atresias and three genitourinary anomalies. In 52 pregnancies in which cocaine use occurred throughout the pregnancy, six babies developed seizures (no known causes), two developed cerebral infarctions, and six had genitourinary anomalies. The results of studies conducted by the Chasnoff group indicate that cocaine is a powerful teratogen. There were congenital malformations in 11% of all pregnancies of cocaine-using mothers (23 malformed infants/203 infants), an exceptionally high incidence. As many as 10% of all children may suffer from some type of abnormal development, and less than 10% of these may be due to environmental factors, including drugs. The incidence of cocaine use during pregnancy ranged from 9.8% to 25% (average 14%) in a survey of nine hospitals across the United States (Chasnoff, et al., 1989).

The effects of cocaine on fetus may be dose-dependent, and there may be a critical period when fetuses are more susceptible to cocaine. There could also be genetic differences in susceptibility. The mechanism of adverse effects of cocaine on the fetus is not understood. Cocaine exposure may shorten the average gestational age and thus reduce the birth weight or retard fetal growth (Calhoun & Watson, 1991).

Bingol, et al. (1987) reported cocaine increased stillbirths due to abruptio placentae and was associated with five different malformations (10%, N = 50). The effects included exencephaly, interparietal encephalocele, parietal bone defect, hypoplastic right heart syndrome, and transposition of the great vessels. Their sample consisted of 50% black and 50% Hispanic women in New York. The incidence of malformations was higher in polydrug users (including cocaine) than among those using only cocaine. Cocaine use was associated with lower birth weight and smaller head circumference (Oro & Dixon, 1987). The mechanism underlying the growth retardation associated with cocaine has not been established, but it is probably associated with malnutrition, hypoxia, and neuroendocrine changes. The frequency and dose of cocaine use during pregnancy may determine the magnitude of growth retardation. Other factors frequently associated with cocaine use, such as poverty, homelessness, lack of prenatal care, and poor nutrition, increase the incidence of such conditions as pneumonia, phlebitis, septicemia, hepatitis, endocarditis, meningitis, and convulsions, among others (Kandall, 1991).

There are several reports that suggest that cocaine does not cause malformations in fetuses (Madden, *et al.*, 1986; Calhoun & Watson. 1991). Chouteau, *et al.* (1988) found that cocaine use did not increase the incidence of abruptio placentae or premature rupture of membranes in exposed women (N=143). In most other studies (Zuckerman, *et al.* 1989), cocaine did not increase the incidence of malformation or teratogenicity. Lutiger, *et al.* (1991) reviewed 20 published reports concerning the relationship between gestational cocaine use and pregnancy outcome and found that very few adverse reproductive effects (genitourinary malformations, birth weight, gestational age, head circumference, length) could be shown to be significantly associated with cocaine use. They concluded that a variety of adverse reproductive effects commonly associated with maternal use of cocaine may be caused by other factors associated with cocaine use.

Heroin and Other Opiates

Opiates are a group of alkaloids isolated from opium, an extract prepared from the unripe seeds of the poppy plant, *Papaver somniferum.* Opiates in varying forms, including morphine and, after 1898, heroin, could be purchased from pharmacists, local stores and even by mail order. In the 1880s, Sears-Roebuck offered two ounces of laudanum for 18 cents, or one and a half pints for two dollars (Krivanek, 1988). At the same period, pure alcohol cost 75 cents a quart. Morphine and codeine constitute 10 and 0.5% of the weight of dried opium, respectively. A number of semi-synthetic opiates are formed by relatively simple pharmacological modifications of the natural opium alkaloids. Heroin is morphine with two acetyl groups (Table 1). Once ingested or injected, the acetyl groups are quickly stripped away, and morphine is recreated. A variety of totally synthetic drugs with morphine-like actions were developed, among them methadone, whose chemistry is quite different from opiates.

Morphine and its derivatives are more effective when given parentaerally than after oral administration. Opiates are absorbed by the gastrointestinal tract and readily metabolized in the liver. All opiates act on the gastrointestinal tract, markedly decreasing the peristaltic movements and generally increasing the tone of the intestine. Heroin has a predominantly depressing effect on brain, mind and mood, *i.e.*, drowsiness, mental clouding, sedation and lethargy. The majority of people experience warmth, well-being, peacefulness and contentment, which is often accompanied by a dream-like state, introspection and sleep. Opiates depress the activity of the brain's respiratory centers and have some excitatory effects, such as the stimulating the brain's vomiting center. The major medical action of the opiates is analgesia, which is usually achieved at doses smaller than those that produce significant sedation or respiratory depression. The analgesia produced by opiates is unique because sensory abilities are not altered. In other words, pain is still present and felt, but it no longer bothers the individual. The greatest problem with the use of opiates is the addiction and tolerance.

There are an estimated 500,000 heroin addicts in the United States; as many as 300,000 are women, who are responsible for at least 20,000 or more deliveries per year. The number of heroin users may be underestimated because heroin use is illegal (Dattel, 1990). Addicts experience severe sweating, headaches, abdominal pain, diarrhea, and general discomfort and agitation during opiate withdrawal. The fetus must also make a biochemical adaptation to opiates, which are bound to opiate receptors in various body tissues, including the central nervous system. Maternal withdrawal from opiate use is not recommended during pregnancy because of concomitant fetal withdrawal and resultant fetal death. The opiate supply to the fetus ends abruptly with delivery. The newborn baby metabolizes opiates bound to tissues and eventually experiences symptoms of withdrawal, or neonatal abstinence syndrome (NAS). The infant's metabolism eventually adjusts to the absence of the opiate (Zuckerman & Brenahan, 1991). The neonatal mortality and morbidity attributable to maternal heroin use is not known (Gilbody, 1991). Infants exposed prenatally to opiates tend to have smaller head circumference than infants who are not exposed. However, when other confounding factors are considered, head circumference was not affected by addiction to narcotics alone (Zuckerman & Brenahan, 1991). The use of narcotics has not been associated with congenital malformations and has accelerated fetal lung maturity (Dattel, 1990).

Wilson (1989) found no difference in the cognitive performance of children 3-5 years of age that had been prenatally exposed to heroin and children in a control group; nor were there any differences in preschool behavior, preschool neurologic function, or in grade placement and behavior in elementary school. The heroin-exposed children might have disadvantages due to parenting and home environment because only 2 of 27 children were with their biological mothers when they entered preschool. Postnatal environment may have been more important than *in utero* heroin exposure.

Other Drugs of Abuse

The overall incidence of the nonmedical uses of prescription drugs such as barbiturates, and benzodiazepines may exceed the use of opiates and other narcotics. Heroin users frequently use barbiturates or similar substances. Even alcoholics use a variety of depressants to relieve discomfort associated with withdrawal. Drugs like barbiturates or benzodiazepines can be addictive and may be used during pregnancy. There are no definitive studies on the malformations induced by these drugs, although babies born to users exhibit a withdrawal syndrome as these chemicals cross the placenta. Barbiturates are potent inducers of a variety of liver enzymes even following *in utero* exposure. The implications associated with the use of these prescription drugs are not known.

Psychedelic drugs such as LSD (lysergic acid diethylamide) and phencyclidine also produce strong biochemical changes in the central nervous system, but it is not known if their use during pregnancy affects the fetus. The data that are available are inconclusive, or complicated by confounding factors including other drugs, malnutrition or disease.

Conclusion

A variety of substances that are not necessary nutrients are consumed during pregnancy and may have a profound outcome on the health of the offspring. Nicotine and alcohol, the two most widely abused and legal substances, are known to be teratogenic. Much less is known about the other substances of abuse. The recommended practice should be to avoid any prescription medication during pregnancy unless it is prescribed by a physician. It is also wise to avoid any other non-prescription medications, to limit caffeine intake, and to avoid alcohol or tobacco.

References

Aaronson, L. S., and Macnee, C. L. (1989). Tobacco, alcohol, and caffeine use during pregnancy. *J. Obstet. Gynecol. Neonatal Nurs.* 18:279-287.

Abel, E. L. (1985). Effects of prenatal exposure to cannabinoids. Pages 20-33 *in* T. M. Pinkert, ed., *Current Research on the Consequences of Maternal Drug Abuse.* National Institute of Drug Abuse, Washington, D. C.

Abel, E. L., and Sokol, R. J. (1991). A revised conservative estimate of the incidence of FAS and its economic impact. *Alcohol Clin. Exp. Res.* 15:514-524.

Adams, E. H., Gfroerer, J. C., and Rouse, B. A. (1989). Epidemiology of substance abuse including alcohol and cigarette smoking. *In* D. E. Hutchings, ed., *Prenatal Abuse of Licit and Illicit Drugs. Ann. NY Acad. Sci.* 562:14-20.

Al-Hachim, G. M. (1989). Teratogenicity of caffeine; a review. *Eur. J. Obstet. Gynecol. Reproduct. Biol.* 31:237-247.

Alpert, J. J., and Zuckerman, B. (1991). Alcohol use during pregnancy: What is the risk? *Pediatr. Rev.* 12:375-379.

Anonymous (1987). Fetal alcohol syndrome. Pages 80-96 *in Sixth Special Report to the U.S. Congress on Alcohol and Health.* U. S. Dep. Health & Human Services, Washington, D. C.

Barbour, B. G. (1989). Is fetal alcohol syndrome completely irreversible? *Amer. J. Matern. Child Nurs.* 14:44-46.

Barr, H. M., and Streissguth, A. P. (1991). Caffeine use during pregnancy and child outcome: A 7-year prospective study. *Neurotoxicol. Teratol.* 13:441-448.

Benowitz, N. L. (1991). Importance of nicotine metabolism in understanding the human biology of nicotine. Pages 19-24 *in* F. Adlkofer and K. Thurau, eds., *Effects of Nicotine on Biological Systems.* Birkhauser-Verlag, Berlin.

Berger, A. (1988). Effects of caffeine consumption on pregnancy outcome. A review. *J. Reproduct. Med.* 33:945-956.

Bingol, N., Fuchs, M., Diaz, N., Stone, R. K., and Gromisch, D. S. (1987). Teratogenicity of cocaine in humans. *J. Pediatr.* 110:93-96.

Calhoun, B. C. and Watson, P. T. (1991). The cost of maternal cocaine abuse: I. Perinatal cost. *Obstet. Gynecol.* 78:731-734.

Chasnoff, I. J., Chisum, G. M., and Kaplan, W. E. (1988). Maternal cocaine use and genitourinary tract malformations. *Teratology* 37:201-204.

Chasnoff, I. J., Griffith, D. R., MacGragor, S., Dirkes, K., and Burns, K. A. (1989). Temporal patterns of cocaine use in pregnancy: Perinatal outcome. *J. Amer. Med. Assoc.* 261:1741-1744.

Chasnoff, I. J. (1989). Drug use and women: Establishing a standard of care. *In* D. E. Hutchings, ed., *Prenatal Abuse of Licit and Illicit Drugs.* Ann. *NY Acad. Sci.* 562:208-210.

Chasnoff, I. J., Burns, W. J., Schnoll, S. H., and Burns, F. A. (1985). Cocaine use in pregnancy. *New Engl. J. Med.* 313:666-669.

Chouteau, M., Namerow, P. B., and Leppert, P. (1988). The effect of cocaine abuse on birth weight and gestational age. *Obstet Gynecol.* 72:351-354.

Cohen, M. M. Jr. (1990). Syndromology: An updated conceptual overview. VII. Aspects of teratogenesis. *Intern. J. Oral. Maxillofac. Surg.* 19:26-32.

Dattel, B. J. (1990). Substance abuse in pregnancy. *Semin. Perinatol.* 14:179-187.

Day, N. L., and Richardson, G. A. (1991). Prenatal alcohol exposure: A continuum of effects. *Semin. Perinatol.* 15:271-279.

Dicke, J. M. (1989). Teratology: Principles and practice. *Med. Clin. North Amer.* 73:567-582.

Dow-Edwards, D. L. (1991). Cocaine effects on fetal development: A comparison of clinical and animal research findings. *Neurotoxicol. Teratol.* 13:347-353.

Farrar, H. C., and Kearns, G. L. (1989). Cocaine: Clinical pharmacology and toxicology. *J. Pediatr.* 115:665-675.

Freud, S. (1884). On Cocaine. Pages 151-163 *in* J. Strausbaugh and D. Blais, eds., *The Drug User Documents: 1840-1960.* Blast Brooks, Inc., New York.

Fried, P. A. (1989). Postnatal consequences of maternal marijuana use in humans. *In* D. E. Hutchings, ed., *Prenatal Abuse of Licit and Illicit Drugs. Ann. N. Y. Acad. Sci.* 562:123-132.

Fried, P. A. (1991). Marijuana use during pregnancy: Consequences for the offspring. *Semin. Perinatol.* 15:280-287.

Gilbody, J. S. (1991). Effects of maternal drug addiction on the fetus. *Adverse Drug React. Toxicol. Rev.* 10:77-88.

Hayes, J. S., Lampart, R., Dreher, M. C., and Morgan, L. (1991). Five-year follow up of rural Jamaican children whose mothers used marijuana during pregnancy. *West Indies Med. J.* 40:120-123.

Hollister, L. E. (1986). Health effects of cannabinoids. *Pharmacol. Rev.* 38:1-20.

Hutchings, D. E. (1990). Preface. *In* D. E. Hutchings, ed., *Prenatal Abuse of Licit and Illicit Drugs. Ann. NY Acad. Sci.* 562:xi-xii.

Hutchings, D. E., Brake, S. C., and Morgan, B. (1989). Animal studies of prenatal Δ^9-tetrahydrocannabinol: Female embryolethality and effects on somatic and brain growth. *In* D. E. Hutchings, ed., *Prenatal Abuse of Licit and Illicit Drugs. Ann. NY Acad. Sci.* 562:133-144.

Jones, K. L., and Smith, D. W. (1973). Recognition of the fetal alcohol syndrome in early infancy. *Lancet* (7836): 999-1001.

Kandall, S. R. (1991). Perinatal effects of cocaine and amphetamine use during pregnancy. *Bull. NY Acad. Med.* 67:240-255.

Khoury, M., Gomez-Farias, M., and Mulinare, J. (1989). Does maternal cigarette smoking during pregnancy cause cleft lip and palate in offspring. *Amer. J. Dis. Child* 143:333-337.

Krivanek, J. (1988). *Heroin, Myth and Reality.* Allen & Unwip, Winchester, MA. 260pp.

Levy, M., and Koren, G. (1990). Obstetric and neonatal effects of drugs of abuse. *Emerg. Asp. Drug Abuse* 8:633-652.

London, E. D. (1991). Glucose metabolism: An index of nicotine action in the brain. Pages 239-248 *in* F. Adlkofer and K. Thureau, eds., *Effects of Nicotine on Biological Systems.* Birkhauser-Verlag, Berlin.

Lutiger, B., Graham, K., Einarson, T. R., and Koren, G. (1991). Relationship between gestational cocaine use and pregnancy outcome: A meta-analysis. *Teratology* 44: 405-414.

MacGregor, S. N. , Keith, L. G., Chasnoff, I. J., Rosner, M. A., Chisum, G. M., Shaw, P., and Monogue, J. P. (1987). Cocaine use during pregnancy: Adverse perinatal outcome. *Amer. J. Obstet. Gynecol.* 157:686-690.

Madden, J. D., Payne, T. F., and Miller, S. (1986). Maternal cocaine abuse and effect on the newborn. *Pediatrics* 77:209-211.

Martin, B. R. (1986). Cellular effects of cannabinoids. *Pharmacol. Rev.* 38:45-74.

McIntosh, I. D. (1984). Smoking and pregnancy: Attributable

risks and public health implications. *Can. J. Publ. Health* 75:141-148.

Muther, T. F. (1988). Caffeine and reduction of fetal ossification in the rat: Fact or artifacts? *Teratology* 37:239-247.

Nash, J. E. and Persaud, T. V. (1988). Embryopathic risks of cigarette smoking. *Exp. Pathol.* 33:65-73.

Novello, A. C. (1990). Surgeon General's report on the health benefits of smoking cessation. *Public Health Rep.* 105: 545-548.

Oro, A. S., and Dixon, S. D. (1987). Perinatal cocaine and methamphetamine exposure: Maternal and neonatal correlates. *J. Pediatr.* 111:571-578.

Schenker, S., Becker, H. C., Randall, C. L., Phillips, D. K., Baskin, G. S., and Henderson, G. I. (1990). Fetal alcohol syndrome: Current status of pathogenesis. *Alcohol Clin. Exp. Res.* 14:635-647.

Smith, G. M., Patrick, J., and Sinervo, K. R. (1991). Effects of ethanol exposure on the embryo-fetus: Experimental considerations, mechanisms and the role of prostaglandins. *Can. J. Physiol. Pharmacol.* 69:550-569.

Sokol, R. J., and Clarren, S. K. (1989). Guidelines for use of terminology describing the impact of prenatal alcohol on the offspring. *Alcohol Clin. Exp. Res.* 13:597-598.

Streissguth, A. P., Aase, J. M., Clarren, S. K., Randels, S. P., LaDue, R. A., and Smith, D. F. (1991). Fetal alcohol syndrome in adolescents and adults. *J. Amer. Med. Assoc.* 265:1961-1967.

Streissguth, A. P., Sampson, P. D., and Barr, H. M. (1989). Neurobehavioral dose-response effects of prenatal alcohol exposure in humans from infancy to adulthood. *In* D. E. Hutchings, ed., *Prenatal Abuse of Licit and Illicit Drugs.* Ann. NY Acad. Sci. 562:145-158.

Tittmar, H. G. (1990). What's the harm in just a drink? *Alcohol* 25:287-291.

Voorhees, C. V. (1989). Concepts in teratology and developmental toxicology derived from animal research. *In* D. E. Hutchings, ed., *Prenatal Abuse of Licit and Illicit Drugs.* Ann. NY Acad. Sci. 562:31-41.

Waldorf, D., Reinarman, C., and Murphy, S. (1991). *Cocaine Changes.* Temple University Press, Philadelphia. 326pp.

Watkinson, B., and Fried, P. A. (1985). Maternal caffeine use before, during and after pregnancy and effects upon offspring. *Neurobehav. Toxicol.* 7:9-17.

Wiggins, R. C., Rolsten, C., Ruiz, B., and Davis, C. M. (1989). Pharmacokinetics of cocaine: Basic studies of route, dosage, pregnancy and lactation. *Neurotoxicology* 10:367-381.

Wilson, G. S. (1989). Clinical studies of infants and children exposed prenatally to heroin. *In* D. E. Hutchings, ed., *Prenatal Abuse of Licit and Illicit Drugs.* Ann. NY Acad. Sci. 562:183-194.

Zuckerman, B., and Brenahan, K. (1991). Developmental and behavioral consequences of prenatal drug and alcohol exposure. *Pediatr. Clin. North Amer.* 38:1387-1406.

Zuckerman, B., Frank, D. A., Hingson, R., Amaro, H., Levenson, S. M., Kayne, H., Parker, S., Vinci, R., Aboague, D., Fried, L. E., Cabral, H., Timperi, R., and Bauchner, H. (1989). Effects of maternal marijuana and cocaine use on fetal growth. *New Engl. J. Med.* 320:762-768.

Index

Index

(+)-thermopsine
  See quinolizidine alkaloids
(-)-anagyrine
  See quinolizidine alkaloids
(-)-thermopsine
  See quinolizidine alkaloids
1-methyluric acid 358
  See also paraxanthine
1-methylxanthine 358
  See also paraxanthine
11-*cis* RA 174
11-*cis* RAL
  See 11-*cis* retinal
11-cis retinal 134
  See also retinal
13-*cis*-4-oxo RA 163
13-*cis* RA 152, 163, 169, 172, 174-181,
2-acetylaminofluorene 112-113, 115, 119-
  120, 126-127, 132
2-ethylpiperidine
  See piperidine alkaloids
2-methylpiperidine
  See piperidine alkaloids
2-propylpiperidine
  See piperidine alkaloids, coniine
3-hydroxyacetaminophen 120
3-methylcholanthrene 114-117, 123, 128,
  133
3,4-didehydroRA 155
3,4-didehydroretinol 155
3′,5′,-cyclic adenosine monophosphate
  (cAMP) 287
3,5,3′-triiodothyronine (T3) 234
3,5,3′,5′-tetraiodothyronine (T4) 234
4-oxo RA 174
4-oxo-retinol 151
5′-iodothyronine deiodinase 233, 255
5,6-epoxyretinoic acid 153, 201, 215
6-aminonicotinamide 24, 39, 52, 66, 69
9-*cis* RA 174, 184
9-*cis* retinoic acid 135

A

α-carotene 137
α-chaconine 316
α-naphthoflavone 114
α-solanine 316
abortions
  premature 350
  spontaneous 5, 24, 28, 136, 177-178,
  355, 358
abuse 351
  See also substances of abuse

Accutane 135-136, 177-178
  See also isotretinoin
acetaldehyde 149, 151, 353, 356
acetaminophen 120, 127, 132
acetate 47, 52, 147, 171, 195, 200, 208,
  270, 353
acetonitrile 339, 348
acid phosphatase 87
acitretin 182
acrodermatitis enteropathica 49, 66, 70
acrylonitrile 339
active transport 21-22, 110, 281
acyl-CoA-retinol:acyltransferase (ARAT)
  140-143
acyl-transfer reaction 190
addictive substances 349
adenosine 287, 358
adrenocortical hormones 146
adrenal glands 344
AFB₁
  See aflatoxins
aflatoxins
  aflatoxin B₁ (AFB₁) 271-272, 274-275
  aflatoxin B₃ 276
  aflatoxin M₁ 276
  aflatoxin M₂ 276
AFP
  See alpha feto-protein
agenesis
  See malformations
aipim
  See cassava
alcohol 60, 146, 149
  See also substances of abuse
alcoholism 353
alcohol dehydrogenase 149, 194-199, 201-
  202, 207-209, 212, 219, 224, 228, 353
alcohol-related birth defects (ARBD) 7,
  354, 357
aldehyde oxidase 151
aliphatic nitrites 339
alkaline phosphatase 87
all-*trans* 3,4-didehydroRA 155
all-*trans* RA 152, 163, 171, 173-176, 179-
  181
all-*trans* retinoic acid (RA) 134-136, 147-
  148, 149-152, 191-192
all-*trans* retinol 145, 196
  See also holo-RBP
allantoic placenta 109
almonds 335-336, 344
  bitter 334, 336
alpha feto-protein 239

amelia (absence of limbs)
  See malformations
amino acids 12, 21-22, 39, 41, 48, 53-57,
  64, 70, 125, 127, 235, 270, 333, 337
  arginine 54, 61-62
  isoleucine 54
  leucine 54
  lysine 54, 57
  methionine 48, 54-55, 61, 240-243,
  245-247, 250, 260, 263, 267
  phenylalanine 54, 56-57, 65, 67, 277,
  281, 303
  threonine 54, 56, 64
  tryptophan 33, 48-49, 51-54, 56-57, 61,
  64-66, 69-72, 364
  tyrosine 55-57, 64-65
  valine 54
ammodendrine
  See piperidine alkaloids
Ammodendron 320
amniotic band defect
  See malformations
amygdalin
  See cyanogenic compounds
amyotrophic lateral sclerosis 237
Anabaena flos-aquae 245
anabasine
  See piperidine alkaloids
anagyrine
  See quinolizidine alkaloids
anal atresia
  See malformations
analgesia 367
anemia 7, 27, 29-31, 73-77, 82-83, 86-89,
  98-99, 102-107
anencephaly
  See malformations
ankle clonus 338
ankylosis
  See malformations
anophthalmia
  See malformations
antiepileptic drugs 8
antinutrients
  See nutrients
antithyroid action of cassava 339
  See also antithyroid effect of cyanide
antithyroid effect of cyanide 338
  See also antithyroid effect of cassava
aorta, overriding
  See malformations
aortic arch, interrupted
  See malformations
aortic stenosis
  See malformations
Apgar scores 24, 358, 364
apoptosis 190, 194, 213

apo-RBP 146, 162
apricot
  See Rosaceace
arachidonic acid 287, 300, 308
ARAT
  See acyl-CoA-retinol:acyltransferase
ARBD
  See alcohol related birth defects
arginine
  See amino acids
arotinoids 180
ascorbic acid
  See vitamins, vitamin C
Aspergillus 270, 274, 277, 282-283, 304
  aculeatus 273, 283
  clavatus 273
  flavus 273-274, 282
  fumigatus 273
  ochraceus 283, 304
  parasiticus 273-274
  terreus 282
ataxia
  See cyanide intoxication
atoxic neuropathy 332
auricular aplasia
  See malformations
autonomic ganglion 359
axial skeletal disorders 339

B

β-carotene 137-138, 152, 160
β-glucosidase 336
β-naphthoflavone 114
bamboo 335, 341, 345-346
Bamboo arundinacea
  See bamboo
barbiturates 368
  See also substances of abuse, prescription drugs
beans 58, 335-336, 345, 357
  black lima beans 335
  wild lima beans 335
behavioral aberrations 351
  See also developmental anomalies
behavioral effects 5, 364
benzaldehyde 336
  See also mandelonitrile
benzo(a)pyrene 112, 115-116, 121, 127,
  130-131
benzodiazepine(s) 358, 368
  See also substances of abuse, prescription drugs
benzoylecgonine
  See cholinesterases, metabolites
benzyloxyphenoxazone 114, 125
benzylselenocyanate 251

beriberi 23, 40
bilateral cryptorchidism
   See malformations
bilateral hydronephrosis
   See malformations
bioavailable iron
   See iron, bioavailable
biological half-life for Δ^9-THC 361
biotin
   See vitamins
birth weight 1, 5, 18-19, 23-24, 27-28, 30,
   33, 39, 45, 52, 62, 73, 85-90, 92-95, 97,
   106, 274, 343, 345, 355, 358, 360, 362,
   364-366, 371
   low 1, 18-19, 28, 85, 345, 358
bitter almonds
   See almonds, bitter
bitter cassava
   See cassava, bitter varieties
black cherry, wild 341
black lima beans
   See beans
bladder 344
blastocyst 12, 19, 109, 257
blood nicotine 359
bone fusions 22-23, 84, 88, 99, 110, 140,
   171, 182, 246, 286-287, 289-291, 339,
   342, 346
bowel infarction
   See malformations
brachygnathia
   See malformations
brain 16, 19, 22, 31, 34, 41, 49-50, 55, 82,
   88, 106, 167, 170, 176, 183, 188-189,
   196, 214, 216, 235, 255, 272-273, 276,
   285, 337, 353, 358-359, 363, 367, 372
brominated biphenyls 146

C

caffeine
   See substances of abuse
calcium
   See minerals
caloric intake 2, 332
cannabidiol 361
cannabinoids 354, 361-362, 369, 371-372
   teratogenic effects of 16, 21, 27, 40, 68,
   112, 136, 170, 186, 189, 195, 209-210,
   247, 279, 281, 303, 308, 348, 361
   See also marijuana
cannabinol 361, 372
cannabis
   See substances of abuse
Cannabis salvia
   See marijuana
carbamezapine 8

carbohydrates 12, 19, 21, 67, 278, 308,
   332, 353
carbon dioxide
   See cigarette smoke
carbon monoxide
   See cigarette smoke
carcinogens 359
   See also cigarette smoke
cardiac arrhythmias
   See cocaine use, clinical manifestations
cardiac hypertrophy 31
cardiomyopathy 230, 235
Carica 320
carotenes 137
   See also α- and β-carotenes
carotenoids 134, 137-140, 160, 218, 223
cashew nuts 48, 56
cassava 332-334, 336-339, 341-348
   "bitter varieties" 333-334, 342
   consumption 338-339, 343, 345
   "sweet" 333, 342
Cassia 320
cataracts 42, 45-72, 168, 171, 248, 256
   hypocalcemic 58
   juvenile 45, 58
   senile 42, 45, 47, 71
catecholamine 324, 331, 363
cebocephalia
   See malformations
cellular retinol-binding protein (CRBP)
   140, 145, 163, 200, 217-218, 228
Cephalosporium 291
cephalothoracophagus
   See malformations
cerebellar hypoplasia
   See malformations
cerebellum, hypoplastic
   See malformations, cerebellum
chaetoglobosin A
   See cytochalasins
chaconine (α) 316
cherry
   See Rosaceace
chlorcyclizine 112, 131
chokecherry 337
cholesterol 20, 36, 72, 139, 141, 198, 228
cholesteryl ester hydrolase 142, 206
choline chloride 54
cholinesterases 363
   metabolites 363
chondrodystrophy
   See malformations
chromosomal aberrations 6
chylomicrons 141-142, 197, 223-224
cigarette smoke 359
   carbon dioxide 86, 353, 359
   carbon monoxide 118, 359

cigarette smoke (continued)
  nicotine 359
  nitrogen oxides 359
  polycyclic aromatic hydrocarbons 359
ciliary body hyperplasia 168
citreoviridin 273
citrinin 271, 273, 282-283
citroxanthin 137
Claviceps paspali 273
Claviceps purpurea 273, 283
cleft lip
  See malformations
cleft palate
  See malformations
club feet
  See malformations
clubfoot
  See malformations, club feet
"Coca Cola" 363
coca plant 362-363
cocaine
  See substances of abuse
  half-life of 363
cocaine use, clinical manifestations 363
  cardiac arrhythmias 363
  convulsions 358, 363, 366
  euphoria 363
  hyperglycemia 363
  hyperpyrexia 363
  hypertension 363
  mydriasis 363
  tachycardia 363
codeine
  See substances of abuse
cognitive performance 368
Collidium 320
coloboma
  See malformations
congenital abnormalities
  See malformations, congenital
congenital cataract
  See malformations
congenital infections 352
congenital malformations 9, 21, 23-25, 28-29, 31, 46, 49, 60, 95, 109, 171, 209, 230, 253, 310-312, 327, 339-341, 343-344, 352, 358, 365, 368
  See malformations, congenital
coniine
  See piperidine alkaloids
coniceine (γ) 319
Conium 310, 319, 323, 327-330
  maculatum 319, 323, 327-330
connective tissue 20
convulsions
  See cocaine use, clinical manifestations

copper
  See minerals
cortico-spinal tracts, lesions in 338
corticosterone 288-290, 300
Council on Foods and Nutrition 75, 102
cowpeas 48, 56
crack
  See also cocaine
cranial extrusion
  See encephalocoele
craniofacial alterations
  See teratology
CRBP
  See cellular retinol-binding protein
creatine kinase 249
crooked calf disease
  See malformations
crotocin
  See trichothecenes
cryptoxanthin 137
Cupid's bow
  See fetal alcohol syndrome
curly tail
  See malformations
cyanide 332-333, 335-348, 359
cyanide in blood 344
cyanide intoxication 29, 31, 268, 342
cyanide-containing foods 332
cyanogenic compounds
  amygdalin 334-336, 340, 342, 344-345, 347-348
  cyanogenic glycosides 333-337, 344, 346-347
  linamarin 333-336, 341-347
  lotaustralin 334, 336
  thiocyanates 8, 333, 337-341, 344
cyanogenic glycoside
  See cyanogenic compounds
cyclocephaly
  See malformations
cyclopamine
  See Veratrum alkaloids
cyclopia
  See malformations
cyclopiazonic acid 273
cycloposine
  See Veratrum alkaloids
Cylindrocarpon 291
cynomolgus monkey
  See monkey
cystic fibrosis 35, 237, 268
cyt.P450 151, 153
cytochalasins 271, 273, 296, 305
  chaetoglobosin A 296
  cytochalasin D 296, 307
  cytochalasin E 296

cytochrome oxidase 337
cytochromes 111-112, 118-119, 125

D

Δ^9-*trans*-tetrahydrocannabinol (Δ^9-THC)
  361, 372
  See also biological half-life of and maternal blood concentrations of
Δ^8-THC 361
Δ^9-*trans*-tetrahydrocannabinolic acid
  (THC acid) 361
deermouse, mutant 150
demethylation 114-115, 358
demissidine
  See solanidane alkaloids
deoxynivalenol
  See trichothecenes
developmental anomalies 351
  See also malformations and teratology
developmental toxicology 351-352
  See also teratology
diacetoxyscirpenol (DAS)
  See trichothecenes
diaphragmatic hernia 28, 344
Dichroa 320
dietary factors 6, 376
diethylstilbestrol 8
dihydroisocoumarin 277
  See also ochratoxin A
dimethylsulfoxide (DSMO) 285
diosgenin
  See spirosolane alkaloids
dioxins 117, 146
DNA 13-14, 47, 49-50, 116, 231-234, 237,
  248, 250-251, 256, 258-259, 262-263,
  265-267, 269, 275, 280
dopamine 83, 285, 364
dopaminergic pathways 364
drug dependence 350
drug exposure 352, 364
Duboisa 320
dysarthria 9
dysmorphogenesis 21, 110, 113, 122, 125,
  156, 177, 222
  embryonic 21, 110
dyspnea 29, 342
  See cyanide intoxication

E

ecgonine methyl ester 363
ectopic cell death 182, 189
ectrodactyly
  See malformations
embryolethality
  See teratology

embryonic dysmorphogenesis
  See dysmorphogenesis
embryonic implantation 6
encephalocoele
  See malformations
endocytosis 142, 147
endoplasmic reticulum 146, 203
enterocytes 139-141
environmental pollutants 8
  lead 9-10, 266
  methylmercury 9, 249, 263
enzymatic isomerization 152, 223
enzyme inhibitors 6
epicanthal folds (eye skin folds)
  See fetal alcohol syndrome
epinephrine 358
ergotoxins 273
erythropoiesis 75, 78, 82
Erythroxylon coca
  See coca plant
essential fatty acids
  See fatty acids, essential
essential lipids
  See lipids, essential
estrogens 121, 304
ethoxyphenoxazone 114-116
ethoxyresorufin 114, 127, 131
ethyl alcohol 353
  See also substances of abuse, alcohol
Etretinate 136, 181-182, 196, 205, 211,
  220-221
  See also Tigason
euphoria
  See cocaine use, clinical manifestations
exencephaly
  See malformations
exophthalmos
  See malformations
eyes, absence of
  See anophthalmia
eyes, small
  See microphthalmia

F

facial dysmorphia
  See malformations
facial malformations
  See malformations, facial
FAS
  See fetal alcohol syndrome
fatty acids
  free 20
ferritin 75-84, 88, 90-92, 96-98, 101, 103-
  107, 199
ferrous calcium citrate 97
ferrous fumarate 97

ferrous gluconate 97
ferrous sulphate 91, 97
fetal alcohol syndrome 354, 364, 370, 372-373
  Cupid's bow 355
  epicanthal folds 355
  fetal hypoxia 356
  midfacial hypoplasia 355
  palpebral fissures 355
  philtrum 355
fetal hypoxia
  See fetal alcohol syndrome
fetal ossification 359
fetal protein synthesis 21
fetal resorption 23, 29, 31, 274, 278, 285, 358, 361-362
fibrinoid necrosis 87-88
fingernail hypoplasia
  See teratology
folate
  See vitamins
  See also vitamins, folic acid
folic acid
  See vitamins
fortified dairy products 100
free fatty acids
  See fatty acids, free
freebasing 363
  See also cocaine
frontonasal mesenchyme 184-185
fumitremorgens A and B 273
furanopiperidine 314
fusarenon-X
  See trichothecenes
Fusarium 270, 273, 291, 294, 301, 304

G

γ-carotene 137
γ-coniceine 319
galactokinase 60
galactose
  See monosaccharides
galactose epimerase 60
galactosemia 60, 71
generally recognized as safe (GRAS) 357
genetalia (external) 344
genetic anomalies 5
genetic mutations
  See mutations, genetic
Genista 320
genitourinary malformations
  See malformations, genitourinary
genitourinary tract 28, 364, 370
geotaxis 285
glucocorticoids 287-288, 290

glucose
  See monosaccharides
glucose-6-phosphate dehydrogenase 290
glucosidase (β) 336
glutathione 51, 59, 64, 71, 121-122, 127, 230, 232-235, 237-238, 248, 251-252, 254-255, 258, 261-262, 265, 267-269
glutathione conjugation 121-122
glutathione peroxidase 59, 230, 232-235, 237-238, 252, 254-255, 258, 261-262, 265, 267-268
glutathione reductase 51, 233
glycogen 19-20, 62, 281, 305
glycogenesis 281
glycogenolysis 281
goitre 249, 346
Goldenhar's syndrome
  See malformations
Golgi apparatus 146
growth 1, 5, 8, 12-19, 25, 27, 30-31, 34, 36-37, 41, 53-55, 66, 70, 72, 85, 87, 90, 104-105, 110, 134, 148, 180, 187, 195, 215, 224-225, 237, 239, 246-248, 253, 264, 270, 275-276, 278, 280, 285, 291, 295-296, 302, 341, 350-352, 354, 356, 360, 362, 364-365, 372, 374
  retardation 1, 13, 31, 85, 105, 110, 180, 239, 248, 275-276, 280, 295, 341, 351-352, 354, 360, 362, 364-365

H

harelip
  See malformations
head circumference 358
heart 15, 20, 22, 30, 46, 55, 144, 167, 170, 172, 176, 183, 189, 230, 243, 245-246, 273, 276, 358, 365
hematocrit 75, 78, 81, 86, 89, 91, 98, 158
hematopoiesis 30, 70
hemodynamics 159
hemoglobin 7, 29, 73-74, 79, 82, 85-86, 89, 101, 105-106
heroin
  See substances of abuse
high-risk categories 4
Hoeniscium sp. 273
holo-RBP 144-147, 159, 161-162, 167
  See also all-trans retinol
homeobox genes 183, 193
  See also Hox genes
horseshoe kidney
  See malformations
Hox genes 183, 187-188, 193
HT-2 toxin
  See trichothecenes

Hydrangea 320
hydrocephaly
    See malformations
hydrocortisone 287, 289
hydrocyanic acid 333, 336
hydrogen cyanide
    See prussic acid
hydronephrosis
    See malformations
hydroureter
    See malformations
hydroxocobalamin 337
hydroxycotinine, trans-3'-
    See trans-3'-hydroxycotinine
hydroxynitrile lyase 336
    See also benzaldehyde
hyperestrogenic syndrome 294
hypergalactosemia 60
hyperglycemia
    See cocaine use, clinical manifestations
hyperplasia 13, 15, 133, 168, 190, 313
hyperpyrexia
    See cocaine use, clinical manifestations
hypertension 87, 101, 244
    pregnancy-induced (PIH) 244
hypertrophy 13, 15, 31, 59, 66, 86
hypervitaminosis A 46, 169-172, 204, 209-210
hypocalcemia 28, 59, 66
hypocalcemic cataract
    See cataracts, hypocalcemic
hypocalcemic tetany 57
hypoglycemia 60, 62
hyponatremia 30
hypoplasia
    See malformations, hypoplasia
hypoplasia of the aorta
    See malformations, aorta, hypoplasia
hypoplasia of the telencephalon
    See malformations, telencephalon, hypoplasia
hypoplastic genital papilla
    See malformations
hypoplastic right heart syndrome
    See malfromations
hypothermia
    See cyanide intoxication
hypoxia 87-88, 190, 356, 365
hystrine
    See piperidine alkaloids

I

Idjwi Island 337
ileal atresias
    See malformations

illicit compounds (drugs) 349, 351
    See also cannabis, cocaine, opiates
impaired skeletal ossification 343
imperforate anus
    See malformations
industrial chemicals 351
infertility 27, 294
insecticides 339
interparietal encephalocele
    See malformations
intracellular repair 352
intrauterine growth retardation 237, 239, 351, 360, 362
    See also developmental anomalies
iodine 8, 30, 259, 337-338
    See also minerals
iron
    bioavailable 98
    nonheme 99, 102, 107
    See also minerals, iron
iron absorption 78, 96, 98-99, 101-102
iron deficiency
    See anemia
iron index 80
iron intake 73, 77-78, 90, 92, 96, 98, 101
iron metabolism 78, 80
iron status 73, 75, 78, 80-82, 86, 91, 94, 96-98, 100-101, 105-106, 108
iron supplementation 7, 82-83, 88, 90-91, 93-96, 98, 100, 103, 107
iron transfer 80
iron transport 101
ischemic decidual necrosis 84
isoleucine
    See amino acids
isotretinoin 177
    See also Accutane

J

jaws, retarded
    See malformations
jejunal atresia
    See malformations
jerveratrum steroidal alkaloids 313-314, 324-325
jervine
    See Veratrum alkaloids
jervine analogs 314

K

Keshan disease 235-237, 268
kidney 344
kinked tail
    See malformations
konzo 338

konzo (continued)
  See also myelopathy and spastic para-
    peresis
Kupffer cells (of liver) 143
kyphoscoliosis
  See malformations
kyphosis
  See malformations

L

L-methionine 48, 55, 260
L-tryptophan 48-49, 51, 53-54, 56
lactation 2-3, 23, 47-48, 56-57, 66, 83, 156,
  195, 226, 241-243, 252, 262, 266, 273-
  274, 341, 374
laetrile 334, 340
  See also cyanogenic compounds, amyg-
    dalin
laudanum
  See heroin
laurate 142
lead
  See environmental pollutants
lecithin-retinol:acyltransferase (LRAT)
  140, 142
lens 42-44, 46-47, 49-65, 67-69, 71, 248,
  256
leucine
  See amino acids
lima beans
  See beans, lima
limbs, absence of
  See amelia
limbs, small size
  See phocomelia
linamerase 336
  See also β-glucosidase
linamarin
  See cyanogenic compounds
linoleate 21, 142
Liparia 320
lipids, essential 20
liver 20, 22-23, 28-32, 54-55, 58, 62-63,
  74, 80-81, 91, 96, 113, 116, 118, 126,
  130-131, 134, 137, 139, 141-147, 149-
  152, 154, 157, 160, 162-163, 165-167,
  169, 190-191, 195-202, 204-209, 212,
  214-221, 224, 226, 228, 233, 235, 239,
  241, 243, 245, 247, 249, 255, 265, 272,
  275-276, 280-281, 289-290, 301-302,
  305, 308, 344, 353, 364, 367-368
lotaustralin
  See cyanogenic compounds
low protein diet 279, 343
LRAT
  See lecithin-retinol:acyltransferase

LSD 368
  See lysergic acid diethylamide
lumbar vertebrae
  See malformations
Lupinus 310-311, 317, 319-321, 324, 327,
  329-330
  caudatus 317, 320
  formosus 321-322, 324, 327, 329
  sericeus 317, 321
lyase 336
lysergic acid diethylamide (LSD)
  See substances of abuse, psychedelic
    drugs
lysine
  See amino acids

M

Macaca fascicularis 175, 207, 247, 267
macronutrients
  See nutrients
magnesium
  See minerals
malformations
  abruptio placentae 364-366
  agenesis (ureter) 171; (renal) 278-279,
    285; (ribs) 342
  amelia 8
  amniotic band defect 364
  anal atresia 171
  anencephaly 29, 35, 47, 170, 269, 274,
    296
  ankylosis 171, 341, 347
  anophthalmia 28, 39, 46, 49-50, 52, 60,
    64, 168, 171, 230, 245, 278-279, 285,
    313
  aorta, hypoplasia 178
  aorta, overriding 171
  aortic arch, interrupted 178
  aortic stenosis 171, 281
  auricular aplasia 171
  bilateral cryptorchidism 364
  bilateral hydronephrosis 364
  bowel infarction 364
  brachygnathia 170
  cebocephalia (cebocephaly) 313-314
  cephalothoracophagus 343
  cerebellar hypoplasia 177
  cerebellum, hypoplastic 293
  chondrodystrophy 30
  cleft lip 29-30, 47, 170, 283, 360, 372
  cleft palate 23-24, 27, 46, 50-51, 131,
    170-171, 173, 176-178, 210, 249, 282-
    290, 293, 295, 297, 305, 308, 314, 320,
    323, 330, 358, 360
  club feet 29-30, 47, 364
  coloboma 171

malformations (continued)
congenital 9, 21, 23-29, 31, 35, 38, 45-47, 49, 60, 70, 95, 109, 171, 209, 230, 253, 310-312, 327, 339-341, 343-344, 352, 358, 360, 365, 368
congenital cataract 42, 45, 52-53, 60-63, 171
crooked calf disease 317, 319, 321-324, 327, 329-331
curly tail 30, 279
cyclocephaly 171
cyclopia 313
ectrodactyly 358
ectopic kidney 279
encephalocele 170-171, 230, 314, 339, 343, 365
exencephaly 24, 29, 47, 170-171, 175, 275, 280-281, 285, 291, 293, 295, 314, 329, 339, 343, 365
exophthalmos 171
eyelids, open 275, 283, 291, 295
facial 23, 207, 224, 280, 313
facial cleft 280
facial dysmorphia 170
genitourinary 28, 174, 364-366, 370
Goldenhar's syndrome 172
harelip 314
horseshoe kidney 364
hydrocephaly 23-24, 26, 30, 36, 38, 41, 50-51, 60, 72, 171, 177, 213, 278-280, 282, 293, 295, 343
hydronephrosis 168, 171, 279, 285, 295, 364
hydroureter 171
hypoplastic genital papilla 171
hypoplastic right heart syndrome 365
ileal atresias 364
imperforate anus 364
interparietal encephalocele 365
intestines (protrusion of) 275
jejunal atresia 364
kinked tail 29
kyphoscoliosis 171
kyphosis 171
lordotic exencephaly 343
lumbar vertebrae 293
mandibular ankylosis 171
mandibular hyperplasia 313
median cleft mandible 171
meningocele 171
meningoencephalocele 171
microcephaly 28, 39, 171, 175, 341, 364
micrognathia 27, 30, 171, 177, 279
micromelia 27
microphthalmia 28, 46-47, 49-52, 56, 60, 64, 168, 171, 173, 230, 245, 279, 281, 285, 355
oligodactyly 171
omphalocele 24, 278-279
open eyes 50, 175, 278
otoliths 31
phocomelia 8
pinnae 295
polydactyly 30, 280
prune-belly syndrome 364
pulmonary hypoplasia 171
renal agenesis 285
retarded jaws 291
retinoid embryopathy 169
retrolental fibroplasia 47
rib fusions 171
scoliosis 29, 47, 171
spina bifida 8, 170-171, 175, 194, 269, 330
supernumary ribs 342
syndactyly 23, 29-30, 50-51, 170-171
telencephalon, hypoplasia 280
testis, cryptorchid 279
tracheo-esophageal fistula 285
transverse distal limb reduction 364
truncus arteriosus communis 178
umbilical hernia 29, 171, 295
ureter agenesis 171
ventricular septal defect 171, 178
ventricular spinal defect 281
vertebrae, absent 171
malnutrition
See nutrition
malonate 270
mandelonitrile 336
See also benzaldehyde
mandibular ankylosis
See malformations
mandibular hyperplasia
See malformations
mandioca
See cassava
manganese
See minerals
Manihot esculenta
See cassava
manioc
See cassava
marijuana 360
See substances of abuse
maternal blood concentrations of Δ^9-THC 361
maternal-fetal conflicts 350
mean corpuscular volume 81
meclizine 112
median cleft mandible
See malformations

meningocele
  See malformations
meningoencephalocele
  See malformations
mental retardation 5, 9, 60, 343
mercury 9-10, 249, 257-258, 263, 266
  poisoning 9-10
metalloenzymes 49, 337
metatarsal bones 343
  See also impaired skeletal ossification
methionine
  See amino acids
methoxyphenoxazone 114-115
methylfolate 50-51
methylmercury
  See Environmental pollutants
methylxanthines 117
mevalonate 270
microcephaly
  See malformations
micrognathia
  See malformations
micromelia
  See malformations
micronutrients
  See nutrients
microphthalmia
  See malformations
midfacial hypoplasia (underdeveloped midface)
  See fetal alcohol syndrome
Minamata disease 5, 9-10
minerals 2-4, 12, 29, 41, 70, 104-105, 238
  calcium 4-5, 30-31, 50, 52, 58-59, 63, 65, 67, 71, 97, 100, 107, 250, 268, 333
  iodine 4, 8, 30, 33, 259, 268, 337-338
  iron 2, 4-10, 29-31, 33-34, 40, 45, 68-70, 73-84, 86-108, 122, 193, 245, 248, 253, 257, 259-262, 264, 266-267, 272, 297, 299-306, 326-327, 329, 333, 336, 347-348, 352, 357, 365, 368
  magnesium 4, 30, 33, 107
  manganese 30-31
  potassium 30, 341
  selenium 4, 7, 33, 52, 59-60, 68-72, 230-269
  sodium 30, 44, 56, 59, 65, 68, 70, 240, 246-248, 250-251, 255, 258, 264-269, 339-340, 346, 363
  zinc 4-5, 26, 31-33, 35-36, 39-40, 46, 49-50, 64, 68-70, 94-96, 101-105, 107, 199, 239-240, 257, 259, 261, 266, 269
mirror-image duplication 187
misinformation (in the literature) 2
mitochondria 14, 51-52, 234, 250, 252, 261, 268, 281, 290, 302, 304, 337

monkey
  cynomolgus 175-176, 207-208
monooxygenases 112
monosaccharides 60
  galactose 60, 62, 64, 71
  glucose 12, 19, 21, 35, 60, 62-65, 67, 72, 281, 290
  xylose 60
monosodium glutamate 56
morphine
  See substances of abuse
muldamine
  See Veratrum alkaloids
muscular dystrophy 249
mutations
  genetic 6
mycotoxins 270-272, 274, 285, 291, 293, 295-297, 301, 307-308
  See also cytochalasins, rubratoxins, trichothecenes, zearalenone
mydriasis
  See cocaine use, clinical manifestations
myelopathy 338
  See also konzo
myristate 142
Myrothecium 291

N
N-acetylhystrine
  See piperidine alkaloids
N-formimino-L-glutamate 25
N-methylammodendrine
  See piperidine alkaloids
N-methylanabasine
  See piperidine alkaloids
N-methyljervine 314-315
N-methylmethiodide 314
N-methylpelletierine
  See piperidine alkaloids
naphthoflavones 117
  See also α- and β-naphthoflavone 114
NAS 367
  See also neonatal abstinence syndrome
National Research Council 1-4, 7, 10, 27, 32, 38, 77, 90, 98, 105, 230, 235, 252, 263
neonatal abstinence syndrome
  See substances of abuse, withdrawal
neosolaniol
  See trichothecenes
nephrotoxin 283
nervous system 16, 20, 24-25, 39, 49, 148, 177, 202, 214, 273, 353-354, 356, 358-359, 367, 369
neural tube defects
  See teratology

neurotransmitters 83
NHANES 74-75, 77, 105
niacin
    See vitamins
Nicotiana 310, 319-320, 323, 326, 328-
    330, 359
    glauca 320, 323, 328-329
    tabacum 320, 326, 359
nicotine
    See pyridine alkaloids
nitriles 339, 348
nitrogen oxides
    See cigarette smoke
nivalenol
    See trichothecenes
non-dietary factors 349
nonheme iron
    See iron
noradrenaline 83
norchlorcyclizine 112
norepinephrine 358
NRC
    See National Research Council
nuclear receptors 71, 136, 148, 183-184,
    192-193, 219
    RARα 148, 184--186
    RARβ 148, 184-186
    RARγ 148, 184-186
    RXR 148, 184, 186, 213-214
nuclear transcription factors 6
nutrients
    antinutrients 17
    deficiencies 13, 17-18, 22
    macronutrients 12, 17
    micronutrients 12, 14, 17, 22, 267
nutrition 1-3, 5, 12, 15, 33, 36-37, 40, 45-
    46, 63-64, 67, 71, 87, 103-106, 113, 117,
    122, 124-125, 141, 161, 201, 209, 218,
    222, 226, 238, 249, 258-259, 263-264,
    296-297, 360
    deficiencies 2, 5
    maternal 1, 9, 11, 21, 36, 39, 73-74,
    82-83, 85-86, 88, 103, 105-106, 156,
    169, 204, 222, 226, 239, 249, 259, 263,
    268, 289, 329, 360-362, 367, 369-370,
    372-374
    quality 1
nymphomania 294

O
O-debenzylation 114-115
O-deethylation 114-115
O-depentylation 114-115, 118-119
OA
    See ochratoxin A
ochratoxin 277, 280-281, 301, 303-304

ochratoxin A (OA) 271-273, 277, 280,
    297-308
oleate 21, 142
oligodactyly
    See malformations
omphaloc(o)ele
    See malformations, omphalocele
open eyes
    See malformations
opiates
    See substances of abuse
opium
    See substances of abuse
optic atrophy, inherited 337
organogenesis 6, 109-114, 117, 121-123,
    125, 129, 133, 154-157, 164, 166, 168,
    173-174, 183, 189-190, 193, 200-202,
    218, 247, 272, 275, 292, 294, 352, 356
organoselenium compounds 251, 260
osteomalacia 28
otoliths
    See malformations

P
p-methoxybenzeneselenol 251
packed cell volume 79, 93-94, 104
palatogenesis 286-287
palmitoleate 142
palpebral fissures (small eye openings)
    See fetal alcohol syndrome
pancreas 344
pantothenic acid
    See vitamins
Papaver somniferum
    See poppy plant
paraperesis 338, 346
parathyroid 59, 66
paraxanthine 358
    See also 1-methylxanthine
parenchymal cells (of liver) 141-145, 166,
    197, 205
pattern formation 187
patulin 273
PCV
    See packed cell volume
peach
    See Rosaceace
peach pits 337
pellagra 24, 70
penicillic acid 273
Penicillium 270, 273, 277, 282-283, 295,
    307
    citreoviride 273
    citrinum 273, 282
    cyclopium 273
    oxalicum 273, 283, 307

Penicillium (continued)
  purpurogenum 295
  rubrum 273, 295
  urticae 273
  viridicatum 273
penitrems A, B, and C 273
pentoxyphenoxazone 114-115, 118, 129
pernicious anemia 27
pesticides 351
pharmaceuticals 351
phencyclidine
  See substances of abuse, psychedelic drugs
phenobarbital 118, 128, 130
phenoxazone 114-116, 118-119, 125, 129, 133
phenoxazone ethers 114, 119, 133
phenylalanine 54, 56-57, 65, 67, 277, 281, 303
  See also amino acids
phenytoin 8
philtrum, underdeveloped (upper lip depression)
  See fetal alcohol syndrome
phocomelia (limbs of small size)
  See malformations
Phoma sp. 273
Phoma terrestris 283
Phomosis sp. 273
phosphodiesterase 118, 358
phospholipase A$_2$ 190, 287, 290
phospholipids 20
phosphorylase-β-kinase 281
photoisomerization 152
physical tolerance 350
phytate 50, 99, 105
PIH
  See hypertension, pregnancy-induced
pinnae, malformed
  See malformations, pinnae
piperidine alkaloids 311, 319-324
  2-ethylpiperidine 320
  2-methylpiperidine 320
  ammodendrine 321-322, 324
  anabasine 319-321, 323, 328-329
  γ-coniceine 319, 323
  coniine 319-320, 323
  hystrine 321
  N-acetylhystrine 321
  N-methylammodendrine 321
  N-methylanabasine 321
  N-methylpelletierine 321
Pithomyces chartarum 273
placental transport 160
plum
  See Rosaceae

poisonous plants 310-312, 325
  See also Conium, Lupinus, Nicotiana, Solanum, Veratrum
polychlorinated biphenyls 113
polycyclic aromatic hydrocarbons
  See cigarette smoke
polydactyly
  See malformations
polyhalogenated biphenyls 117
polynuclear aromatic hydrocarbons 117
polyphenol 99
ponderal index 358
poppy plant 366
potassium
  See minerals
potassium cyanide 341
preeclampsia 260
premature abortion
  See abortions
premature delivery 364
prescription drugs
  See substances of abuse
propionitrile 339
Prosopis 320
prostaglandin 84, 132, 244, 287, 356, 373
prostaglandins 356, 373
prostanoid 21, 35
protoporphyrin 75-76, 82
protrusion of intestines
  See malformations, intestines, protrusion of
provitamin A 134, 137
prunasin 336, 345, 348
prune-belly syndrome
  See malformations
Prunus amygdalus
  See almonds
Prunus serotina
  See black cherry, wild
prussic acid 333, 342
psoriasis 180-181
psychedelic drugs
  See substances of abuse
psychomotor dysfunctions 7
ptosis (drooping eyelids)
  See fetal alcohol syndrome
pulmonary hypoplasia
  See malformations
Punica 320
Pyrenochaeta terrestris 283
pyridine alkaloids 319
  nicotine 319-320, 325, 349-350, 359, 370, 372
pyridoxal
  See vitamins, vitamin B$_6$
pyruvate 270

Q

quinolizidine alkaloids 311, 317-318, 321-323, 325
  anagyrine 321-324, 327
  (-)-anagyrine 317-318
  (+)-thermopsine 318
  (-)-thermopsine 318

R

RA
  See all-*trans* retinoic acid
rachitogenic diet 50
RAL 148-151
  See also retinal, retinaldehyde, and 11-*cis* RAL
RAR genes 185
RARα
  See nuclear receptors
RARβ
  See nuclear receptors
RARγ
  See nuclear receptors
RBP
  See retinol binding protein
RDA
  See Recommended Dietary Allowances
recalcitrant cystic acne 135, 177
Recommended Dietary Allowance 3, 10, 18, 32-33, 38, 77, 105, 230, 235, 263
renal agenesis
  See malformations, angenesis (renal)
resorufin 114, 118, 127, 130-131
retin-A 179
retinal 47, 134, 137-139, 144, 147, 201, 208-209, 211, 216-217, 219
  See also 11-*cis* retinal
retinal reductase 138
retinaldehyde 137, 147
retinoic acid 6, 121, 125-126, 129, 134-136, 138-139, 153, 168, 192, 195-196, 198-223, 225, 228, 258, 326
retinoid embryopathy
  See malformations
retinoid homeostasis 159
retinoid metabolism 154, 201
retinol 33, 107, 125, 129, 134-136, 138-152, 154-168, 171, 179-180, 193, 196-209, 211-226, 228
retinol binding protein 144-147, 167, 200, 209, 226
retinol dehydrogenase 149, 212
retinol esterification 141-142, 144, 166, 220
retinol oxidation 149-150, 215
retinoyl-β-glucuronide 153
retinyl acetate 147, 171, 195, 200, 208

retinyl ester hydrolase 142-143, 146, 199
retinyl esters 139-146, 157, 160-161, 163-164, 166, 171, 204
retinyl palmitate 141-142, 197, 206, 219
retinyl stearate 141
retrobulbar neuritis 337
retrolental fibroplasia
  See malformations
rib fusions
  See malformations
riboflavin
  See vitamins
ribosomes 14
rickets 28, 36, 57
risk assessment of drug use 262, 351
rock 363
  See also cocaine
Rosaceace 335
  apricot 335, 340, 347
  cherry 335, 337, 348
  peach 335, 337, 344
  plum 335
Rubella 42
rubratoxins 271, 273, 295
  rubratoxin A 295
  rubratoxin B 272, 295, 301-302
RXR
  See nuclear receptors
RXR genes 186, 214

S

sacrocaudal vertebrae 343
  See also impaired skeletal ossification
schikimate 270
scoliosis
  See malformations
secalonic acid 271
secalonic acid D 272-273, 283, 289-290, 297, 299-300, 302-305, 307
Sedum 320
selenate 243-247, 251, 257-258, 260, 262, 266
selenite 59-60, 64-65, 67-68, 70-71, 231, 240-241, 243, 245-248, 250-251, 255-260, 262-269
selenium
  bioaccumulation 248
  deficiency 59, 235-237, 249, 251-255, 263, 268
  metabolism 232
  placental transfer 243
  status 233, 235-238, 243, 249, 251-253, 259, 262, 265
  supplementation 252
  toxicosis 70, 248
  See also minerals

seleno-deiodinase 249
selenoamino acid 232
selenocarrageenan 248
selenocysteine 230, 232-235, 242, 249,
    255, 261, 263
selenomethionine 240-243, 245-247
selenoproteins 230, 232-236, 250, 253-
    254, 256, 259, 262-263, 265, 267
selenotrisulfide 250
serotonin 83, 258, 287, 308, 364
sertoli cells 144, 147, 196, 223
serum urate 89-90
sodium
    See minerals
sodium nitrile 339
sodium selenite 59, 65, 70, 240, 246-248,
    250-251, 255, 258, 264-266, 269
sodium thiosulfate 339-340
solanidane alkaloids 314
    demissidine 315-316
    solanidine 314-317
solanidine
    See solanidane alkaloids
solanine (α) 316
Solanum 314, 327, 329
solasodine
    See spirosolane alkaloids
sorghum plants 337
Sorghum vulgare 335
spastic paraperesis 338, 346
spastic peresis 338
spermatogenesis 234, 252, 268
spina bifida
    See malformations
spirosolane alkaloids 314
    solasodine 314-315, 329-330
    tomatidine 314-315, 330
spleen 344
spontaneous abortions
    See abortions, spontaneous
sporidesmins 273
Stachybotrys 291
stearate 141-142
stellate cells (of liver) 142-145, 166, 197,
    205, 226, 228
sterigmatocystin 273
sternebrae 278-279, 343
    See also impaired skeletal ossification
steroid hormones
    See hormones
steroids 48, 159, 314
stillbirth 6, 23-24, 29, 52, 83-84, 178, 292,
    355, 360, 364-365
structural defects 5
structural malformations 351
    See also teratology

subclavian artery, retroesophageal right
    See malformations, subclavian artery
substances of abuse
    alcohol 4-5, 7, 41, 60, 134, 146, 149,
        194-199, 201-202, 207-209, 212-213,
        215, 219, 224, 228, 349-350, 353-357,
        362, 364, 366, 368-374
    caffeine 41, 287, 306, 349, 357-359,
        369-370, 373-374
    cannabis 349, 360-361
    cocaine 349-350, 354, 357, 360, 362-
        366, 370-374; half-life 363
    codeine 366
    heroin 350, 354, 366-368, 372, 374
    marijuana 350, 357, 360-362, 364, 371,
        374
    morphine 366-367
    nicotine 349-350, 354, 359
    opiates 349-350, 364, 366-368, 374
    opium 366
    prescription drugs 7, 169, 368
    psychedelic drugs 368-369
    withdrawal (symptoms) 350, 367
Sudan grass 341
sulfur-containing amino acids 57, 333, 337
supernumary ribs
    See malformations, supernumary ribs
supplements 2, 5, 21, 26, 34, 39-40, 61, 90,
    99, 106, 137, 169, 172, 192, 243, 256
    multivitamin-mineral 4
syncytial knots 88
syndactyly
    See malformations

T
T-2 toxin
    See trichothecene mycotoxins
tachycardia
    See cocaine use, clinical manifestations
tapioca
    See cassava
Tegison 135, 180
    See also Etretinte and Tigason
telencephalon
    See malformations
terata induction 323
teratogenicity 35, 126-127, 129-130, 132,
    173, 200, 202, 207, 210-211, 217, 226,
    231, 238, 246, 250, 253-254, 259, 263,
    274, 277-278, 280, 282-286, 289-290,
    292, 296, 298-300, 303, 310, 312, 314-
    316, 319-320, 322-324, 326, 328, 330-
    331, 339-340, 366
teratogens
    See teratology, teratogen(s)

teratology 10-11, 35, 39, 68, 110, 125-126,
   128-131, 194, 203, 207-211, 220-222,
   227, 269, 298-301, 306-307, 326-327,
   329-331, 346, 348, 351, 370-373, 376
   embryolethality 174, 177, 292, 296,
      352, 372
   neural tube defects 8, 21, 24-28, 34,
      38-40, 339
   teratogen(s) 5-6, 16, 21, 24, 27, 31, 35,
      37, 40-42, 46, 51-52, 66, 68, 109, 112,
      122, 124-132, 136, 153, 161, 169-171,
      173-176, 179-180, 182-183, 186-189,
      191-193, 195, 200, 202-204, 207, 209-
      211, 217, 220, 226, 230-231, 238, 245-
      247, 250, 253-254, 259, 263, 265,
      272-300, 303-304, 306, 308, 310, 312-
      331, 339-342, 345, 348, 352-353, 356,
      361, 365-366, 369, 371
   teratogenesis 31, 112, 122, 124, 127-
      129, 131, 170-171, 176, 182-183, 186-
      188, 204, 210, 245, 259, 276, 288, 298,
      303, 352-353, 356, 371
   See also developmental toxicology
testes 344
tetrahydrocannabinol, Δ^9-*trans*-
   See Δ^9-*trans*-tetrahydrocannabinol
Thalidomide 5, 7, 112
theophylline 357
thermopsine
   See quinolizidine alkaloids
thiamin
   See vitamins
thiamine
   See vitamins
thiocyanate excretion 338, 340, 344
thiocyanates
   See cyanogenic compounds
thiomolybdate 31, 36
threonine
   See amino acids
thymus 24, 170, 176, 178, 181, 183
thyroid 24, 48, 59, 66, 145, 234, 236, 249,
   337-339, 341, 344, 346
thyroid deficiency 249
thyroxine 145
Tigason 135-136, 180
   See also Etretinate
tobacco alkaloids
   See piperidine (anabasine)
tomatidine
   See spirosolane alkaloids
toxemia 30, 85
toxicology 10, 65, 128, 196, 257, 269, 303,
   305-307, 327, 329, 331, 345-346, 376
trace substances 3, 7
tracheo-esophageal fistula
   See malformations

trans-3'-hydroxycotinine 359
transferrin 75-76, 78-81, 99, 106, 132, 226
transglutaminase 190, 199, 203, 208, 219,
   222
transthyretin 145, 167, 204, 214, 223
transverse distal limb reduction
   See malformations
tremors
   See cyanide intoxication
Trichoderma 291
trichothecenes (mycotoxins) 273, 291,
   301, 308
   crotocin 291
   deoxynivalenol (vomitoxin) 273, 291,
      301-302, 304
   diacetoxyscirpenol 291, 293
   fusarenon-X 291, 301
   HT-2 toxin 291
   neosolaniol 291
   nivalenol 291-292, 301-302, 304
   T-2 toxin 272-273, 291-292
   type A 271
   type B 271
   vomitoxin (see deoxynivalenol, above)
Trichothecium 291
trimethadione 8, 132
trophoblast 12, 87
truncus arteriosus communis
   See malformations
tryptophan
   See amino acids
TTR
   See transthyretin
tyrosine
   See amino acids

U

umbilical hernia
   See malformations
undernutrition
   See nutrition
ureter 344
ureter agenesis
   See malformations, agenesis (ureter)
urinary system 24
uterine glands 12

V

valine
   See amino acids
valproate 8
valproic acid 121
ventricular septal defect
   See malformations
ventricular spinal defect
   See malformations

veratramine
  See Veratrum alkaloids
Veratrum 310, 313-314, 324-326, 328, 331
  californicum 313, 326, 328
Veratrum alkaloids
  cyclopamine 313-314, 325
  cycloposine 313
  jervine 313-315, 324, 326, 331
  muldamine 314
  veratramine 314
vertebrae, absent
  See malformations
Verticimonosporium 291
Vigna sinensis
  See cowpeas
villous fibrosis 87-88
vitamin A
  accumulation 165
  See also vitamins
vitamin B$_{12}$
  See vitamins
vitamin D
  See vitamins
vitamin E
  See vitamins
vitamin K
  See vitamins
vitamins 2-4, 12, 22-23, 25-26, 38, 41, 46,
  48, 51-52, 54, 70, 104, 139, 201, 219,
  333
  biotin 17, 27, 40
  folate 4-5, 8, 25-26, 33-34, 39-40, 50-
  51, 64, 104, 107
  folic acid 8, 25-26, 34, 36, 38, 50, 76,
  97, 102, 105, 107
  niacin 4, 24, 33, 35, 48, 51-52, 54, 56,
  64, 70
  pantothenic acid 4, 27, 52, 64
  riboflavin 4, 23-24, 33, 50-51, 64, 67,
  69, 337
  thiamin 4, 23, 33-34, 38, 51-52, 65, 70,
  357
  thiamine 34, 52, 65, 70, 357
  thiamine deficiency 357
  vitamin A 7, 11, 27-28, 33, 38-39, 46,
  64, 72, 134-143, 145-148, 155-161,
  163-173, 192-197, 199-218, 220-228
  vitamin B$_6$ 24
  vitamin B$_{12}$ 102, 107
  vitamin C 5, 27-28, 33, 37, 51, 61, 68,
  99, 101-102, 107, 258, 333
  vitamin D 5, 28, 33, 58, 107, 172
  vitamin E 29, 33, 35, 47-49, 57, 64-68,
  71-72, 204, 228, 267, 269
  vitamin K 29, 33
vomitoxin
  See deoxynivalenol (trichothecenes)

W

white clover 335
white fat 20
WIC
  See Women, Infants, and Children Program
wild lima beans
  See beans
Withania 320
Women, Infants, and Children Program
  91-92

X

xanthophylls 137, 140
xenobiotic bioactivating enzymes 122
xerophthalmia 134, 168
xylose
  See monosaccharides

Y

yolk sac 109-111, 113-128, 130-132, 163,
  167, 223, 276, 280
yolk sac P4501A1 116
yuca
  See cassava

Z

zearalenone 271, 272, 293-295, 297-299,
  306-307
zinc
  See minerals

PRODUCTION INFORMATION

Typesetting: Pacific Division AAAS, California Academy of Sciences, San Francisco, California. Type was set in Adobe Systems 12pt. Times Roman face using Ventura Publisher DOS-version 3.0 by Xerox Desktop Software, Inc. on an ALR 486/33 microcomputer and printed on an HP LaserJet III® using an HP–Adobe® Postscript® Level 2 cartridge.

Printing and Binding: Braun-Brumfield, Inc., Ann Arbor, Michigan / Richard Thunes, San Francisco, CA. The text is printed on 60# Natural Hi-Bulk acid-free paper that meets the guidelines for permanence and durability established by the Committee on Publication Guidelines and Book Longevity of the Council on Library Resources.

Date of Publication: 31 March 1993.

Place of Publication: San Francisco, California, USA.

Number of Copies (First Printing): 1,000.